COSMETIC DERMATOLOGY
FOR SKIN OF COLOR

COSMETIC DERMATOLOGY FOR SKIN OF COLOR

EDITORS

Murad Alam, MD
Chief, Section of Cutaneous and Aesthetic Surgery
Associate Professor, Department of Dermatology, Otolaryngology, and Surgery
Feinberg School of Medicine, Northwestern University, Chicago, Illinois

Ashish C. Bhatia, MD, FAAD
Director, River North Dermatology & Dermatologic Surgery
DuPage Medical Group, Naperville, Illinois
Assistant Clinical Professor, Department of Dermatology
Feinberg School of Medicine, Northwestern University, Chicago, Illinois

Roopal V. Kundu, MD
Director, Northwestern Center for Ethnic Skin
Adjunct Assistant Professor, Department of Dermatology
Feinberg School of Medicine, Northwestern University, Chicago, Illinois

Assistant Professor, Department of Dermatology
New York University School of Medicine, New York, New York

Simon S. Yoo, MD
Assistant Professor, Department of Dermatology
Feinberg School of Medicine, Northwestern University, Chicago, Illinois

Henry Hin-Lee Chan, MD, FRCP
Honorary Associate Clinical Professor, Division of Dermatology, Department of Medicine
University of Hong Kong, Hong Kong, People's Republic of China

Visiting Scientist, Wellman Center for Photomedicine, Massachusetts General Hospital
Harvard Medical School, Boston, Massachusetts

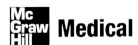 **Medical**

New York   Chicago   San Francisco   Lisbon   London   Madrid
Mexico City   Milan   New Delhi   San Juan   Seoul   Singapore   Sydney   Toronto

Cosmetic Dermatology for Skin of Color

1 2 3 4 5 6 7 8 9 0   CTP/CTP   12 11 10 9 8

ISBN 978-0-07-148776-4
MHID 0-07-148776-X

This book was set in Trade Gothic by Aptara®, Inc.
The editors were Anne M. Sydor and Robert Pancotti.
The production supervisor was Catherine Saggese.
The illustration manager was Armen Ovsepyan.
Project management was provided by Satvinder Kaur, Aptara®, Inc.
The cover designer was Elizabeth Pisacreta.
Cover photographs: Close-up of young woman looking away.
Photo Credit: John Lamb.
China Translation & Printing Services, Ltd. was printer and binder.

This book is printed on acid-free paper.

Library of Congress Cataloging-in-Publication Data

Cosmetic dermatology for skin of color / editors, Murad Alam ... [et al.].
      p. ; cm.
  Includes bibliographical references and index.
  ISBN-13: 978-0-07-148776-4 (hardcover : alk. paper)
  ISBN-10: 0-07-148776-X (hardcover : alk. paper) 1. Surgery, Plastic.
2. Dermatology. 3. Human skin color. 4. Ethnic groups. I. Alam, Murad.
  [DNLM: 1. Cosmetic Techniques. 2. Skin. 3. Ethnic Groups. 4. Skin
Diseases—therapy. 5. Skin Pigmentation—physiology. WR 650 C8336 2009]
  RD118.C67 2009
  617.4'770592—dc22
                                                                    2008037025

DEDICATION

To MP, RT, my parents, Rahat and Rehana, and my sister, Nigar.

—Murad Alam

My sincere gratitude goes to my mother and father, to my two brothers, Vikas and Manish, and especially to my wife, Tania, for supporting me throughout my career and continuing to do so every day. I would also like to thank Dr. Robert Brodell for kindling my interest in dermatology, dermatologic surgery, education, and research. Thanks for your support and for inspiring me always to be a better person, educator, student, and physician. I thank Dr. Thomas Rohrer for inspiring me to be the best dermatologic and cosmetic surgeon that I can be, and for preparing me for the exciting adventure ahead.

I would also like to thank my colleague and partner in practice, Dr. Jeff Hsu and my amazing nurses, MAs, administrative assistant, office coordinator, PAs, NP, histology technician, research staff, and front office staff—all of whom make it possible to have a fulfilling practice as well as a research and academic career. Thank you for making every day fun and exciting!

—Ashish C. Bhatia

To my husband, Som, my children, Nalin and Nayana, my sisters, Neelam and Ronak, and my wonderful parents, Ajit and Kaumudini, who have been "the wind beneath my wings."

—Roopal V. Kundu

To my parents, Young Ho and Seul Hi, who are my inspiration, to my sister, Suzanne, for her encouragement, and to my brothers, Bon and Glen, for their sharpening.

—Simon S. Yoo

I would like to acknowledge my mother, my wife, Shirley, my daughter, Scarlett, and my son, Henry, for their support throughout my career.

—Henry Hin-Lee Chan

CONTENTS

CONTRIBUTORS

Murad Alam, MD   Chief, Section of Cutaneous and Aesthetic Surgery; Assistant Professor, Department of Dermatology, Otolaryngology, and Surgery, Feinberg School of Medicine, Northwestern University, Chicago, Illinois
Chapters 11 and 22

Andrew F. Alexis, MD, MPH   Assistant Clinical Professor, Columbia University College of Physicians & Surgeons, New York, New York; Director, Skin of Color Center, Department of Dermatology, St. Luke's Roosevelt Hospital, New York, New York
Chapter 1

Sonia R. Batra, MD, MSc, MPH   Assistant Clinical Professor, Department of Dermatology, Keck School of Medicine, University of Southern California, Los Angeles, California
Chapter 9

Ashish C. Bhatia, MD, FAAD   Director, River North Dermatology & Dermatologic Surgery, Naperville, Illinois; Assistant Clinical Professor, Department of Dermatology, Feinberg School of Medicine, Northwestern University, Chicago, Illinois
Chapter 8

Tina Bhutani, MD   Resident Physician, Department of Internal Medicine, University of California, San Diego, San Diego, California
Chapter 9

Cheryl M. Burgess, MD, FAAD   Assistant Clinical Professor, Department of Dermatology, Georgetown University Hospital, Washington, DC
Chapter 20

Henry Hin-Lee Chan, MD, FRCP   Honorary Associate Clinical Professor, Division of Dermatology, Department of Medicine, University of Hong Kong, Hong Kong, People's Republic of China; Visiting Scientist, Wellman Center for Photomedicine, Massachusetts General Hospital, Harvard Medical School, Boston, Massachusetts
Chapters 3, 6, 7, 15, and 21

Nicola P.Y. Chan, MBBChir, MRCP   Honorary Associate Clinical Professor, Department of Medicine, University of Hong Kong, Hong Kong, People's Republic of China
Chapter 6

Suneel Chilukuri, MD   Associate Clinical Professor, Department of Dermatology, Baylor College of Medicine, Houston, Texas; Assistant Clinical Professor, Department of Dermatology, Columbia University College of Physicians & Surgeons, New York, New York; Assistant Clinical Professor, Department of

Medicine, Division of Dermatology, Albert Einstein College of Medicine of Yeshiva University, Bronx, New York
Chapter 8

Kee-Yang Chung, MD, PhD   Professor, Department of Dermatology, Yonsei University College of Medicine, Seoul, South Korea
Chapter 13

James C. Collyer, MD   Resident, Department of Dermatology, Feinberg School of Medicine, Northwestern University, Chicago, Illinois
Chapter 16

Zoe Diana Draelos, MD   Investigator, Dermatology Consulting Services, High Point, North Carolina
Chapter 14

Greg J. Goodman, MD   Senior Lecturer, Department of General Practice, Monash University, Clayton, Victoria, Australia
Chapter 18

Joseph F. Greco, MD   Clinical Instructor, Division of Dermatology, Department of Medicine, David Geffen School of Medicine, University of California, Los Angeles, Los Angeles, California
Chapter 23

Rebat M. Halder, MD   Professor and Chairman, Department of Dermatology, Howard University College of Medicine, Washington, DC
Chapter 2

Stephanie G.Y. Ho, MBBS, MRCP   Honorary Clinical Research Associate, Department of Medicine, Division of Dermatology, University of Hong Kong, Hong Kong, People's Republic of China
Chapter 21

Richard H. Huggins, MD   Clinical Research Fellow, Department of Dermatology, Henry Ford Health System, Detroit, Michigan
Chapter 22

Changhuh Huh, MD, PhD   Assistant Professor, Department of Dermatology, Seoul National University Bundang Hospital, Seongnam, Gyeonggi, South Korea
Chapter 3

Taro Kono, MD, PhD   Assistant Professor, Department of Plastic and Reconstructive Surgery, Tokyo Women's Medical University, Tokyo, Japan
Chapter 7

David J. Kouba, MD, PhD Chief of Cosmetic Dermasurgery, Henry Ford Health System, Department of Dermatology, Detroit, Michigan
Chapter 13

Roopal V. Kundu, MD Director, Northwestern Center for Ethnic Skin; Adjunct Assistant Professor, Department of Dermatology, Feinberg School of Medicine, Northwestern University, Chicago, Illinois; Assistant Professor, Department of Dermatology, New York University School of Medicine, New York, New York
Chapters 2 and 10

Diana Leu, MD Dermatology Chief Resident, Department of Dermatology, Feinberg School of Medicine, Northwestern University, Chicago, Illinois
Chapter 5

Susan Leu, MD Resident, Department of Dermatology, University of Michigan, Ann Arbor, Michigan
Chapter 16

Joyce Teng Ee Lim, MD, FRCPI, FAMS Consultant Dermatologist, Department of Dermatologic Laser and Surgery, National Skin Centre, Singapore
Chapter 15

Jennifer Y. Lin, MD Instructor, Department of Dermatology, Harvard Medical School, Boston, Massachusetts
Chapter 15

Ronald L. Moy, MD Professor, David Geffen School of Medicine, University of California, Los Angeles; Director, Moy Dermatology, Los Angeles, California
Chapter 13

Vic A. Narurkar, MD, FAAD Associate Clinical Professor, Department of Dermatology, University of California Davis Medical School, Sacramento, California; Director, Bay Area Laser Institute, San Francisco, California
Chapter 12

Keyvan Nouri, MD, FAAD Professor, Department of Dermatology and Cutaneous Surgery; Director, Mohs, Dermatologic and Laser Surgery; University of Miami Leonard M. Miller School of Medicine, Miami, Florida
Chapter 19

Asha R. Patel, BS Medical Student, Department of Dermatology and Cutaneous Surgery, Leonard M. Miller School of Medicine, University of Miami, Miami, Florida
Chapter 19

Sejal K. Shah, MD Resident, Department of Dermatology, St. Luke's Roosevelt Hospital Center, New York, New York
Chapter 1

Teresa Soriano, MD Associate Clinical Professor, Division of Dermatology, Department of Medicine, David Geffen School of Medicine, University of California, Los Angeles, Los Angeles, California
Chapter 23

Voraphol Vejjabhinanta, MD Postdoctoral Procedural Fellow, Department of Dermatology and Cutaneous Surgery, Leonard M. Miller School of Medicine, University of Miami, Miami, Florida
Chapter 19

Joslyn N. Witherspoon, MD, MPH Clinical Research Fellow, Department of Dermatology, Feinberg School of Medicine, Northwestern University, Chicago, Illinois
Chapter 22

Simon S. Yoo, MD Assistant Professor, Department of Dermatology, Feinberg School of Medicine, Northwestern University, Chicago, Illinois
Chapter 5

Siegrid S. Yu, MD Assistant Professor, Department of Dermatology, Dermatologic Surgery and Laser Center, University of California, San Francisco, San Francisco, California
Chapter 4

Yan I. Zhu, MD, PhD Department of Dermatology, University of Colorado Health Sciences Center, Aurora, Colorado
Chapter 17

PREFACE

More than half of the population of the United States will soon be non-Caucasian. Further, much of the currently burgeoning demand for cosmetic dermatology emanates from Latin America, the Middle East, and the Far East. Fortunately, improvements in technology have made the treatment of pigmented skin more feasible. For instance, long-pulsed Nd:YAG lasers can be used to safely remove hair in darker-skinned patients, and gentler fractionated lasers can resurface the skin of Indian, African American, and Asian persons without a high risk of pigment change.

The purpose of this book is to collate information about cosmetic procedures in pigmented skin. We define "pigmented skin" or "ethnic skin" as any skin darker than the fair Caucasian skin of blondes and redheads. Thus, pigmented skin includes the darker skin of the Mediterranean; of Africa; of indigenous ethnic areas such as those populated by Native American aboriginal peoples; of India and the Near East; of the Middle East; and of the Far East. Of course, many patients have mixed ethnic heritage. Both genetic endowment and environmental factors will influence an individual patient's suitability for certain cosmetic procedures.

To make the text more useful, we have subdivided it into small parts. Most chapters are only 1000 to 2500 words in length and hence can be easily digested in a single, brief sitting. Chapters are organized in categories so that the reader can easily find what is needed.

The first cluster of chapters defines the concept of ethnic skin and clarifies the approach to evaluating and treating cosmetic patients with darker skin. Significantly, a detailed discussion of common adverse events is included in the initial part. Prevention and improvement of such unwanted outcomes is a crucial part of a successful cosmetic practice.

The second part of the book is its heart. This part includes discussions of common cosmetic treatments for skin color and tone in patients with ethnic skin. Primary organization of this material is by the depth, location, and type of skin structure treated rather than by the device or procedure used. We chose this paradigm because, in actual clinical practice, we are confronted with patients who would like the best outcome for their problem, regardless of the technique used. We begin by considering superficial textural and color imperfections. Then we consider treatment of the deeper dermis, including nonablative and ablative resurfacing for improvement of wrinkles and scars. Lastly, we address problems that can occur in areas other than the face, such as excess hair, body contour irregularities, and sagging of the skin. So as not to complicate chapters unnecessarily, when widely divergent modalities are employed for similar indications, we have discussed these in consecutive chapters. For example, in the realm of color improvement, successive chapters examine the use of chemical peels and microdermabrasion for color and texture; lasers and lights for vascular lesions; and lasers and lights for pigment excess. In each chapter in this section, procedures are described in general and then the specific elements relevant to skin of color patients are highlighted. In this manner, readers learn the procedure in its entirety, including techniques that are the same for all patients regardless of ethnicity.

No book on cosmetic dermatology would be complete without a section on cosmeceuticals. Because these constitute a gentle form of noninvasive therapy and because certain cosmeceuticals may be better suited for patients with skin of color, we include a chapter on such topical therapies as a transition to the last part of the book.

In the third section of the book, experts discuss treatments of specific conditions and diagnoses that are likely to afflict those persons with skin of color. Among these problems are melasma, dermatosis papulosa nigra, acne scarring, and postinflammatory hyperpigmentation. The reader who is more interested in a patient's particular condition than in global improvement of skin color or texture can consult these chapters rather than the more general chapters in the second part of the book. Once the reader chooses a particular treatment approach, it may be appropriate to refer to an earlier chapter that provides a detailed explanation on how to proceed step by step.

The fourth and final part of the book summarizes the challenges associated with cosmetic treatments in ethnic skin. The chapters in this section acknowledge that ethnic skin can be separated into subtypes. We asked notable experts in their specialties to consider patients of different ethnic and racial types, including African, Latino, Far Eastern, and Indian patients. Such patients are in some ways similar, and in other ways different, in their cosmetic dermatology needs.

We hope you find this book useful.

ACKNOWLEDGMENTS

This book would not have been possible were it not for the vision of Anne M. Sydor, the commissioning editor, whose kind words and energy subsequently propelled the project toward completion. Satvinder Kaur and Robert Pancotti provided indispensable help by copyediting the manuscript and preparing the text and illustrations for publication. Throughout the process, the McGraw-Hill staff made our work on this book a pleasure.

We would also like to thank Jillian Havey, the Northwestern University research associate, who shepherded this book through obstacles on a day-to-day basis. Jillian communicated with contributors, reassured editors, managed files and versions, and in general vigorously prevented errors of omission or commission. We wish Jillian well as she returns to medical school and we look forward to welcoming her in the future as a valued colleague in the field of dermatology.

Thanks also to Natalie Kim, who reviewed the final version, corrected overlooked errors and ensured consistent quality in the text and images.

COSMETIC DERMATOLOGY
FOR SKIN OF COLOR

CHAPTER 1

Defining Skin of Color

Sejal K. Shah, MD, and Andrew F. Alexis, MD, MPH

Ethnic skin, or *skin of color,* refers to the broad range of skin types and complexions that characterize individuals with darkly pigmented skin, including (but not limited to) persons of African, Asian, Latino, Native American, and Middle Eastern descent (Figure 1.1). Differences in structure, function, and cultural practices in individuals with skin of color contribute to variations in the prevalence, clinical presentation, and impact on quality of life of numerous skin conditions. Understanding these differences is paramount in the treatment of persons with skin of color, especially in the context of cosmetic dermatology. Failure to recognize these differences can result in incorrect assumptions about an individual patient's standards of beauty as well as potentially disfiguring treatment complications. A thorough understanding of ethnic variations in skin structure and function, cultural practices, and responses to treatment is essential to safely and effectively treat the entire spectrum of patients who seek cosmetic dermatologic procedures. In this chapter, the clinical and cultural nuances that characterize skin of color are discussed. The challenges of defining or classifying skin of color are also addressed.

DEFINING SKIN OF COLOR—ISSUES AND CONTROVERSIES

When defining *skin of color*, the concepts of "race" and "ethnicity" are often invoked. The terms "race" and "ethnicity" are sociopolitical constructs that are poorly defined and are often used interchangeably or as an all-inclusive label, "racial/ethnic." However, it is important to note that the terms have very different connotations. Historically, *Homo sapiens* have been classified into three to six racial taxons since the 18th century, before the development of genetics and evolutionary biology.[1] The "modern" races included Caucasoid (Europeans, Arabs, Indians, Pakistanis), Mongoloid (Asians), Australoid (Australian Aborigines), Congoid or Negroid (Africans, Afro-Caribbeans, African Americans), and Capoid (Kung San tribe of Africa).[2,3] These divisions were traditionally based on phenotypic characteristics, geographic origin, and even psychological impressions.[1] Thus, the classification of individuals according to "race" is arbitrary and subjective, lacking a biologic basis. In essence, it is a method of classifying diverse populations into socially or politically defined categories. Although genetic studies reveal that genetic variation corresponds to geographic origin, or our concept of "race," if an individual's ancestors are from one particular region, 85% to 90% of genetic variation is found within racial groups and only 10% to 15% is found between groups.[4–7] As such, some authors have argued against the use of racial classifications in biomedical literature.[8] Ethnicity, on the other hand, identifies individuals and populations on the basis of shared social variables such as religion, language, diet, and customs. Ethnic groups are dynamic, and boundaries between groups are often not precise.[1] Because ethnicity encompasses multiple variables, not all group members may adhere to all the aspects of one particular group, so the group characteristics may not describe all members.

Both race and ethnicity are often narrowly defined for population research or surveillance purposes. In the United States, for example, federal statistics on race and ethnicity are collected by the U.S. Census Bureau using a minimum of five racial categories—American Indian or Alaska Native, Asian, black, or African American, Native Hawaiian or Other Pacific Islander, and white, while ethnicity is specified as "Hispanic or Latino" and "not Hispanic or Latino."[9] Although these categories are self-identified by individuals and more than one racial group can be selected by a given individual, this list does not include all the ways individuals classify themselves.

For the purposes of this chapter, specification of race or ethnicity will be used to group individuals who share common skin and hair characteristics as well as cultural practices. Categorization of race or ethnicity in no way implies that there is genetic homogeneity among members of a particular racial or ethnic group, nor is it intended to ignore the myriad biologic and cultural variations within each group.

DEMOGRAPHIC TRENDS IN PERSONS WITH SKIN OF COLOR

The geographic distribution of populations considered to have skin of color is extremely wide. It includes, but is not limited to, large populations in the Americas (North, Central, and South America), the Caribbean, Africa, Asia, and the Middle East, as well as immigrant populations in Europe and beyond. As such, people with skin of color constitute the majority of the world's population. Geographic regions where people of color predominate are shown in Figure 1-2.

In the United States, census projections predict that people of color (those who identify themselves as African American, Asian and Pacific Islander, Hispanic/Latino, American Indian, Eskimo, and Aleut) will constitute approximately 50% of the U.S. population by 2050 (Figure 1.3).[9] Contributing to this demographic shift are immigration patterns. In 1960, most immigrants to the United States were from Europe; whereas by 2000, most immigrants were from Asia or Latin America.[9]

With these demographic trends in mind, it will be increasingly important for dermatologists to recognize clinical and cultural differences in patients with skin of color. Moreover, efforts to better define optimal approaches to cosmetic procedures in skin of color will be paramount as a growing proportion of patients requesting cosmetic procedures will have skin of color.

CLASSIFICATION SYSTEMS FOR SKIN OF COLOR

Accurate classification of individuals into clearly defined skin types according to pigmentation or responses to external stimuli is a considerable challenge that remains elusive. The most widely used classification system used by dermatologists is the Fitzpatrick Skin

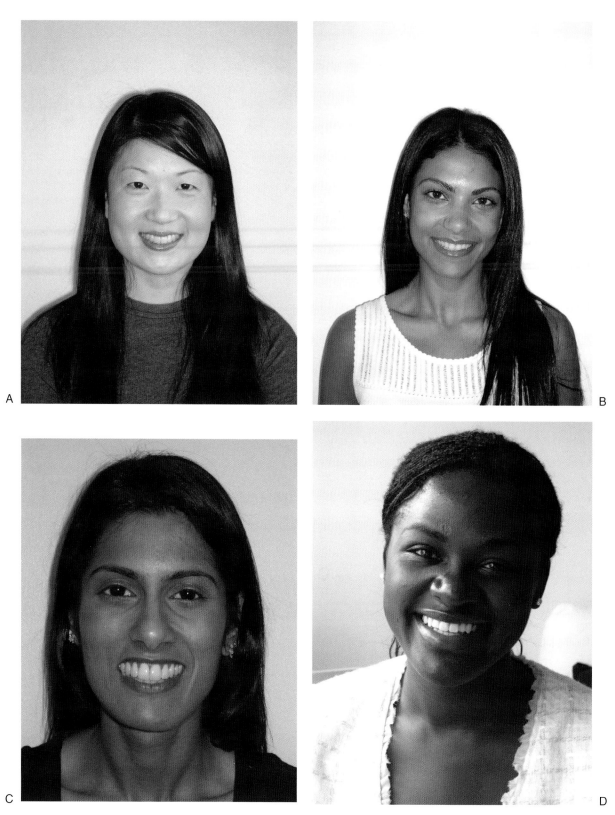

Figure 1.1 *Spectrum of skin of color. (A) Woman of East Asian (Chinese) descent. (Used with permission from Andrew F. Alexis, MD.) (B) Woman of Egyptian descent. (Used with permission from Andrew F. Alexis, MD.) (C) Woman of South Asian (Indian) descent. (D) Woman of West African (Ghanaian) descent. (Used with permission from Andrew F. Alexis, MD.)*

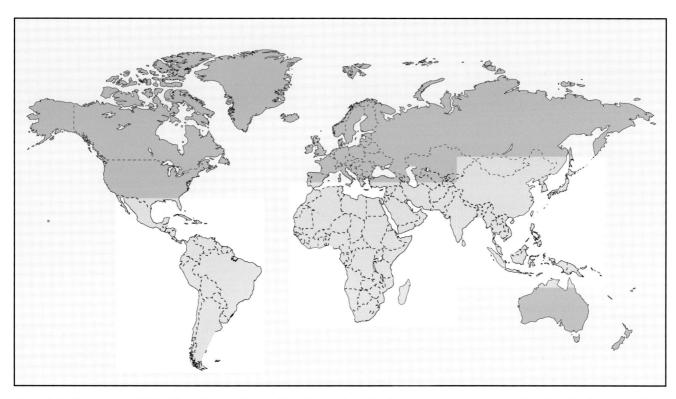

Figure 1.2 *Geographic distribution of populations with skin of color, showing regions where people with skin of color predominate*

Phototype (SPT) system. Devised in 1975, this system was designed to classify an individual's response to ultraviolet radiation (UVR) with respect to burning or tanning ability.[10] Its intended purpose was to help estimate starting doses for phototherapy. In this system, lightly pigmented (i.e., "white" or "melanocompromised") constitutive skin color is characterized as type I through III, while darkly pigmented ("melanocompetent") individuals with brown constitutive skin color are classified as type IV through VI.[11] Light brown skin tone is specified as type IV skin; type V skin is brown in color, and dark brown skin is classified as type VI skin.[11] In this classification system, these darker ("melanocompetent") skin types are characterized by the

ability to easily tan and never burn.[11] When using the SPT system, multiple skin phototypes may exist within one racial group. This reflects not only the variability between races but also the variability within each racial group, as well as the effects of interbreeding.

Although the Fitzpatrick SPT system is a valuable tool because each person can be assigned a skin phototype even if it is difficult to determine racial and ethnic classifications, it has limitations. Studies have found that while this rapid method is able to clearly distinguish differences in minimal erythema dose (MED) between the two extremes of pigmentation, there is considerable overlap of MED values among the six Fitzpatrick skin types.[12,13] Some studies have even shown that for some individuals there is no significant relationship between SPT and MED.[12] Moreover, while the current version of the SPT system considers skin types IV through VI to never burn, individuals with skin of color may still minimally or rarely burn with intense UVR exposure.

In response to these limitations, alternative skin classification systems and skin color charts have been proposed.[14–18] Several studies have suggested the use of a quantitative measure of skin pigmentation, such as chromameters or reflectance spectrometers, especially when administering phototherapy, as these methods more accurately predict MED than do skin phototypes.[12,13,19] Although they produce reliable and reproducible results, these noninvasive tools may not be practical in most clinical settings because of the cost, training, and time issues. It has also been suggested that it may be more appropriate to use a skin classification system based on criteria that are more applicable to individuals with darkly pigmented skin, such as the tendency to develop postinflammatory hyperpigmentation.[3] The Taylor Hyperpigmentation Scale is a visual scale that was developed to quantify the degree of hyperpigmentation, and it may be a useful assessment tool in skin of color.[17] Recently, a new

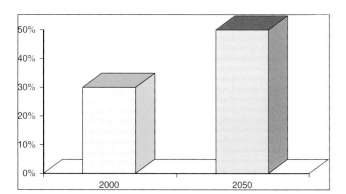

Figure 1.3 *The U.S. Census projections. It is projected that people with skin of color will constitute 49.9% of the U.S. population by 2050.[9] "People with skin of color" means those who identify themselves as black, Asian, Hispanic, American Indian, Alaska native, native Hawaiian, or other Pacific Islander.*

Skin Color Chart based on quantitative measurements of the spectrum of human skin colors in two-dimensional color space (clarity and hue) has been proposed.[14] An ongoing initiative to develop a comprehensive skin classification system that better defines all skin types (including constitutive skin color, response to UVR, tendency to develop dyschromias, propensity to form keloids, and photoaging properties) is being led by the Skin of Color Society.

STRUCTURAL AND FUNCTIONAL DIFFERENCES IN SKIN OF COLOR

A number of structural and functional differences in the skin and hair of darkly pigmented individuals (compared with lightly pigmented populations) have been reported. Many of these differences have important clinical implications. These differences along with their clinical relevance are summarized in Tables 1.1 and 1.2.

CULTURAL DIFFERENCES IN PERSONS WITH SKIN OF COLOR

The standards of beauty conveyed by the U.S. media influence all Americans, regardless of race or ethnicity. However, the cultural background of the individual also plays a role. Many cultures, including those from which individuals with darker skin types originate, value fair, smooth skin with even skin color and texture. In Asian culture, flawless skin free of scars and pigment abnormalities, both hyperpigmentation and hypopigmentation, is a widely held ideal. Accordingly, Asian patients may refuse treatments that cause tanning, such as phototherapy, especially if the face will not be shielded.[31] Individuals of South Asian and Middle Eastern descent often believe that fair skin equals beauty. More than 50% of responders in a community-based survey of Arab Americans viewed very fair or fair skin as visually pleasing; those individuals who had resided in the United States for less than 20 years were twice as likely to hold this opinion. In this same survey, the top five most urgent subjective concerns reported were uneven skin tone, skin discoloration, dry skin, acne, and facial hair.[32] Like several Asian cultures, Hispanic- and African-based cultures place great importance on even skin tone, fair skin, or smooth skin texture. Individuals of these cultural backgrounds may use various topical bleaching or lightening agents to lighten their complexion or correct dyschromias.[3] Many of these agents are obtained without a prescription and may be found in ethnic beauty supply stores.[3] Commonly (especially outside the United States), these products contain superpotent corticosteroids, 2% to 10% hydroquinone, mercury, phenolics, or other unknown chemicals and plant derivatives.[33] Individuals who use these agents can develop dermatologic or medical complications (Table 1.3).

The appearance of one's hair is also a measure of beauty in the black community; women of African descent often equate healthy, full hair with overall health and beauty and devote great amounts of time and money to hair maintenance and styling. A woman may choose a particular hairstyle for ease of maintenance, because she feels that it is acceptable to the dominant culture in society or because she feels it suits her best.[36] Hair care practices that involve the application of chemicals, heat, or traction to the hair and scalp are widespread and generally begin in childhood.

TABLE 1.1 ■ Structural and Functional Differences and Dermatologic Implications[3,20–30]

Structural/Functional Factor	Dermatologic Implication	Examples of Contributing Skin and Hair Care Practices
Increased tyrosinase activity → increased melanin content; larger individually dispersed melanosomes; increased melanosomes; dispersion of melanosomes throughout epidermis	Greater photoprotection, less prominent photoaging, lower incidence of skin cancer	
Labile melanocytes; slower melanin degradation	Dyschromias	Skin-lightening agents
Larger, more numerous, binucleated and multinucleated fibroblasts; fibroblast hyperreactivity; larger mast cell granules; increased tryptase	Greater prevalence of keloids and hypertrophic scarring	Scarification
Curved hair follicle; spiral hair shape (specific to individuals of African descent)	Greater prevalence of pseudofolliculitis	Shaving
Fewer elastic fibers anchoring hair follicles to the dermis; lower hair density; lower breaking stress and breaking extension; flat/elliptical hair shaft predisposed to developing knots and fissures (specific to individuals of African descent)	Greater prevalence of hair breakage and traumatic alopecias	Traumatic hair care practices (e.g., tight braids, "corn rows," chemical relaxers, hot combing, extensions)

TABLE 1.2 ■ **Differences in Hair Characteristics of Persons from Different Descent**[3,21,25]

Descent	Hair Follicle	Hair Morphology and Appearance	Hair Diameter
Caucasian	Ovoid, intermediate between curved and straight; anchored by more elastic fibers	Oval shaft; wavy	Intermediate
Asian	Round, straight	Round shaft; straight	Largest
African	Curved; anchored by fewer elastic fibres	Flat or elliptical shaft; spiral	Smallest

Individuals with skin of color may desire Western structural facial features idealized in the popular culture and media. The desire to change facial features may not only be based on perceived standards of beauty but also fueled by the desire to assimilate into one's adopted culture, as in the case of immigrant groups in North America and Europe. East Asian cultures regard large eyes as aesthetically pleasing. The wide, bright-eyed look is a widely held perception of beauty that suggests a youthful appearance. However, the majority of East Asians have an eyelid structure that does not impart this look; therefore, they often request cosmetic procedures to achieve larger, more open eyes.[37] The nose is another feature that is often surgically altered. People of color may seek a smoother nasal contour while preserving the ethnic characteristic of their natural nose, which has been referred to as the "ethnic" rhinoplasty. Alternatively, some individuals may want to completely eliminate the ethnic features of their natural nose and have a more "Western" nasal contour, which has been reported as a common cosmetic procedure requested by patients of Southeast Asian descent in the United States.[38]

Individuals with skin of color commonly undergo cultural practices to attain culturally specific ideals of beauty. Some of these practices can result in several adverse effects that are relevant to dermatologists (Table 1.3, Figure 1.4).

CLINICAL AND THERAPEUTIC IMPLICATIONS

Differences in skin structure and function, standards of beauty, and cultural practices overlap to produce racial and ethnic variations in cosmetic dermatologic concerns (Figure 1.5). Not only are there variations in epidemiology, clinical presentation, and treatment regimens, but the approach to the patient may also be influenced by cultural nuances in skin of color patients. The cosmetic dermatologist should keep in mind that the demand for specific cosmetic treatments is often influenced by cultural perceptions of what is beautiful or ideal. Dermatologists are, therefore, faced with the challenge of providing services in a culturally sensitive manner. By being aware of the common traditions, beliefs, and practices of various ethnicities, the cosmetic dermatologist can reduce barriers and gain the patient's trust to build good rapport. This cultural competency includes a familiarity with skin and hair care practices as well

as cultural standards of beauty. Before embarking on any particular treatment course, the cosmetic dermatologist should openly discuss the skin condition; skin care history, including prior prescription and nonprescription treatments; therapeutic options that are appropriate for the patient's skin; the risks, benefits, and costs of each, and expectations, of both the patient and the physician. If the patient is requesting a cosmetic surgical procedure, such as a blepharoplasty or rhinoplasty, inquire about his or her motivations (Does the patient want to enhance his or her natural ethnic features? Or does the patient want a more "Western" appearance?). It is often helpful to let the patient point out his or her concerns in a mirror. The patient should be asked about his or her ancestry, as this may not be obvious by simply looking at the patient. In the era of mass marketing and the Internet, patients with skin of color are often misled by product information, especially information based on Caucasian skin. They may develop unrealistic expectations or assume that cosmetic treatments that are available to Caucasian skin are appropriate for their skin. In the initial consultation, the cosmetic dermatologist should discuss these points with the patient and rectify any misconceptions.

Racial and ethnic minorities underwent 21.7% of the 11.5% million cosmetic surgical and nonsurgical procedures performed in the United States in 2006.[40] Common cosmetic concerns in individuals with skin of color that are often rooted in cultural standards include dyschromias, uneven skin texture, hair loss, hirsutism and hair removal, hypertrophic and keloidal scars, and photoaging.[32,39,41,42] A recent study at the Skin of Color Center in New York City retrospectively reviewed charts for diagnoses and race/ethnicity. Dyschromias, alopecias, hirsutism, folliculitis, keloids, and vitiligo were among the top ten most common diagnoses noted in blacks. Dyschromias and alopecias were the second and fourth most common diagnoses, respectively, and neither was observed as top ten diagnoses in Caucasians.[41] Acne, photoaging, facial melasma, hyperpigmentation, and alopecia were among the twelve most common diagnoses reported in 1000 Latino patients treated in a private dermatology practice.[42] A community-based survey of Arab Americans found that acne and melasma were among the five most common self-reported cutaneous diseases based on a prior diagnosis made by a physician.[32] As in other ethnic populations with skin of color, the prevalence of melasma is higher in Asians than in Caucasians.[39]

TABLE 1.3 ▪ Common Cultural Practices and Clinical Implications[3,33–35,39]

Cultural Practice	Definition	Cultures	Why Used	Potential Clinical Implications
Henna	A natural red-orange dye derived from the leaves of the shrub *Lawsonia inermis*	Indian subcontinent, Middle Eastern, African	Dye for hair, skin, fingernails, decorative body art, especially for special occasions such as weddings	Hemolysis caused by oxidation; Contact dermatitis; Allergic reactions that may include shortness of breath and chest tightness
"Black henna"	A black dye containing primarily paraphenylenediamine (PPD), a synthetic aromatic amine, and little or no henna	Began in Africa, India, Arabian Peninsula, and Western countries, especially common in tourist areas	Body art	Severe allergic reactions which may include contact dermatitis with blistering, pruritus, scarring, angioneurotic edema, shock, and lifelong sensitization
Coining	Traditional healing practice in which warm oil or Tiger Balm (topical analgesic) is applied to the skin and a coin or special instrument is rubbed linearly on the skin	Asian	Traditionally used to release "bad wind" or treat "wind illness"; used to treat a variety of illness including febrile illnesses, colds, headache, myalgias, and malaise	Temporary linear ecchymosis and petechiae which may be confused with abuse, especially in children
Cupping	Traditional healing practice in which bell-like suction apparatus or cup with suction is applied to the skin, drawing up the skin "Fire" cupping uses flame in the cup to create suction	Asian	Traditionally used to release "bad wind" or treat "wind illness"; thought to improve circulation in the area; commonly used to treat aches and pains and respiratory conditions	Temporary circular ecchymosis
Moxibustion	Traditional healing practice in which burning mugwort herb, *Artemesia vulgaris,* is placed on acupuncture points; may be accompanied with knives or needles to cut the body and release toxins (scarification)	Asian, African	Traditionally believed to stimulate circulation and strengthen life energy, or *qi*, of the body; used for menstrual cramps, breech presentation fetus, chronic conditions, pain, fatigue, disease prevention, and maintaining health	Burns, blistering, scarring; increased risk of blood-borne diseases if nonsterile knives or needles are used
Skin-lightening agents	Products containing various depigmenting agents such as hydroquinone (in some regions, >4%), class 1 and 2 corticosteroids, mercury, phenolics, caustics, and other unknown plant and chemical derivatives	Asian, African, Middle Eastern	Applied to lighten or even out complexion; practice is often rooted in cultural perceptions of beauty and the ideal image	Effects depend on specific ingredient used; skin atrophy and fragility, telangiectasias, dyschromias, exogenous ochronosis, acne, skin infections; may induce serious systemic complications such as Cushing's syndrome, renal impairment, and neurological problems

(continued)

TABLE 1.3 ■ Common Cultural Practices and Clinical Implications[3,33–35,39] *(Continued)*

Cultural Practice	Definition	Cultures	Why Used	Potential Clinical Implications
Hair styling and maintenance techniques	Braids, microbraids, "corn rows," twists, locks/dreadlocks, weaves/extensions (sewn or glued), tight ponytails, buns, jheri curl, hot comb, pressing, semipermanent or permanent hair dyes, chemical relaxers, rollers, curling irons, hair dryers, pomades, oils, gels	African-based (continental African, African American, Afro-Caribbean)	Used to enhance beauty, improve texture and manageability; because particular style is thought to be accepted by mainstream culture	Traction alopecia, central centrifugal cicatricial alopecia (CCCA, also known as hot comb alopecia or follicular degeneration syndrome), thinning, breakage, contact dermatitis, burns, pomade acne
Threading	Ancient method of hair removal by which unwanted hairs are plucked out using twisted cotton thread	Indian subcontinent, Middle Eastern	Fast method of removing unwanted hair from follicle; unlike tweezing, plucks rows of hair rather than individual hairs	Pain, pruritus, erythema, swelling or puffiness, folliculitis, pigment alterations

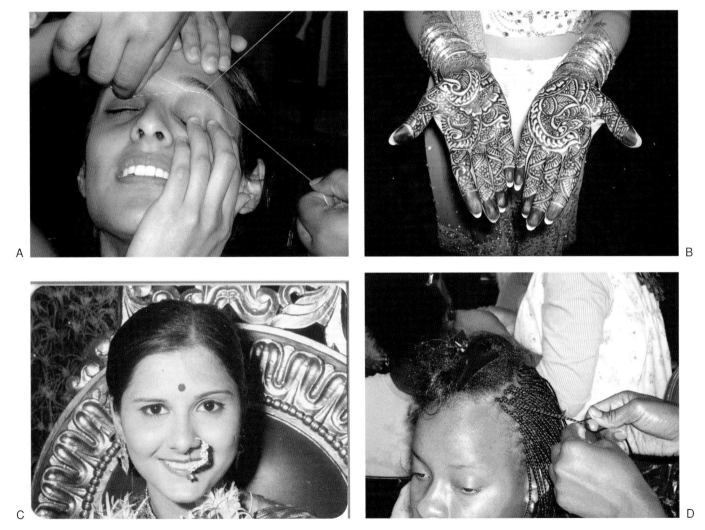

Figure 1.4 *Cultural skin and hair care practices. (A) Threading. (B) Henna. (C) Nasal piercing and bindi ("red dot") on Indian woman. (Used with permission from Sejal Shah, MD.) (D) Hair braiding. (Used with permission from Andrew F. Alexis, MD.) (continued)*

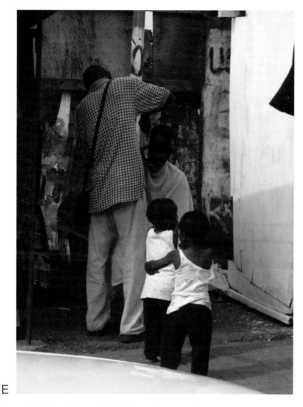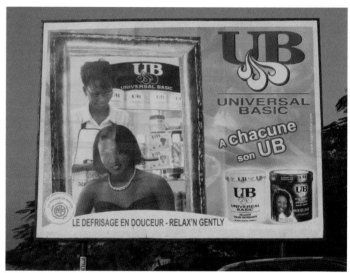

E   F

Figure 1.4 Continued *(E) Street barber in Ghana. (Used with permission from Andrew F. Alexis, MD.) (F) Billboard advertising chemical hair relaxer in Ghana*

Patients with ethnic skin are increasingly requesting procedures that reverse or minimize the signs of photoaging. Although people of all races may develop cutaneous changes as a result of chronic sun exposure as they age, darker skin types appear to be less susceptible, secondary to photoprotection conferred by melanin. Among blacks, photoaging occurs more commonly in African Americans than in Africans and Afro-Caribbeans, which may be because of their more heterogeneous ancestry.[43] In African Americans, the effects of chronic sun exposure include fine wrinkling, variable pigmentation, and dermatosis papulosa nigra (DPN). Photoaging in lighter-skinned Hispanics is similar to that of Caucasians, with wrinkling more common than abnormal pigmentation.[43] Hispanics with darker skin tend to develop features similar to those of South Asians and African Americans.[43] Pigment abnormalities are the primary clinical manifestations of actinic damage in Asians. These include ephelides (freckles), solar lentigines, seborrheic keratoses, mottled pigmentation, and melasma. Wrinkling is often considered to be a less prominent feature of photoaging in Asians, with wrinkles becoming apparent in the fifth decade.[44]

Technological advances have made many cosmetic procedures available to patients with skin of color. A number of laser and light technologies have recently been added to the armamentarium of treatments for patients with skin of color. Additionally, the cosmetics and skin care industry is beginning to develop products that are specifically formulated for and marketed to people of darker skin types. Even with these advances, the cosmetic dermatologist must tailor the cosmetic procedure or topical regimen to patients with skin of color to minimize adverse effects, such as postinflammatory hyperpigmentation and keloid or hypertrophic scar development (Table 1.4). With the proper training, many cosmetic treatments commonly used in persons with lighter skin can be used safely and effectively in persons with darker skin.

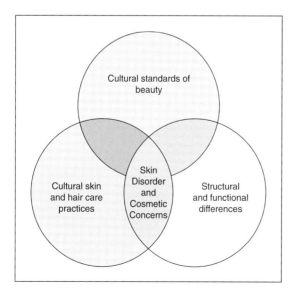

Figure 1.5 *The overlap of structural and functional differences and cultural differences. Differences in structure and function overlap with differences in cultural standards of beauty and skin and hair care practices to produce racial and ethnic variations in cosmetic concerns, skin disorders, and impact on quality of life*

TABLE 1.4 ■ **Cosmetic Procedures in Skin of Color**[43,45–48]

Procedure	Indications	Modifications for Skin of Color	Potential Complications
Chemical peels	Dyschromias, acne, pseudofolliculitis barbae, uneven/rough skin texture, fine lines	Use superficial peels; leave peeling agent on skin just long enough to cause slight burning and redness; typical endpoint (e.g., white frost of trichloroacetic acid [TCA] peel may be inappropriate); consider spot treatments; longer intervals between treatments	*Postpeel dyschromias/postinflammatory pigment changes; dermal scarring including keloids/hypertrophic scars
Microdermabrasion	Textural irregularities and scar removal, dyschromias, acne, early photoaging, fine lines	Avoid overly aggressive technique; use linear strokes at a low setting and one or two passes; typical endpoint of erythema may not be desired; consider spot treatments with additional passes for focal areas	†Postinflammatory pigment changes; dermal scarring including keloids/hypertrophic scars
Laser and light-based procedures	Dyschromias, textural irregularities and scarring, hypertrichosis, photoaging, and benign cutaneous tumors (e.g., DPN)	Conservative treatment parameters; lower energy settings; long wavelength devices; epidermal cooling devices; nonablative techniques; may require more treatments	‡Prolonged erythema, postinflammatory pigment alterations, burns, and scarring including keloids/hypertrophic scars
Botulinum toxin	Improve hyperfunctional facial lines, to achieve youthful relaxed appearance, widen eyes (in East Asian patients)	Treat conservatively; reduce trauma by injecting as few times as possible into skin	Expressionless or paralyzed facial expression; postinflammatory pigment alterations caused by trauma to skin
Injectable filling agents	Volume restoration, facial rejuvenation	Treat conservatively; reduce trauma by injecting as few times as possible into skin	Postinflammatory pigment alterations caused by trauma to skin; lumps/bumps

*Complications are considerably more likely with medium depth and deep peels (risks usually outweigh benefits).
†Dermabrasion should generally be avoided in skin of color as risks usually outweigh benefits.
‡Complications are more likely with ablative devices.

CONCLUSION

The terms "ethnic skin" and "skin of color" refer to the spectrum of skin complexions that would be considered "melanocompetent" or with increased pigmentation and are typically characterized as FSP types IV, V, and VI. Treating skin of color patients can often be challenging for cosmetic dermatologists not only because of structural and functional differences but also because of diverse cultural backgrounds, which include myriad skin and hair care practices and unique perceptions of beauty. These differences produce variations in the prevalence, clinical presentation, and quality of life impact of numerous skin disorders and cosmetic concerns. Moreover, many cosmetic procedures can be associated with potentially disfiguring complications when the nuances of treating pigmented skin are not taken into consideration. Thus, it is essential that the cosmetic dermatologist be familiar with racial/ethnic differences in skin characteristics and cultural practices (as well as their clinical and therapeutic implications) to successfully treat patients with skin of color.

REFERENCES

1. Witzig R. The medicalization of race: scientific legitimization of a flawed social construct. *Ann Intern Med.* 1996;125(8): 675-679.

2. Coon CS. *The Origin of Races.* New York, NY: Alfred A. Knopf, Inc.; 1962.

3. Taylor SC. Skin of color: siology, structure, function, and implications for dermatologic disease. *J Am Acad Dermatol.* 2002; 46(2 Suppl):S41-S62.

4. Bamshad MJ, Wooding S, Watkins WS, et al. Human population genetic structure and inference of group membership. *Am J Hum Genet*. 2003;72(3):578-589.

5. Jorde LB, Wooding SP. Genetic variation, classification and 'race'. *Nat Genet*. 2004;36(11 Suppl):S28-S33.

6. Rosenberg NA, Pritchard JK, Weber JL, et al. Genetic structure of human populations. *Science*. 2002; 298(5602):2381-2385.

7. Shriver MD, Kennedy GC, Parra EJ, et al. The genomic distribution of population substructure in four populations using 8,525 autosomal SNPs. *Hum Genomics*. 2004;1(4):274-286.

8. Kaplan JB, Bennett T. Use of race and ethnicity in biomedical publication. *JAMA*. 2003;289(20):2709-2716.

9. U.S. Census Bureau. http://www.census.gov. 2004. Accessed March 30, 2007.

10. Fitzpatrick TB: the validity and practicality of sun-reactive skin types I through VI. *Arch Dermatol*. 1998;124(6):869-871.

11. Fitzpatrick TB, Ortonne J. Normal skin color and general consideration of pigmentary disorders. In: Freedberg IM, Eisen AZ, Wolff K, et al., eds. *Dermatology in General Medicine*. 6th ed. New York, NY: McGraw-Hill, 2003 pp. 820-821.

12. Damian DL, Halliday GM, Barnetson RS. Prediction of minimal erythema dose with a reflectance melanin meter. *Br J Dermatol*. 1997;136(5):714-718.

13. Westerhof W, Estevez-Uscanga O, Meens J, et al. The relation between constitutional skin color and photosensitivity estimated from UV-induced erythema and pigmentation dose-response curves. *J Invest Dermatol*. 1990;94(6):812-816.

14. de Rigal J, Abella ML, Giron F, et al. Development and validation of a new Skin Color Chart. *Skin Res Technol*. 2007;13(1):101-109.

15. Kawada A. UVB-induced erythema, delayed tanning, and UVA-induced immediate tanning in Japanese skin. *Photodermatol*. 1986;3(6):327-333.

16. Lancer HA. Lancer ethnicity scale (LES). *Lasers Surg Med*. 1988;22(1):9.

17. Taylor SC, Arsonnaud S, Czernielewski J. The Taylor Hyperpigmentation Scale: a new visual assessment tool for the evaluation of skin color and pigmentation. *Cutis*. 2005;76(4):270-274.

18. Taylor S, Westerhof W, Im S, et al. Noninvasive techniques for the evaluation of skin color. *J Am Acad Dermatol*. 2006;54(5 Suppl 2):S282-S290.

19. Dornelles S, Goldim J, Cestari T. Determination of the minimal erythema dose and colorimetric measurements as indicators of skin sensitivity to UV-B radiation. *Photochem Photobiol*. 2004;79(6):540-544.

20. Alaluf S, Atkins D, Barrett K, et al. Ethnic variation in melanin content and composition in photoexposed and photoprotected human skin. *Pigment Cell Res*. 2002;15(2):112-118.

21. Franbourg A, Hallegot P, Baltenneck F, et al. Current research on ethnic hair. *J Am Acad Dermatol*. 2003;48(6 Suppl):S115-S119.

22. Grimes PE, Stockton T. Pigmentary disorders in blacks. *Dermatol Clin*. 1988;6(2):271-281.

23. Kaidbey KH, Agin PP, Sayre RM, et al. Photoprotection by melanin—a comparison of black and Caucasian skin. *J Am Acad Dermatol*. 1979;1(3):249-260.

24. Khumalo NP, Doe PT, Dawber RP, et al. What is normal black African hair? A light and scanning electron-microscopic study. *J Am Acad Dermatol*. 2000;43(5 Pt 1):814-820.

25. Montagna W, Carlisle K. The architecture of black and white facial skin. *J Am Acad Dermatol*. 1991;24(6 Pt 1):929-937.

26. Porter CE, Diridollou S, Holloway Barbosa V. The influence of African-American hair's curl pattern on its mechanical properties. *Int J Dermatol*. 2005;44(Suppl 1):4-5.

27. Sperling LC. Hair density in African Americans. *Arch Dermatol*. 1999;135(6):656-658.

28. Sueki H, Whitaker-Menezes D, Kligman AM. Structural diversity of mast cell granules in black and white skin. *Br J Dermatol*. 2001;144(1):85-93.

29. Wesley NO, Maibach HI. Racial (ethnic) differences in skin properties: the objective data. *Am J Clin Dermatol*. 2003; 4(12):843-860.

30. Wolfram LJ. Human hair: a unique physiochemical composite. *J Am Acad Dermatol*. 2003;48(6 Suppl):S106-S114.

31. Moy JA, McKinley-Grant L, Sanchez MR. Cultural aspects in the treatment of patients with skin disease. *Dermatol Clin*. 2003;21(4):733-742.

32. El-Essawi D, Musial JL, Hammad A, et al. A survey of skin disease and skin-related issues in Arab Americans. *J Am Acad Dermatol*. 2007;56(6):933-938.

33. Ajose FO. Consequences of skin bleaching in Nigerian men and women. *Int J Dermatol*. 2005;44(Suppl 1):41-43.

34. Mahe A, Ly F, Perret JL. Systemic complications of the cosmetic use of skin-bleaching products. *Int J Dermatol*. 2005; 44(Suppl 1):37-38.

35. Traore A, Kadeba JC, Niamba P, et al. Use of cutaneous depigmenting products by women in two towns in Burkina Faso: epidemiologic data, motivations, products and side effects. *Int J Dermatol*. 2005;44(Suppl 1):30-32.

36. Hall CC. Beauty is in the soul of the beholder: psychological implications of beauty and African American women. *Cult Divers Ment Health*. 1995;1(2):125-137.

37. McCurdy JA Jr. Beautiful eyes: characteristics and application to aesthetic surgery. *Facial Plast Surg*. 2006;22(3):204-214.

38. Davis RE. Rhinoplasty and concepts of facial beauty. *Facial Plast Surg*. 2006;22(3):198-203.

39. Lee CS, Lim HW. Cutaneous diseases in Asians. *Dermatol Clin*. 2003;21(4):669-677.

40. The American Society for Aesthetic Plastic Surgery. 11.5 million cosmetic procedures in 2006. http://www.surgery.org/press/news-release.php. 2006. Accessed April 5, 2007.

41. Alexis AF, Sergay AB, Taylor SC. Common dermatologic disorders in skin of color: a comparative practice survey. *Cutis*. 2007;80(5):387–396.

42. Sanchez MR. Cutaneous diseases in Latinos. *Dermatol Clin*. 2003;21(4):689-697.

43. Munavalli GS, Weiss RA, Halder RM. Photoaging and nonablative photorejuvenation in ethnic skin. *Dermatol Surg.* 2005; 31(9 Pt 2):1250-1260.

44. Chung JH. Photoaging in Asians. *Photodermatol Photoimmunol Photomed.* 2003;19(3):109-121.

45. Jackson BA. Cosmetic considerations and nonlaser cosmetic procedures in ethnic skin. *Dermatol Clin.* 2003;21(4):703-712.

46. Jackson BA. Lasers in ethnic skin: a review. *J Am Acad Dermatol.* 2003;48(6 Suppl):S134-S138.

47. Roberts WE. Chemical peeling in ethnic/dark skin. *Dermatol Ther.* 2004;17(2):196-205.

48. Downie JB. Esthetic considerations for ethnic skin. *Semin Cutan Med Surg.* 2006;25(3):158-162.

CHAPTER 2

Evaluation of the Ethnic Skin Patient Presenting for Cosmetic Procedures

Roopal V. Kundu, MD, and Rebat M. Halder, MD

INTRODUCTION

Based on the United States 2000 census data, it is estimated that 50% of the population will be comprised of persons of color by 2050.[1] Ethnic skin, also referred to as skin of color, is primarily composed of Fitzpatrick skin types IV-VI and encompasses many racial and ethnic groups, including but not limited to African Americans, Asians, Hispanics, and Native Americans. Cosmetic procedures have become increasingly popular among these darker-skinned racial and ethnic groups. However, currently the majority of the cosmetic surgical literature is limited to the treatment of nonethnic skin.

A fear of increased pigmentary and scarring complications has made dermatologists and cosmetic surgeons in the United States hesitant to perform elective procedures on persons of color. However, by appreciating the influences of structural and functional differences, such as increased melanin, follicular reactivity, and fibroblast reactivity, on ethnic skin dermatoses,[2,3] these fears can be replaced by a unique skill set to effectively and comfortably treat this patient population. Treatment of ethnic skin patients also requires knowledge of adverse reactions in darker skin, modification of surgical techniques, unique racial differences, and awareness of cultural issues specific to these patient populations.[4] In addition, an understanding and accepting of the norms of different cultures are imperative for the cosmetic surgeon to better treat persons of color who desire cosmetic surgery.

The treatment of common conditions in patients with skin of color can be multi-modal. This section will focus primarily on the initial evaluation of the ethnic skin patient presenting for cosmetic procedures.

STRUCTURAL AND FUNCTIONAL DIFFERENCES IN ETHNIC SKIN TYPES

There are various differences observed in the biology of ethnic skin and hair. These differences are important to consider because they may influence presentation of skin and hair disorders, along with the effects and tolerability of therapeutic interventions.

▪ Melanin

Melanin is the major determinant of color in the skin. The most clinically apparent difference between lightly pigmented and darkly pigmented skin is the amount of epidermal melanin. There is no difference in number of melanocytes between different skin types,[5] but the concentration of epidermal melanin in melanosomes is double in darker skin types compared to lightly pigmented skin

types.[6] It is important to remember that epidermal melanin content is twofold greater in chronically photoexposed skin regardless of ethnicity.[7] In addition, melanosome degradation within the keratinocyte is slower in darkly pigmented skin when compared to lightly pigmented skin. Therefore, although the increased melanin provides protection from the harmful effects of ultraviolet radiation (skin cancer and photoaging), it also makes darkly pigmented skins more vulnerable to postinflammatory dyspigmentation.

▪ Stratum Corneum

The stratum corneum is the outermost layer of skin functioning as the principal barrier tissue to prevent water loss from the body and provide mechanical protection. It has been found that the stratum corneum of black skin has a greater number of cell layers and higher lipid content than that of white skin. Although, the thickness of the stratum corneum is similar in both subgroups,[8] the more compact stratum corneum may influence the effectiveness of topical therapies, along with cosmetic interventions such as superficial chemical peels and microdermabrasion, in black skin.

▪ Dermis

The dermis is a dense fibroelastic connective tissue, composed of collagen fibers, elastic fibers, and glycosaminoglycans. Asian and black skin have thicker and more compact dermis than white skin, with the thickness being proportional to the degree of pigmentation.[9] This likely contributes to the lower incidence of facial rhytids in Asians and blacks. This may also lead to the propensity toward hypertrophic scarring as well in these groups.

▪ Fibroblast

The major cell type of the dermis is the fibroblast, which synthesizes the main structural elements of the dermis. Fibroblasts are more numerous, larger, and more multinucleated in black skin than white skin.[3] Fibroblast reactivity, likely influenced by mast cell induction and decreased collagenase activity, can lead to abnormal scarring, specifically hypertrophic scar, and keloid formation.

▪ Hair Follicle

The hair follicle is one of the most proliferative cell types in the human body distributed over the entire skin surface, except for the palms and soles. There have been several racial differences found in hair.[10] Asian hair is round, straight, and has the largest cross-sectional area. Black hair is spiral with a flattened elliptical shape, more brittle, more susceptible to breakage and spontaneous knotting when compared to whites. These differences may lead to propensity for pseudofolliculitis barbae (Figures 2.1 and 2.2), acne keloidalis, and central centrifugal cicatricial alopecia in black patients.

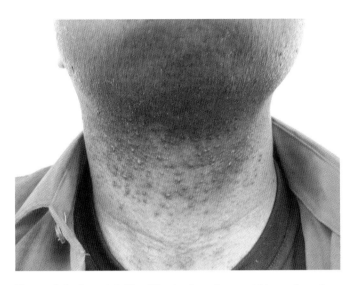

Figure 2.1 *Pseudofolliculitis barbae in an African American male. Hyperpigmented macules and papules on the neck*

RACIAL DIFFERENCES IN AGING

With advancing years, an aged appearance often is a presenting complaint for the white population. This group is often affected with secondary effects of photoaging: fine lines, deep furrows, hyperpigmentation, and age spots. Because skin of color is less susceptible to sun-induced photodamage,[11] these clinical manifestations of aging are less severe and typically occur 10 to 20 years later than those of age-matched white counterparts. In Fitzpatrick phototypes IV-VI, the initial complaints of aging are often different than lighter-skinned counterparts, with more concern about development of uneven skin color and loss of subcutaneous fat. Younger patients in the ethnic skin population also may more frequently present with unhappiness regarding their uneven skin color, postinflammatory hyperpigmentation, scarring, or excessive hair growth (Figures 2.3 and 2.4).

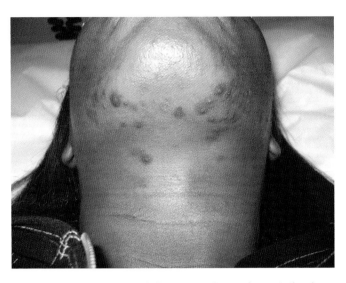

Figure 2.3 *Acne with postinflammatory hyperpigmentation in an African American female. Erythematous papules and hyperpigmented macules along the jawline*

■ Extrinsic Aging

Extrinsic aging relate to environmental exposures, health and lifestyle. These factors are controllable and related to individual habits such as sun exposure, tobacco use, diet, and exercise.

■ Photoaging

Cumulative exposure to sun is the most important factor in aging of the skin for lighter skin types and is responsible for the majority of unwanted aesthetic effects in this subgroup. Ethnic patients of Fitzpatrick types III-IV or those of mixed ethnicity may also suffer from dermatoheliosis. In darker skinned patients, pigmentary changes are common features of photoaging.[12] The common clinical signs of photoaging in these patients include lentigines, keratosis, rhytids, telangiectasias, and loss of elasticity.

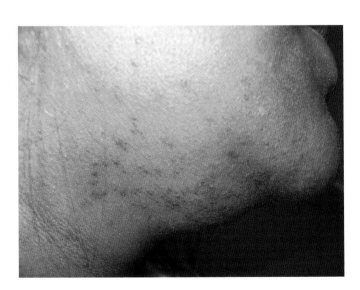

Figure 2.2 *Pseudofolliculitis barbae in an African American female. Hyperpigmented papules and coarse terminal hairs on the cheek and neck*

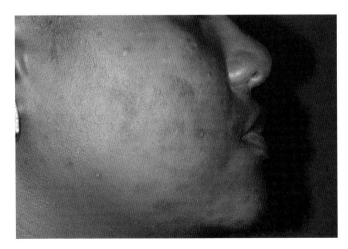

Figure 2.4 *Postinflammatory hyperpigmentation in an African American female. Hyperpigmented macules over the cheek and chin*

Smoking, Alcohol, Poor Nutrition

Other external factors such as smoking, excessive use of alcohol, and poor nutrition can also contribute to premature skin aging regardless of skin type.

Intrinsic Aging

Over the last century, life expectancy has nearly doubled, leading individuals expecting to be productive well beyond the seventh decade of life along with a strong desire to maintain a youthful appearance. Intrinsic aging reflects the genetic background of an individual and results from the passage of time. It is uncontrollable and inevitable. Intrinsically aged skin is typically smooth and unblemished, with exaggerated expression lines, fat atrophy with soft tissue redistribution, and bone remodeling. It is commonly accepted that people of color exhibit less severe intrinsic facial aging when compared to their lighter-skinned counterparts; however, there is a paucity of literature discussing the relationship between facial morphology in darker-pigmented persons and the aging face.

PATIENT SELECTION FOR COSMETIC PROCEDURES

Identifying the Chief Complaint and Anatomic Defect

Detailed patient interviews to clearly identify the chief concerns of the patient, diagnose the primary anatomic defect, and determine the patient's treatment objective is important to ensure a satisfactory outcome. Many ethnic skin patients are concerned most by postinflammatory hyperpigmentation, and less so by the inciting factor such as acne or eczema. Improving the dyschromia will create a satisfied patient for the short-term, but the inciting dermatoses must also be adequately treated for long-term benefit. Along with clearly identifying the patient's primary complaint and achieving the correct medical diagnosis, it is also important to correctly match the appropriate therapeutic procedure to the particular anatomic defect. Failure to do so will often lead to mediocre or possibly disastrous results and unhappy patients. For example, ethnic skin patients with deep pitted and rolling scars may be better candidates for subscision with fillers or laser surgery, instead of deep chemical peels or dermabrasion which may lead to further scarring and dyspigmentation over the short- or long-term.

Obtaining Pertinent History

After discussing the chief complaint, a thorough review of past medical history, current medications (including over-the-counter and alternative treatments, recent isotretinoin use, photosensitizing medications), allergies (including contact), social history (exercise, alcohol, tobacco, and drug use), family history (scarring), and review of symptoms should be conducted.

The patient's individual beauty care routine should be discussed with special attention given to specific cultural habits and practices that the patient follows for their skin, hair, and nail care regimens. For example, it is common practice for African American women to use toners and astringents containing alcohol and/or witch hazel to help treat acne, along with over-the-counter bleaching creams containing hydroquinone for their postinflammatory hyperpigmentation. Lastly, it is important to discuss routine sun protection habits, since many patients of color do not practice sun avoidance or use daily sun protection.

Physical Examination

A thorough physical examination of not only the primary anatomic defect, but also the remainder of the skin should be completed, with special focus for signs of abnormal scarring or poor healing. For facial evaluations, the patient should remove all makeup, moisturizers, and topical medications prior to evaluation. A mirror can be a useful simple tool to help the patient point directly to his/her problem areas. In addition, the physician can also use the mirror to demonstrate potential effects of cosmetic interventions (i.e., improvement of rhytids and scarring).

Obtaining Consent

Obtaining consent with a clear outline of risks and benefits is essential prior to beginning any cosmetic procedure, especially in persons of color because of the higher risk of untoward effects, particularly postinflammatory hyperpigmentation and scarring. The main reasons for poor patient satisfaction are unrealistic expectations, a lack of understanding postprocedure skin care, and short-term complications, such as postinflammatory hyperpigmentation. The consent process for procedures in ethnic skin will be outlined in Chapter 4.

Photography

Standardized digital photography can be a great asset to demonstrate potential effects of treatments during the consent process. It can also be utilized to show a patient his/her own before and after photographs. It is imperative to standardize the lighting, patient positioning, and frame of the photograph for a good comparison.

PSYCHOLOGICAL ASPECTS OF COSMETIC DERMATOLOGY

Body dissatisfaction is considered a potent risk for the development of eating disorders and can contribute to depression.

Body Dysmorphic Disorder

Body dysmorphic disorder (BDD) is a psychiatric disorder defined as preoccupation with an imagined or slight defect in appearance.[13] This preoccupation causes impairment in social, occupational, or other important areas of functioning and daily living. These patients may often request and undergo unnecessary cosmetic procedures. Most BDD patients are dissatisfied with dermatological treatment and, even if the outcome is objectively acceptable, they do not worry less about their appearance afterwards. BDD is relatively common in cosmetic practice, yet it remains under-recognized.

It is important that dermatologists screen for BDD. A simple and reliable set of questions that dermatologists can ask to diagnose BDD has been published.[14] Clinical experience suggests that once

BDD is diagnosed, it is best to openly tell patients that they have a body image problem known as BDD and provide a list of resources for them. Treatment is best given by a health professional experienced in treating these patients, who may be a psychiatrist or dermatologist with an interest in psychocutaneous disease.

PHYSICIAN–PATIENT COMMUNICATION

Patients of color are often seeking guidance from a physician who has firsthand knowledge and experience treating problems that are common to their skin. Physicians treating skin of color should identify their interest in darker pigmented skins to the patient and discuss their professional experience. This will allow the physician to quickly make a personal connection with the patient carving a path for an open, trusting relationship.

When pursuing more high-risk cosmetic interventions or those with prolonged healing time, the physician may consider a built-in waiting period when the patient is under initial medical management for several months. This waiting period provides an opportunity to assess the rate of progression of disease and more importantly, allows the clinician time to assess patient desires, expectations, and willingness to comply with postprocedural care. All these behavioral factors are critical in determining the ultimate success of a procedure.

EXCLUSION CRITERIA

Not all patients are appropriate candidates for cosmetic interventions. Patients treated with isotretinoin within the previous 6 months, a predisposition to keloid or hypertrophic scarring, recent suntan, and those with unrealistic expectations should be excluded. Procedures on pregnant and nursing women or those trying to get pregnant should be avoided.

END-OF-VISIT COUNSELING

Regardless if the patient decides to pursue a cosmetic procedure or not, it is important to discuss the tools to develop a lifelong healthy skincare regimen, with particular attention to sun protection and avoidance of smoking and excessive alcohol. Most people of color do not feel it is necessary for them to wear sun protection because of their innate pigment and lower risk of skin cancer; however, daily sun protection with a minimum of SPF 15 should be strongly encouraged to help limit and prevent uneven skin color, postinflammatory hyperpigmentation, and extrinsic aging. For patients with dyschromia, guidance on cosmetic camouflage options to use prior to and posttreatment, such as CoverFx© and Dermablend®, which have a large palette of colors to help closely match skin tone, should be offered. This attention to detail will hopefully lead to not only better treatment outcomes, but also a long-term physician–patient relationship.

SUMMARY

The reasons to undergo cosmetic procedures are always personal, psychological, and closely linked to body image. It is important for the dermatologist to understand that appearance matters in our society; however, it is only one component of overall self-esteem. Studies have shown that improving physical attractiveness positively affects personality and interpersonal interactions.[15] The cosmetic dermatologist can play a unique role in patient's lives by not only providing them with services to impart a more youthful and beautiful appearance, but also by educating patients on techniques to prevent aging and avenues to further develop a healthy psyche.

REFERENCES

1. Taylor SC. Skin of color: biology, structure, function, and implications for dermatologic disease. *J Am Acad Dermatol.* 2002; 46:S41.

2. Richards GM, Oresajo CO, Halder RM. Structure and function of ethnic skin and hair. *Dermatol Clin.* 2003;21:595.

3. Montagna W, Carlisle K. The architecture of black and white facial skin. *J Am Acad Dermatol.* 1991;24:929.

4. Moy JA, McKinley-Grant L, Sanchez MR. Cultural aspects in the treatment of patients with skin disease. *Dermatol Clin.* 2003;21:733.

5. Staricco RJ, Pinkus H. Quantitative and qualitative data on the pigment cells of adult human epidermis. *J Invest Dermatol.* 1957;28:33.

6. Iozumi K, Hoganson GE, Pennella R, et al. Role of tyrosinase as the determinant of pigmentation in cultured human melanocytes. *J Invest Dermatol.* 1993;100:806.

7. Alaluf S, Atkins D, Barrett K, et al. Ethnic variation in melanin content and composition in photoexposed and photoprotected human skin. *Pigment Cell Res.* 2002;15:112.

8. Weigand DA, Haygood C, Gaylor JR. Cell layers and density of Negro and Caucasian stratum corneum. *J Invest Dermatol.* 1974;62:563.

9. Montagna W, Giusseppe P, Kenney JA. The structure of black skin. In: Montagna W, Giusseppe P, Kenney JA, eds. *Black Skin Structure and Function.* San Diego, CA: Academic Press; 1993:37.

10. Vernall DG. A study of the size and shape of cross sections of hair from four races of men. *Am J Phys Anthropol.* 1961;19:345.

11. Kaidbey KH, Agin PP, Sayre RM, et al. Photoprotection by melanin—a comparison of black and Caucasian skin. *J Am Acad Dermatol.* 1979;1:249.

12. Chung JH, Lee SH, Youn CS, et al. Cutaneous photodamage in koreans: influence of sex, sun exposure, smoking, and skin color. *Arch Dermatol.* 2001;137:1043.

13. American Psychiatric Association. *Diagnostic and Statistical Manual of Mental Disorders.* 4th ed. Washington, DC: American Psychiatric Association; 1994.

14. Dufresne RG, Phillips KA, Vittorio CC, et al. A screening questionnaire for body dysmorphic disorder in a cosmetic dermatologic surgery practice. *Dermatol Surg.* 2001;27:457.

15. Patzer GL. Improving self-esteem by improving physical attractiveness. *J Esthet Dent.* 1997;9:44.

CHAPTER 3

Potential Adverse Effects After Procedures in Ethnic Skin

Henry Hin-Lee Chan, MD, FRCP, and Changhuh Huh, MD, PhD

INTRODUCTION

Complications can arise in any cosmetic procedure, and appropriate consultation prior to any treatment to obtain informed consent is of utmost importance. This chapter concerns the potential complications of common cosmetic procedures that are performed on Asian patients. Procedures that are discussed here include chemical peels, laser therapy, radio frequency (RF), botulinum toxin, and fillers.

CHEMICAL PEEL, ABLATIVE, AND FRACTIONAL RESURFACING

Chemical peeling, especially medium depth and deep peels, are in many ways similar to ablative resurfacing and have similar potential complications, so they are discussed together. Plasma skin resurfacing and fractional resurfacing are new technologies that are considered to be nonablative but do have results that are compatible to ablative resurfacing. The complications of these procedures are also discussed.

Absolute contraindications of chemical peels and ablative resurfacing are rare and include previous history of keloid, autoimmune disease, pregnancy, and current oral isotretinoin intake. Prior to any ablative procedure, a careful inspection to detect any scars, excoriation, or inflammation is necessary. For chemical peel, the peeling agent can penetrate deep into even undetectable scars, causing unexpected worsening of the scar. Petroleum jelly should be applied onto the scar and sensitive areas such as the canthus and vermilion border.

Temporary reactions that occur after ablative procedures are expected consequences, and appropriate explanations to the patient are important to avoid any unnecessary misunderstanding. To minimize permanent or long-lasting complications, physicians must understand the properties of the peel agent and, in cases of ablative laser resurfacing, be familiar with the laser device and parameters, select the proper patients, and detect early signs of complications.

◼ Pain

Patients often complain of a tingling, itchy feeling or pain after chemical peel or ablative resurfacing. For patients undergoing superficial chemical peel who experience excessive pain, the peeling agents should be immediately and completely removed by thorough washing. For deep peel and ablative resurfacing, a nerve block and topical anesthetic reduce the pain during the procedure. Oral analgesic is usually adequate for postoperative pain control.

◼ Erythema/Edema

In general, erythema is a normal, inevitable reaction that can occur after chemical peel, fractional resurfacing, and ablative resurfacing. Depending on the type of procedure, erythema disappears spontaneously within several hours to days. Patients should be informed that such a reaction is temporary and inevitable for such treatment. Excessive erythema can be associated with a greater risk of postinflammatory hyperpigmentation (PIH), and in cases of deep peel and ablative resurfacing, scarring can develop.

Measures to minimize erythema include avoidance of spicy food and alcohol, sunlight exposure, fragrant cosmetics (some contain photosensitizer), tretinoin use, and frequent repetitive peels. Topical antioxidant to reduce free radicals can also be helpful to minimize the erythema.

For persistent erythema (lasting longer than 1 week), low-potency topical steroid with twice-daily application can be useful. Potent topical steroids are reserved for more severe cases, and triamcinolone intralesional injection is required for the nodular erythema. Pulsed dye laser in conjunction with topical steroid can also be used for the treatment of persistent erythema.

Edema is extremely rare after superficial peels, so allergic reaction to the chemical agent must be considered in the case of significant edema. For fractional resurfacing and plasma skin resurfacing, edema lasting 2 to 4 days is expected. Nonsteroidal anti-inflammatory medication can be used to reduce postoperative edema and thereby reduce the downtime associated with fractional resurfacing. For ablative procedure such as deep chemical peel and laser skin resurfacing, edema tends to last several days. However, because the downtime associated with such procedures is usually related to the duration of cutaneous reepithelization, the degree of edema is not usually a main concern.

◼ Pigmentary Changes

PIH is the most important and common complication that can occur after chemical peel, fractional resurfacing, and ablative procedures. Obtaining proper informed consent is important, but measures to avoid PIH can improve the clinical outcome. Factors that contribute to PIH include skin type, recent sun exposure, and degree of inflammation, especially at the epidermal–dermal junction.

In general, the darker the skin type, the more likely it is that PIH can occur. While Fitzpatrick skin type is the only universal means to classify skin phototype, it is not very accurate when applied to skin of color patients. Detailed questioning regarding the patient's tendency to tan or burn is necessary to get a better understanding of the patient's phototype. Previous history of color change after minor injuries such as insect bite or acne is another way to assess the patient's phototype. For patients who are prone to develop PIH, a more conservative approach should be adapted.

Preoperative measures to minimize PIH include sun avoidance and use of sun protection at least 2 weeks before any such procedure and avoidance of photosensitizing agents such as tetracycline or oral contraceptives. As for the sunscreen, physical sunscreen and avoidance are preferable to chemical sunscreen because the latter can lead to irritation.

The preoperative use of bleaching agents is more controversial; a previous study indicated that recent suntan is more significant in the development of PIH and the use of bleaching agents preoperatively was shown to be less significant.[1]

In general, superficial chemical peels using 20% to 30% alpha-hydroxy acid for 3 to 5 minutes are usually very safe with a low risk of PIH. Depending upon the degree of erythema, the operator can alter the concentration and exposure time after the first treatment. For fractional resurfacing, previous studies indicate that while both energy and density are important in the determination of the risk of PIH, density is of particular importance and should be adjusted to about half of that used in Caucasians[2] (Figure 3.1). In general, the duration of edema should be no longer than 2 days and of erythema no longer than 1 week. For laser resurfacing and plasma skin resurfacing, PIH is a definite risk unless one uses energy that induced very superficial injury similar to that observed in superficial peel (Figure 3.2). Among Asians, laser resurfacing or plasma skin resurfacing can be used in the treatment of atrophic acne scar or surgical scar, especially among male patients. If the whole face is treated, increased pigmentation often mimics a suntan and is usually well accepted by male patients provided that prior informed consent is given. For ablative procedures, feathering is important to avoid marked demarcation lines between treated and untreated area.

Strict sun avoidance should be encouraged for at least 4 weeks postoperatively. Bleaching agents can be used postoperatively to prevent the development of PIH, but timing is important to avoid further irritation, which can increase the likelihood of PIH. The generally accepted optimal time for the posttreatment is 1 week after exfoliation of crust.

If PIH develops, most cases tend to resolve within 6 months to 1 year; rarely, some last for years. Treatments of PIH include the use of bleaching agents such as Kligman's formula, which consists of hydroquinone, topical steroid, and tretinoin. Detailed use of bleaching agents is discussed in Chapter 5. In addition to topical bleaching agents, the use of superficial peels, microdermabrasion, or low-energy large-spot size 1064-nm Nd:YAG laser treatment can be helpful.

Delayed permanent hypopigmentation that occurs after laser resurfacing and deep peel is widely reported in light-skinned patients and tends to be less common in Asians. Up to now, no such cases have been reported in patients treated with fractional resurfacing or plasma skin resurfacing.

Unlike laser resurfacing or deep peels, fractional resurfacing and plasma skin resurfacing can also be used in areas off the face. The risk of pigmentary changes increases in off-face use and lowering of the energy is important to reduce such risk.

▨ Scarring

Scarring is extremely rare with superficial peels but more common with deeper peels or laser resurfacing, especially in cases complicated by superimposed infection. Scarring should not occur in fractional resurfacing except in cases of bulk tissue heating, whereby the lack of cooling combined with consecutive passes in a small anatomical area leads to a significant elevation in skin temperature[3] (Figure 3.3). Plasma skin resurfacing is not known to cause scarring except in cases of infection. In general, for ablative procedures, if

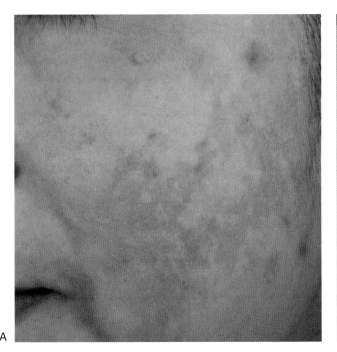
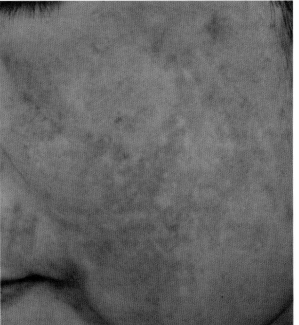

Figure 3.1 *(A) Before treatment and (B) PIH after the use of fractional laser resurfacing for the treatment of melasma*

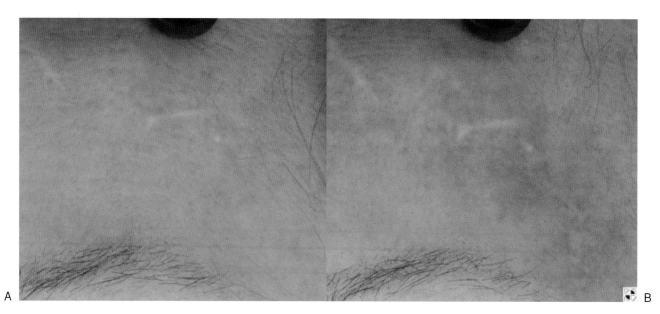

Figure 3.2 *(A) Before treatment and (B) PIH after the use of plasma skin resurfacing (4 J/cm²) for atrophic scar*

wound healing is not completed by 2 weeks postoperatively or if persistent erythema develops, early intervention should commence to prevent or minimize scar development.

Hypertrophic scarring is more common on certain areas of the face, like the perioral area, neck, chest, and hand and special caution is needed especially around eye lesions, where ectropion can develop. Patients who have been taken isotretinoin also have an increased risk for scar development, and this medication should be stopped at least 6 months preoperatively.

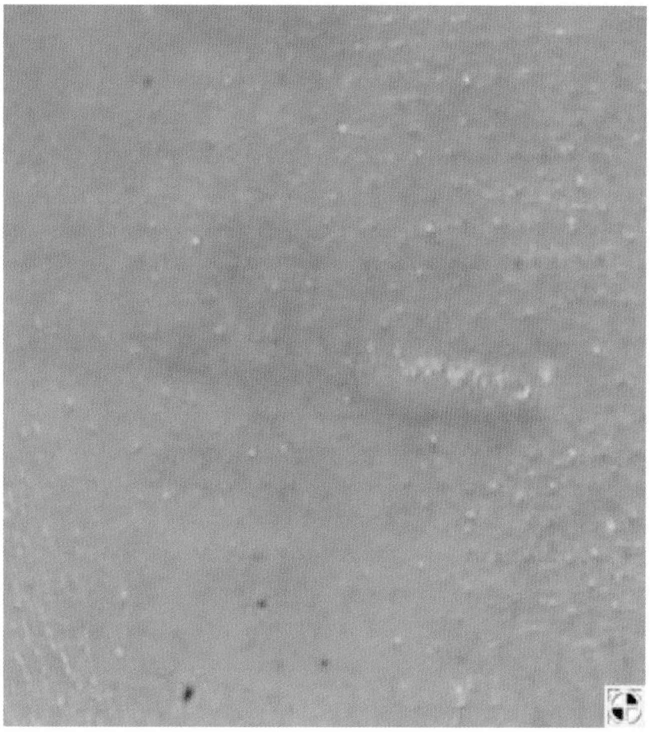

Infections

Infection is also an uncommon complication, but when it occurs, early detection and prompt treatment are most important to prevent scar formation.

Most bacterial superinfections are caused by poor wound care management, so this can often be avoided by providing the patient with clear and explicit postoperative care instructions. If this occurs, a culture sample should be taken and the patient treated with appropriate oral antibiotics immediately to prevent further complications.

For patients who undergo deep chemical peel, fractional resurfacing, plasma skin resurfacing, and laser resurfacing, systemic antiviral agents (e.g., aciclovir, valaciclovir, or famciclovir) and systemic antibiotic (cefuroxime) should be commenced 48 hours before laser surgery and until complete re-epithelization occurs. Herpetic infection after these procedures is hard to diagnose because epidermis is removed so blister formation is not common. Sometimes painful erythema or necrosis is the only symptom. To differentiate bacterial and herpetic infection, the time sequence of pain and erythema may be helpful. If pain exists prior to erythema, herpetic infection should be suspected, because pain only develops in bacterial infection.

Acne/Milia

Acne or perioral acneiform dermatitis can occur after the chemical peel, fractional resurfacing, or ablative resurfacing. This is particular common among acne scar patients, and in the author's (H.C.) experience, it would be best to commence 2 weeks of antibiotic to prevent reactive acne in these patients postoperatively.

Milia formation occurs frequently and is easily treated. The use of appropriate postoperative skin care product, lotion, or gel rather

Figure 3.3 *Atrophic scar in the forehead after fractional resurfacing when cooling was not used*

than ointment can prevent milia development. Milia tends to develop 3 to 6 days postoperatively and disappears spontaneously in 6 to 12 weeks. Topical use of tretinoin and other keratolytic agents can reduce formation of milia and light superficial scrubs can also be helpful for multiple or smaller lesions. Comedone extraction can be performed, if necessary.

Eye Injury

Eye injury can occur during the peeling procedure. Corneal abrasion and conjunctivitis have been reported from trichloroacetic acid (TCA) during peeling. Risk can be minimized by diligence during the procedure the use of protective ophthalmic ointment and eye guards. If peeling agent accidentally spills into the eye, it must be rinsed out with water and steroid-containing eye drops applied as soon as possible.

For laser procedure, a metal eye shield can be used to avoid laser injury. The operator and assistants should also wear the appropriate eye protection to avoid occupational injury.

Systemic Absorption

Some deep peels like phenol may cause a systemic side effect like cardiac arrhythmia, which is potentially fatal and electrocardiographic monitoring is therefore necessary. To prevent those systemic reactions to chemical agents, patients must be fully hydrated before the treatment and treatment must be divided by cosmetic unit, with the appropriate time intervals.

Salicylate toxicity is also well-known systemic intoxication caused by salicylic acid. It usually begins with tinnitus and vertigo and may progress to deafness or anaphylactic shock when excessive doses are used. The procedure lesion must be less than 50% of body surface with 20% salicylic acid. Lesolucynol, a component of Jessner's solution, also may cause hypothyroidism when used on a long-term basis. It is also associated with hepatic toxicity and may cause methemoglobinemia-induced jaundice.

For laser procedure or plasma skin resurfacing, systemic absorption of topical anesthetic occurs if a large area is treated. Potent topical lidocaine (30%) can potentially be absorbed, leading to systemic issues, and this is best avoided.

PIGMENT LASER

The most common complication associated with the use of pigment laser in Asian skin is PIH. As mentioned earlier, sun exposure should be avoided at least 2 weeks before the laser procedure and for 4 weeks after. In addition to skin types and sun exposure, the risk of PIH depends on the type of lesions and setting of the laser/intense pulsed light source (IPL).

For freckles and lentigines, previous studies indicated that while Q-switched (QS) laser can be most effective, requiring only one or two treatment sessions, the risk of PIH can be as high as 5% to 10%, especially in cases of lentigo.[4,5] Such a high incidence of PIH is proposed to be related to the photomechanical effect of QS laser, which can lead to an excessive degree of inflammation. Long-pulsed laser (millisecond domain) can also be used for the treatment of freckles and lentigines. The risk of PIH is lower, estimated to be approximately 1%; this is largely because of the lack of photomechanical effect. More recently, compression to empty the blood vessels and, in doing so, reduce competing chromophobes has been found to be effective in further reducing the risk of PIH in both long-pulsed and QS lasers when used in the treatment of lentigines.[6,7]

QS lasers are well established as the gold standard for the treatment of dermal melanocytic lesions such as nevus of Ota or Hori's macules.[8,9] Both PIH and hypopigmentation can occur after laser treatment. Pigmentary disturbances are particularly common among patients with Hori's macules, and most experience PIH after the first two or three QS lasers treatment[10] (Figure 3.4). Hypopigmentation can also occur when QS ruby is used, and in cases of nevus of Ota, the risk of hypopigmentation can be as high as 16%.[11] More recent study has indicated that the use of air-cooling in conjunction with QS laser for the treatment of Hori's macules can increase the risk of PIH.[12]

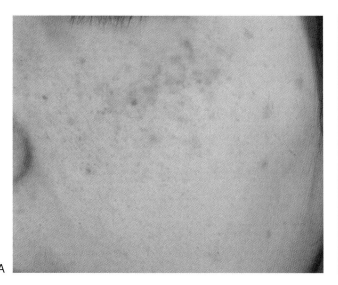
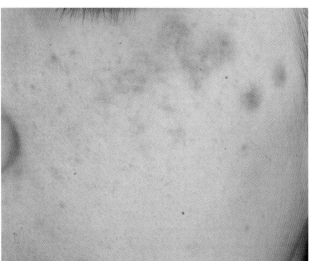

A

B

Figure 3.4 *(A) Before treatment and (B) PIH after treatment with QS ruby for Hori's macules*

LASER-ASSISTED HAIR REMOVAL

Nanni and Alster[13] looked at the adverse effects experienced by 900 patients who underwent laser-assisted hair removal and found that skin type has a direct impact on the risk of unwanted side effects. Factors that are important to reduce adverse reactions among dark-skinned patients during laser-assisted hair removal include the following:

- Effective epidermal cooling
- Long pulse duration
- Long wavelengths
- Sun protection and avoidance
- Prophylactic bleaching program
- Topical steroid application postlaser surgery

Long-pulsed ruby is one of the first used for hair removal with pigmentary changes that ranged from 37% to 83% in skin type IV or V patients. Short-pulsed duration (1 ms) was associated with a higher risk of complication compared with longer pulse duration (20 ms).[14] For long-pulsed alexandrite laser, Garcia et al.[15] looked at 150 patients with skin type IV to VI and found a low complication rate (2% compared with 37% in a previous study) when a 10-day prophylactic bleaching program (2% HQ/glycolic acid at night plus sun block) was used. Not surprisingly, skin type VI patients had the highest risk of adverse effects (two of two).

Another study looked at dark-skinned patients treated with alexandrite laser for hair removal and found postinflammatory complications to be common, with the initial development of hyperpigmented rings, to be followed later by thin wafer-like crust and then subsequent hypopigmentation.[16]

A study that investigated the efficacy and complications of long-pulsed diode and long-pulsed Nd:YAG lasers in hair removal from skin type III and IV patients showed that long-pulsed Nd:YAG laser was associated with significantly greater pain immediately after surgery and a more protracted treatment time.[17] Transient adverse effects were erythema and perifollicular edema. One patient developed hypopigmentation at week 6, which resolved by week 36. These findings were further confirmed by Alster et al.,[18] who examined 20 dark-skinned patients treated with long-pulsed Nd:YAG lasers, which were found to be safe and effective. Battle et al.[19] suggested that for effective hair removal from dark-skinned patients, including those with skin types V and VI, very long pulses (20–200 ms) are necessary to improve clinical efficacy without a significant increase in the risk of adverse effects. Using a very long-pulsed diode laser, they found that transient pigment changes, the most common side effect, were further reduced.[19]

A recent study that looked at 28 Koreans who were treated with four sessions of IPL indicated minimal adverse effects with a clearance rate of up to 80%.[20] A combination of bipolar RF and IPL has been used effectively for hair removal. At 6 months after four treatment sessions, the clearance rate ranged from 40% to 85% and the results did not show any dependence in terms of skin color.[21] Mild erythema was observed in 20% of patients, and hyperpigmentation in 8%.

Paradoxical hypertrichosis after laser epilation is an uncommon phenomenon in which patients observe increased hair growth at sites of untreated areas close to the previously treated laser epilation areas. The estimated prevalence is approximately 0.6%.[22] It is more common in persons of darker skin phototypes (IV) with black hair. This paradoxical effect is most common after the use of IPL and alexandrite lasers and has been considered to be activation of dormant hair follicles by suboptimal fluencies.[23] The application of an ice pack to the adjacent area immediately after laser hair removal can reduce the risk of paradoxical hypertrichosis.

VASCULAR LASERS

Asian patients with more melanin in the epidermis are at a higher risk of adverse effects such as vesiculation and pigmentary changes. Furthermore, with the epidermal melanin acting as a competing target chromophore for hemoglobin, higher fluence may be necessary to produce the desirable clinical end point. A study in Singapore looked at 36 Chinese patients with port wine stain who were treated with pulsed dye lasers, and transient PIH was seen in all subjects.[24] Another study reported that while dark-skinned patients with port wine stain could benefit from pulse dye lasers, adverse effects were not uncommon and affected 12% of their subjects.[25] Other European series found a much lower degree of pigmentary change when patients with lighter skin types were treated.[26]

The use of skin cooling in conjunction with vascular laser has dramatically improved the clinical efficacy and reduced adverse effects. Cryogen cooling with pulsed dye laser was examined in the treatment of port wine stains in skin types III and IV and was found to be effective with reduced adverse effect compared to pulsed dye laser alone.[27] However, for skin types V and VI, epidermal protection could not be achieved even at the lowest radiant exposure (8 J/cm^2).[28] A variable pulse 532-nm Nd:YAG laser equipped with contact cooling with a water glass chamber was comparatively ineffective when used in the treatment of port wine stains in skin types III and IV but was used effectively for the treatment of facial telangiectasia.[29] There are only limited data on the optimal cooling parameters and efficacy of other cooling devices such as air-cooling for the treatment of vascular lesions when used in dark-skinned patients.

The most common transit adverse effects following the use of vascular lasers are swelling and redness when subpurpuric dose is used. For the treatment of port wine stain, a purpuric dose is necessary, and while skin cooling has reduced the risk of adverse effect, pigmentary changes can still occur but are usually transient, especially for facial lesions. For the treatment of leg telangiectasia, if a purpuric dose is used, then hemosiderin deposition can lead to prolong increase in pigmentation. Among all the vascular lasers, a long-pulsed 1064-nm Nd:YAG laser can result in more serious complication if used inappropriately. Pulse staking with this laser can lead to bulk tissue heating with disastrous consequences, including blister and scar formation.

RF AND FOCUSED ULTRASOUND

These devices induce deep dermal and subcutaneous injury and are therefore independent of skin type. Nonetheless, the use of monopolar RF can induce linear erythema caused by cryogen

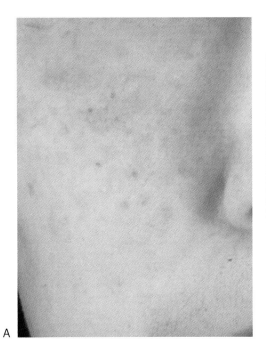
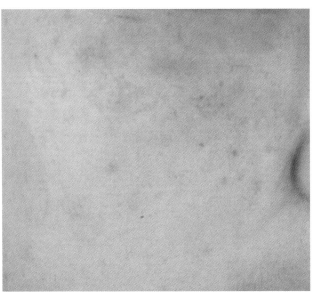

A

B

Figure 3.5 *(A) Before treatment and (B) Swelling and linear erythema after treatment with monopolar RF*

injury (Figure 3.5). Such linear erythema can result in PIH. Tissue irregularity and fat atrophy were reported when high-energy monopolar RF was used, but a change in treatment approach using low energy and multiple passes significantly reduced such adverse effects.[30] The use of bipolar RF with light source or laser can result in blister and scar formation if the operator failed to ensure adequate contact of both electrodes to the skin surface (Figure 3.6).

Focused ultrasound has been used for body contouring. Treatment over bony area must be avoided to prevent reflection of ultrasonic energy to the skin surface causing blister and subsequent scar formation.

BOTULINUM TOXIN

Since botulinum toxin is widely used for treatment of wrinkle, many physicians broaden its indications to other applications including hyperhidrosis and the treatment of masseteric hypertrophy. Complications from the use of botulinum toxin (Botox) injections occur infrequently and are transient, reversible, and, in most cases, technique dependent.[31]

▓ Edema

Edema is not uncommon after botulinum toxin injection in Asians. From the author's (C.H.) experience, the degree of edema appears to be related to the volume of injection and increase when higher dilutions are used. The exact cause of edema is uncertain but lymphatic insufficiency caused by muscle paralysis and eyebrow ptosis are considered to be important factors.

▓ Bruising

Bruising is most common in the upper face, especially in crow's feet. The avoidance of aspirin, NSAIDs, and garlic at least 10 days prior to treatment can reduce the risk of bruising. Topical anesthetic such as EMLA or the application of an ice bag before injection-induced vasoconstriction can further reduce the risk of bruising. Topical vitamin K can be used to hasten the resolution of bruises.

▓ Undesirable Paralysis of Muscle

Although doses and injection points should be individualized, in general, lower doses should be used in Asians compared to Caucasians.

Figure 3.6 *Scar after bipolar RF with light source*

A typical dose regimen for Asians is 6 to 8 U for crow's feet, 10 to 16 U for glabella, and 6 to 10 U for the forehead to start; doing so will reduce the risk of complications such as eyebrow ptosis. In the upper face, the most serious side effects are ptosis and, very rarely, diplopia or ectropion.

Ptosis develops as a result of the diffusion of botulinum toxin through the orbital septum to the levator palpebral muscle. Excessive paralysis of the frontalis can also induce eyebrow ptosis.

When ptosis develops, the application of 0.5% iopidine eye drops (mydriatic agent) can affect Muller's muscle and improve ptosis by elevating the eyebrow.[32] Another common complication for Asian people is excessive elevation of the lateral eyebrow. Inadequate treatment of the lateral frontalis is the main reason; if this occurs, an additional injection of 1 to 1.5 U on the lateral frontalis will amend the condition. The most serious complication seen in the upper face is diplopia, which can last 4 to 8 weeks.[33]

Complications associated with botulinum toxin in the lower face are more common and include asymmetrical smiling and dribbling. In general, lower face injection does not produce the same degree of patient satisfaction as does upper face injection, and therefore other therapeutic options, such as fillers or ablative resurfacing should be considered either as an alternative or used in combination with botulinum toxin.

One of the popular indications for cosmetic botulinum toxin therapy in Asia is to reduce the masseter muscle volume to narrow the face.[34] Botulinum toxin blocks the movement of masseter muscle and results in disuse atrophy. The most common complication of this procedure is overdosing, which can result in difficulty in mastication.[35] Partial reactive hypertrophy of the masseter muscle, caused by partial paralysis, can also occur.

Injection into the platysma can also be associated with dysphagia and difficulties in flexing the neck and nodding.[36]

In the treatment of hyperhidrosis, small muscle weakness of the hands can be troublesome.[37] Residual hyperhidrosis and asymmetries have also been reported, which can be amended by repeat treatment 2 weeks after the initial injection.

Systemic Adverse Effects

The use of botulinum toxin is reported to have unmasked underlying myasthenia gravis in one patient; therefore, its use is contraindicated in patients with myasthenia gravis, systemic lupus erythematosus, and other autoimmune diseases.

Antibody Formation

Antibody to botulinum toxin can develop after repeat injection, especially when a high dose is used in medical rather than cosmetic treatment.[38] In general, a lower-dose treatment regimen, such as less than 100 U per treatment session, and increased treatment interval to more than 1 month can reduce the risk of antibody production. The possibility of antibody production arises among patients who fail to improve after subsequent injection. As there are seven serotypes of botulinum toxin, an alternative serotype can be used in patients who have developed antibody to a particular serotype of botulinum toxin.

SOFT TISSUE AUGMENTATION

Most of the complications associated with the use of fillers are preventable and depend on factors including operator technique, sterility of the procedure, type of fillers, and patient's general condition. Adverse reactions to fillers can be classified as acute or delayed reaction. Acute reactions include pain, erythema, edema, and bruise.[39] Such a reaction is common and can be reduced by taking the appropriate measures. Delayed complications are less common and include infection, local necrosis, migration of filler material, and chronic foreign body granuloma formation.

Pain

To minimize pain during the procedure, topical anesthetics or nerve block can be used. Application of an ice pack before injection may also be helpful.

Bruising

To avoid bruising, the patients must not take aspirin or other NSAIDs at least 3 days before and after injection. The use of a cross-polarized magnifying lens can also assist the operator in the identification of small capillaries and, in doing so, reduce the chances of bruising. If bruising develops, the use of vitamin K cream can also be helpful.

Surface Irregularity

It is commonly seen in superficial injection, with the fan technique, and with overcorrection. This surface deformity can last several weeks or months depending on the type of filler. To avoid this, proper massage to mold the shape must be applied after injection. The advantage of hyaluronic acid is that it is not permanent and the use of hyaluronidase (Hyalase) could correct this issue.[40]

Infection

Infection associated with filler injection is uncommon but can lead to serious consequences. Strict aseptic technique is necessary. Once open, the filler should be used as soon as possible. In the author's (H.C.) practice, if the filler is not completely used during the initial treatment, patients are advised to return the next day for potential further injection once the initial swelling subsided. Although a study suggested that stored nonanimal, stabilized hyaluronic acid gel syringes remained sterile at room temperature as long as 9 months after initial patient injection,[41] in the author's (H.C.) practice, hyaluronic acid gel syringes are disposed within 24 hours after opening. For patients who develop significant pain and swelling after injection, a skin swab should be taken and a broad-spectrum antibiotic such as cefuroxime should be commenced.

Necrosis/Blindness

Local necrosis is an uncommon occurrence but can occur when filler is injected into a blood vessel. Factors that contribute to the development of tissue necrosis include anatomical site, density of

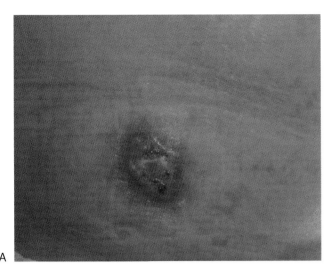
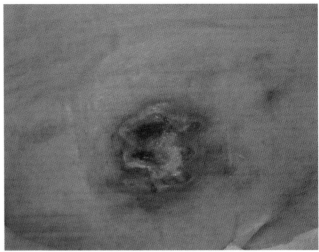

A B

Figure 3.7 *(A) and (B) Ulceration and wound infection after focused ultrasound for body contouring*

the filler, and the injection technique. Anatomical sites that are more prone to such adverse effects include the tip of nose and glabella.[42] In terms of density, the thicker the filler, the more likely it is that this can develop. Operator skill is also important; the filler should be injected when the operator withdraws the needle. In the event that filler is injected into a vessel, local blanching can be observed and patients often complain of sharp pain. If this occurs, immediate massage is necessary to reduce the risk of tissue necrosis. Other useful measures include the application of a warm pack and nitroglycerin paste to enhance local tissue perfusion. Hyaluronidase and low-molecular-weight heparin injection may also be helpful.

Blindness has been reported during periorbital filler injection.

Allergic Reaction

An allergic reaction to filler material can occur and depends on the type of filler. A skin allergy test is necessary if bovine collagen is used. Newer nonpermanent fillers such as hyaluronic acid carry a much lower risk of allergic reaction and do not require regular skin testing. Rarely, allergic reaction has been reported with these new fillers and intralesional steroid, or hyaluronidase injection can be most effective in the treatment of such complication.

Granuloma

Since autologous fat was used as a filler by Dr. Neuber in 1893, many materials have been developed to augment soft tissue. Paraffin was very popular in the early 20th century, but it was prohibited before 1920s in Western countries because of foreign body granuloma formation and paraffin migration into other tissues. Granuloma formation has been reported with a wide range of fillers, especially synthetic injectable facial fillers, with a permanent effect (Figure 3.7). A combination of moderate foreign body reaction, fibrosis, and, in some cases, bacterial infection has been reported after injection with such permanent filler.[43] According to the literature, inflammatory nodules can occur no later than 1 year after injection with polyacrylamide hydrogel but up to 6 years after injection of

combination gels (Artecol) and up to 28 years after injection of silicone gel.

Granuloma may involute with time or after triamcinolone intralesional treatment. Isotretinoin, minocycline, or doxycycline can also improve the condition.

REFERENCES

1. West TB, Alster TS. Effect of pretreatment on the incidence of hyperpigmentation following cutaneous CO_2 laser resurfacing. *Dermatol Surg.* 1999;25:15-17.

2. Chan HH, Manstein D, Yu CS, Shek S, Kono T, Wei WI. The prevalence and risk factors of postinflammatory hyperpigmentation after fractional resurfacing in Asians. *Lasers Surg Med.* 2007;39:381-385.

3. Laubach H, Chan HH, Rius F, Anderson RR, Manstein D. Effects of skin temperature on lesion size in fractional photothermolysis. *Lasers Surg Med.* 2007;39:14-18.

4. Chan HH, Fung WKK, Ying SY, et al. An in vivo trial comparing the use of different types of 532 nm neodymium: yttrium-aluminum-garnet (Nd:YAG) lasers in the treatment of facial lentigines in oriental patients. *Dermatol Surg.* 2000;26:743-749.

5. Wang CC, Sue YM, Yang CH, Chen CK. A comparison of Q-switched alexandrite laser and intense pulsed light for the treatment of freckles and lentigines in Asian persons: a randomized, physician-blinded, split-face comparative trial. *J Am Acad Dermatol.* 2006;54:804-810.

6. Kono T, Manstein D, Chan HH, Nozaki M, Anderson RR. Q-switched ruby versus long-pulsed dye laser delivered with compression for treatment of facial lentigines in Asians. *Lasers Surg Med.* 2006;38:94-97.

7. Kono T, Groff WF, Chan HH, Sakurai H, Nozaki M. Comparison study of a Q-switched alexandrite laser delivered with versus without compression in the treatment of dermal pigmented lesions. *J Cosmet Laser Ther.* 2007;9:206-209.

8. Chan HH, Leung RS, Ying SY, et al. A retrospective study looking at the complications of Q-switched alexandrite (QS Alex) and Q-switched neodymium: yttrium-aluminum-garnet (QS Nd-YAG) lasers in the treatment of nevus of Ota. *Dermatol Surg.* 2000;26:1000-1006.

9. Kunachak S, Leelaudomlipi P. Q-switched Nd: YAG laser treatment for acquired bilateral nevus of Ota-like maculae: a long-term follow-up. *Lasers Surg Med.* 2000;26:376-379.

10. Kono T, Nozaki M, Chan HH, Mikashima Y. A retrospective study looking at the long-term complication of Q-switched ruby laser in the treatment of nevus of Ota. *Lasers Surg Med.* 2001;29:156-159.

11. Polnikorn N, Tanrattanakorn S, Goldberg DJ. Treatment of Hori's nevus with the Q-switched Nd:YAG laser. *Dermatol Surg.* 2000; 26:477-480.

12. Manuskiatti W, Eimpunth S, Wanitphakdeedecha R. Effect of cold air cooling on the incidence of postinflammatory hyperpigmentation after Q-switched Nd:YAG laser treatment of acquired bilateral nevus of Ota like macules. *Arch Dermatol.* 2007;143:1139-1143.

13. Nanni CA. Laser assisted hair removal: side effects of Q-switched Nd:YAG, long-pulsed ruby, and alexandrite lasers. *J Am Acad Dermat.* 1999;41:165-171.

14. Elman M, Klein A, Slatkine M. Dark skin tissue reaction in laser assisted hair removal with a long-pulse ruby laser. *J Cutan Laser Ther.* 2000;2:17-20.

15. Garcia C, Alamoudi H, Nakib M, Zimmo S. Alexandrite laser hair removal is safe for Fitzpatrick skin types IV-VI. *Dermatol Surg.* 2000;26:130-134.

16. Weisberg NK, Greenbaum SS. Pigmentary changes after alexandrite laser hair removal. *Dermatol Surg.* 2003;29:415-419.

17. Chan HH, Ying SY, Ho WS, Wong DS, Lam LK. An in vivo study comparing the efficacy and complications of diode laser and long-pulsed neodymium: yttrium-aluminum-garnet (Nd:YAG) laser in hair removal among Chinese patients. *Dermatol Surg.* 2001;27:950-954.

18. Alster TS, Bryan H, Williams CM. Long-pulsed Nd: YAG laser-assisted hair removal in pigmented skin. *Arch Dermatol.* 2001;137:885-889.

19. Battle EF Jr, Suthamjariya KK, Alora MB, Palli K, Anderson RR. Very long-pulsed (20-200 ms) diode laser for hair removal on all skin types. *Laser Surg Med.* 2000;(Suppl 12):85.

20. Lee JH, Huh CH, Yoon HJ, Cho KH, Chung JH. Photoepilation results of axillary hair in dark-skinned patients by IPL: a comparison between different wavelength and pulse width. *Dermatol Surg.* 2006;32:234-241.

21. Sadick NS, Laughlin SA. Effective epilation of white and blond hair using combined radiofrequency and optical energy. *J Cosmet Laser Ther.* 2004;6:27-31.

22. Alajlan A, Shapiro J, Rivers JK, MacDonald N, Wiggin J, Lui H. Paradoxical hypertrichosis after laser epilation. *J Am Acad Dermatol.* 2005;53:85-88.

23. Lolis MS, Marmur ES. Paradoxical effects of hair removal systems: a review. *J Cosmet Dermatol.* 2006;5:274-276.

24. Goh CL. Treatment response of port wine stains with the flash-lamp-pulsed dye laser in the national skin centre: a report of 36 patients. *Ann Acad Med Singapore.* 1996;25:536-540.

25. Sommer S, Sheehan-Dare RA. Pulsed dye laser treatment of port-wine stains in pigmented skin. *J Am Acad Dermatol.* 2000;42:667-671.

26. Boixeda P, Nunez M, Perez B, et al. Complications of 585 nm pulsed dye laser therapy. *Int J Dermatol.* 1997;36:393-397.

27. Chiu CH, Chan HH, Ho WS, Yeung CK, Nelson JS. Prospective study of pulsed dye laser in conjunction with cryogen spray cooling for treatment of port wine stains in Chinese patients. *Dermatol Surg.* 2003;29:909-915.

28. Tunnell JW, Chang DW, Johnston C, et al. Effects of cryogen spray cooling and high radiant exposures on selective vascular injury during laser irradiation of human skin. *Arch Dermatol.* 2003;139:743-750.

29. Chan HH, Chan E, Kono T, Ying SY, Ho WS. The use of variable pulse width frequency double neodymium: YAG 532 nm laser in the treatment of Port wine stain in Chinese. *Dermatol Surg.* 2000;26:657-661.

30. Dover JS, Zelickson B; 14-Physician Multispecialty Consensus Panel. Results of a survey of 5700 patient monopolar radiofrequency facial skin tightening treatments: assessment of a low-energy multiple-pass technique leading to a clinical end point algorithm. *Dermatol Surg.* 2007;33:900-907.

31. Klein AW. Complications and adverse reactions with the use of botulinum toxin. *Semin Cutan Med Surg.* 2001;20:109-120.

32. Wollina U, Konrad H. Managing adverse events associated with botulinum toxin type A: a focus on cosmetic procedures. *Am J Clin Dermatol.* 2005;6:141-150.

33. Aristodemou P, Watt L, Baldwin C, Hugkulstone C. Diplopia associated with the cosmetic use of botulinum toxin a for facial rejuvenation. *Ophthal Plast Reconstr Surg.* 2006;22: 134-136.

34. Choe SW, Cho WI, Lee CK, Seo SJ. Effects of botulinum toxin type A on contouring of the lower face. *Dermatol Surg.* 2005;31:502-507.

35. Ahn KY, Kim ST. The change of maximum bite force after botulinum toxin type a injection for treating masseteric hypertrophy. *Plast Reconstr Surg.* 2007;120:1662-1666.

36. Brandt FS, Boker A. Botulinum toxin for the treatment of neck lines and neck bands. *Dermatol Clin.* 2004;22:159-166.

37. Glass GE, Hussain M, Fleming AN, Powell BW. Atrophy of the intrinsic musculature of the hands associated with the use of botulinum toxin-A injections for hyperhidrosis: a case report and review of the literature [Epub ahead of print January 17, 2008]. *J Plast Reconstr Aesthet Surg.* PMD: 18203669.

38. Yablon SA, Brashear A, Gordon MF, et al. Formation of neutralizing antibodies in patients receiving botulinum toxin type A for treatment of poststroke spasticity: a pooled-data analysis of three clinical trials. *Clin Ther.* 2007;29:683-690.

39. Duranti F, Salti G, Bovani B, Calandra M, Rosati ML. Injectable hyaluronic acid gel for soft tissue augmentation. A clinical and histological study. *Dermatol Surg.* 1998;24:1317-1325.

40. Hirsch RJ, Brody HJ, Carruthers JD. Hyaluronidase in the office: a necessity for every dermasurgeon that injects hyaluronic acid. *J Cosmet Laser Ther.* 2007;9:182-185.

41. Bellew SG, Carroll KC, Weiss MA, Weiss RA. Sterility of stored nonanimal, stabilized hyaluronic acid gel syringes after patient injection. *J Am Acad Dermatol.* 2005;52:988-990.

42. Glaich AS, Cohen JL, Goldberg LH. Injection necrosis of the glabella: protocol for prevention and treatment after use of dermal fillers. *Dermatol Surg.* 2006;32:276-281.

43. Christensen L, Breiting V, Janssen M, Vuust J, Hogdall E. Adverse reactions to injectable soft tissue permanent fillers. *Aesthetic Plast Surg.* 2005;29:34-48.

Siegrid S. Yu, MD

INTRODUCTION

The process of obtaining informed consent is fundamental to the practice of modern medicine. Within the realm of cosmetic surgery and elective procedures, the ability to openly and effectively discuss risk and benefit is particularly crucial for building patient rapport and optimizing outcome. Patients who are well informed make more knowledgeable decisions, formulate more realistic expectations, and often enjoy greater satisfaction. When treating ethnic skin, the physician should recognize the physiologic differences in skin with darker pigmentation and discuss the anticipated response to cosmetic and laser procedures. In this setting, varying cultural models also need to be taken into consideration in order to ensure comprehensive patient understanding and full informed consent.

GOALS OF INFORMED CONSENT

The process of consultation and obtaining informed consent offers the opportunity to create a relationship whereby the patient learns to trust that the physician with offer the most appropriate therapy to the best of his or her ability. The physician should then also be confident that this trust is based on the provision of the most accurate and best available evidence. In cosmetic dermatology, the provider is faced with the additional complexity of variable individual expectations and frequent misinformation. Prior to consultation, the patient may have already been influenced by erroneous or misleading information acquired from numerous nonprofessional sources, including other lay persons as well as media and press focused on consumer-directed advertising. Additional goals of the informed consent process therefore also include patient education and identification of potential concerns and problems.[1] Solid clinical acumen, expert technical skill, and the best intentions often cannot substitute for good rapport, generated by an open preoperative discussion with the patient. Finally, the cosmetic dermatologist must also accept that he or she has heightened ethical obligations in the setting of performing elective, life-enhancing interventions, rather than medically necessary or life-saving procedures.[2]

ELEMENTS OF INFORMED CONSENT

Informed consent is a fundamental principle of modern medicine, a well-recognized ethical obligation of health care providers. The foundation of informed consent was formulated in 1914 by New York Justice Benjamin N. Cardozo, who stated: "Every human being of adult years and sound mind has a right to determine what shall be done with his body, and a surgeon who performs an operation without the patient's consent commits an assault for which he is liable in damages."[3] The term *informed consent* was coined in case law in 1957 and published in *A Patient's Bill of Rights* in 1972 by the American Hospital Association.

The concept of informed consent states that not only is it required that patients give permission for a particular treatment but also the permission must be based on a demonstrated understanding of the nature, consequences, and alternatives of the proposed intervention. Patients are entitled to a discussion of the specific risks, benefits, options, and alternatives of a procedure, including the possibility of no treatment. Five fundamental elements comprising informed consent are disclosure, understanding, voluntariness, competence, and finally consent.[4] It is important that the health care provider discloses the necessary information regarding the diagnosis and treatment in plain, concise, nontechnical, unbiased, and nonjudgmental terms.[5] The patient then should demonstrate an understanding of the discussion, followed by the fundamental right to make a decision regarding treatment, including the refusal of treatment. Finally, in order for the informed consent to be legally and morally valid, the patient must be legally competent, and the consent must be given voluntarily.[6]

Patients may significantly vary from one another with regard to personality, level of education, information processing, and capacity to understand the presented information. While some individuals are content with understanding the basic principles of their care, others may feel compelled to comprehensively investigate every detail. Although these individual patient characteristics need to be taken into consideration for effective communication and informed consent, guidelines for the content of discussion do exist. Some states use the *reasonable physician standard* in which the physician has a duty to disclose information that any reasonable physician would disclose under similar circumstances.[7] However, the national trend is to use the *reasonable patient standard*, which asserts that the physician must disclose anything to which a reasonable person in the patient's position would attach significance in his or her decision-making process. This includes discussion of rare, but important complications that may cause a reasonable patient to decline elective surgery.

There is very little literature reviewing informed consent from the patient's perspective and examining what patients consider important in this process. In one cohort undergoing elective plastic and reconstructive surgery procedures, the following were categorized as essential for discussion prior to consenting for surgery: the opportunity to ask questions and change their mind, the risks of treatment (including not only the common side effects but also the uncommon, but serious side effects), the benefits of treatment, an estimate of how the treatment will affect them specifically, whether the treatment is experimental, and success rate.[8] Within the realm of cosmetic dermatology, patient expectations are particularly difficult to assess unless there is a directed conversation regarding his or her specific goals.

CULTURAL AND PSYCHOSOCIAL CONSIDERATIONS

By 2050, it is projected that 50% of U.S. residents will be non-Caucasian.[9] As physicians increasingly encounter multicultural and multiethnic patients, it is important to recognize how cultural context shapes the relationship of the patient, the physician, and in many cases the patient's family in medical decision making. Culturally sensitive care encompasses recognition and understanding of not only ethnically diverse populations and cultural patterns, but also how social and economic factors come into play. When interacting with diverse ethnic populations, the challenge may lie in communication and demonstration of empathy and understanding of the patient's perspective. Clearly, informed consent may be compromised when language or cultural barriers are unrecognized. Awareness of these issues will improve the physician–patient relationship and will likely positively impact patient compliance and satisfaction.

Ethnic skin also has structural and physiologic differences from Caucasian skin. These distinctions account for variations in response to ultraviolet light exposure and alternate clinical manifestations of photoaging. The response to cosmetic treatment modalities also differs in patients of darker skin pigmentation, and this needs to be recognized by the cosmetic and laser surgeon. For example, the baseline epidermal melanin content is increased in darker-skinned patients and the melanocytes are more reactive to inflammatory stimuli. Patients with ethnic skin are therefore predisposed to unintended postprocedural pigmentary alteration, the most common treatment sequelae being postinflammatory hyperpigmentation. This is particularly true if the treatment area is a sun-exposed location, such as the face.[10] The consent process for procedures in ethnic skin should address these differences in treatment response in order to establish realistic patient expectations.

In the United States, the concept of informed consent is based on the fundamental belief in individual autonomy and was developed over the past few decades in order to protect the rights of the patient.[11] In contrast to this individualistic model, a more social and family-based framework plays a greater role in other countries and among some cultural groups in the United States.[12] Different ethnicities and cultural systems have varying beliefs about individual autonomy, with conceptions of decision-making capacity sometimes embedded within the intricacies of family ties or even community relationships. In some communities, personhood is not defined as an individual but rather as one's family.[13] These cultures are more collectivist than individualist, where the goal is to maintain harmony and further the objectives of the group, rather than any one single person. This may sometimes translate to a patient feeling obligated to telling the physician what he or she thinks the physician wants to hear. In cultures where it is thought to be inappropriate to share feelings with nonfamily members, severity of discomfort, fear, or insecurity may be underreported.

The literature regarding optimizing rapport and patient understanding with specific ethnicities and cultures in the United States is sparse. Although a discussion of a few general guidelines in this regard may be helpful, it is also important to recognize that there is a risk in making assumptions about an individual's information needs and preferences based on perceived ethnicity, socioeconomic background, and other like factors. Cultural references are general, and patients who share a particular heritage may still have diverse values depending on their economic and educational levels, religious affiliations, date of immigration, and English-speaking skills.

Whenever appropriate, the physician should take into account varying cultural models to ensure full patient understanding. Studies have indicated that African American patients may have a higher rate of distrust with the traditional, established medical system. There are several well-documented studies documenting disparities in medical care in this group, and these factors may influence African Americans' approach to medical decision making and their needs for information regarding their health care.[14] From the African American patient's perspective, elements identified as important for development of trust include honesty and interpersonal skills such as patience and kindness. In one study, African American patients older than age 50 supported mutual decision making in conjunction with their physician and thought that imparting more information provided reassurance and helped alleviate fears. A study comparing informed consent between Caucasian and minority (Latino and Asian) patients showed a statistically significant difference in physician behavior in disclosure of elements of informed consent. This included a more limited discussion of risks and benefits, pain or discomfort, and necessary length of treatment compared to discussion with Caucasian counterparts.[15] Awareness of this potential tendency is helpful for providing equitable care. In general, Latino and Asian cultures are less individualistic, and these patients may look more toward the physician for guidance in selecting appropriate therapy. In this setting, the physician may also need to involve family members in the medical decision-making process. Caregivers should be attuned to the patient's communication style and relationship with any family members who may accompany them to the consultation visit. In any situation, it is helpful to ask the patient questions in an open-ended fashion in order to determine which factors are important in their decision-making process.

IMPROVING INFORMED CONSENT

Optimizing physician–patient communication promotes the development of a trusting relationship. Patients who are well informed make more knowledgeable decisions, formulate more realistic expectations, and often enjoy greater satisfaction. There are numerous factors that contribute to a successful, instructive consent process. Studies examining the recall and retention of the informed consent discussion support the common perception that patients frequently forget the majority of the disclosed information given during a preoperative consultation. Patients typically demonstrate less than 50% short-term (2 weeks) and longer-term (months) retention of these oral conversations, and the overall recall rate of potential risks and complications ranges from 29% to 48%.[16,17] Patients with a university or higher level of education have higher levels of recall.[17] Studies have shown that this relatively low rate of recall and retention can be statistically significantly increased with the addition of printed material outlining surgical risks.[17]

With patients with limited English-speaking ability, trained medical interpreters should be used. The use of bilingual staff, family members, or visual prompts places the patient at risk for misunderstanding and the physician at risk for medical malpractice suits. Verification of the patient's understanding is crucial, particularly if cultural or language barriers exist. An effective way of verifying comprehension is by asking the patient to repeat key points of the discussion in his or her own words.

Several studies investigated the issue of race and ethnicity and trust in a physician. When given an opportunity, it appears that patients tend to choose physicians with the same racial and ethnic background as themselves.[18] Racial concordance in a patient-physician relationship is associated with higher levels of patient trust, satisfaction, and active participation in medical decision making.[19] The following strategies are suggested for health care providers who provide cross-cultural care[20]:

1. Investigate what your patient already knows.

2. Learn about the cultural traditions of the groups you are working with.

3. Pay close attention to body language, lack of response, or feelings of tension that may signify that the patient or family is in conflict but is hesitant to communicate this conflict.

4. Ask open-ended questions to elicit more information regarding your patient's assumptions and expectations.

5. Remain nonjudgmental when provided with information that reflects values that differ from your own.

6. Give the patient the opportunity to ask questions first; then address the family.

7. Always inform the patient that the medical team will be available for further conversation.

8. As in any medical encounter, documentation should be complete and accurately reflect the conversation.

In summary, the process of obtaining informed consent is crucial for building patient rapport and optimizing outcome in cosmetic dermatology. Patients who are well informed and trusting of their physician often enjoy greater satisfaction. When performing procedures in ethnic skin, the physician should recognize the physiologic differences in skin with darker pigmentation and discuss the anticipated response to cosmetic and laser procedures in order to set realistic patient expectations. The addition of printed material improves the recall and retention of the surgical risk discussion. Finally, varying cultural models need to be taken into consideration in order to ensure comprehensive patient understanding and full informed consent.

REFERENCES

1. McGillis ST, Stanton-Hicks U. The preoperative patient evaluation: preparation for surgery. *Dermatol Clinics*. 1998;16(1): 1-15.

2. Cantor J. Cosmetic dermatology and physician's ethical obligations: pore than just hope in a jar. *Semin Cutan Med Surg*. 2005;24:155-160.

3. Armstrong AP, Cole AA, Page RE. Informed consent: are we doing enough? *Br J Plast Surg*. 1997;50:637-640.

4. Creedon R. Cultural considerations and surgical consent. *JPP*. 2006;16(10):505-509.

5. Brazell NE. The significance and application of informed consent. *AORN J*. 1997;65:377-386.

6. Ward CM. Consenting to surgery. *Br J Plast Surg*. 1994;47: 30-34.

7. Brazell NE. The significance and applications of informed consent. *AORN J*. 1997;65(2):377-380, 382, 385-386.

8. O'Brien CM, Thorburn TG, Sibbel-Linz A, et al. Consent for plastic surgical procedures. *J Plast Reconstr Aesthet Surg*. 2006;59:983-989.

9. Day JC. Population projections of the United States by age, sex, race, and Hispanic origin. 1995-2050 (Current Population Reports, P-25-1130). Washington, DC: U.S. Government Printing Office.

10. Handley JM. Adverse events associated with nonablative cutaneous visible and infrared laser treatment. *J Am Acad Dermatol*. 2006;55(3):482-489.

11. Kirsch M. The myth of informed consent. *Am J Gastroenterol*. 1995;3:588-589.

12. Ruhnke GW, Wilson SR, Akamatsu T, et al. Ethical decision making and patient autonomy—a comparison of physicians and patients in Japan and the United States. *Chest*. 2000;118:1172-1182.

13. Creedon R. Cultural considerations and surgical consent. *JPP*. 2006;16(10):505-509.

14. Torke AM, Corbie-Smith G, Branch WT. African Amercian patient's perspectives on medical decision making. *Arch Intern Med*. 2004;164:525-530.

15. Simon CM, Kodish ED. Step into my zapatos, doc. *Perspect Biol Med*. 2005;48(1):S123-S148.

16. Leeb D, Bowers DG, Lynch JB. Observations on the myth of "informed consent." *Plast Reconstr Surg*. 1976;58:280-282.

17. Makdessian AS, Ellis DA, Irish JC. Informed consent in facial plastic surgery. *Arch Facial Plast Surg*. 1994;6:26-30.

18. LaVeist TA, Nuru-Jetter A. Is doctor-patient race concordance associated with greater satisfaction with care? *J Health Soc Behav*. 2002;43:296-306.

19. Cooper LA, Roter DL, Johnson RL, et al. Patient-centered communication, ratings of care, and concordance of patient and physician race. *Ann Intern Med*. 2003;139:907-915.

20. McLaughlin LA, Braun KL. Asian and Pacific Islander cultural values: considerations for health care decision making. *Health Soc Work*. 1998;23(2):116-126.

CHAPTER 5

Epidermal and Color Improvement in Ethnic Skin: Microdermabrasion and Superficial Peels

Diana Leu, MD, and Simon S. Yoo, MD

Increasingly, patients with ethnic skin are seeking out cosmetic procedures to provide epidermal and color improvement to their skin. According to the American Society for Aesthetic Plastic Surgery, 11.7 million cosmetic procedures were performed in 2007. Of these, procedures on ethnic patients comprised 21%, an increase from 14% in 1997. Hispanics account for 9%, African Americans 6%, Asians 5%, and all other non-Caucasians 2%. Among ethnic minorities, the most frequently requested procedures were Botox, wrinkle fillers, chemical peels, and microdermabrasion.[1] Based on the 2000 U.S. Census and interim data, the U.S. Census Bureau has projected an increase in the percentage of Asians, Hispanics, and African Americans from 30.6% to nearly 50% by 2050.[2] As this portion of the population increases, the cosmetic dermatologist will need to better understand the unique needs of patients with darker skin types.

Pigmentary disorders are one of the most common dermatologic conditions seen in African Americans, Hispanics, and Asians.[3] These include postinflammatory hyperpigmentation, hypopigmentation, and melasma. Acne is the most common dermatologic diagnosis seen in blacks and Hispanics at 27.7% and 20.4%, respectively. In a study of African female acne, biopsies of acne lesions showed a high degree of histologic inflammation compared to clinical inflammation which may explain the frequency of postinflammatory hyperpigmentation in darker skinned individuals.[4] Other causes include many inflammatory diseases from papulosquamous disorders to vesiculobullous disorders. For darker phototypes, care needs to be exercised so that therapies utilized to treat dyschromia and epidermal texture do not create more problems.

Current medical treatment for dyschromias such as postinflammatory hyperpigmentation and melasma include prescription therapies such as retinoids, hydroquinone, azelaic acid, and alpha-hydroxy acids. However, these therapies often require many months of diligent usage to realize improvement and concentrations need to be titrated slowly to try to prevent development of an irritant dermatitis. In patients with skin of color, irritant dermatitis can easily lead to postinflammatory hypopigmentation or hyperpigmentation. Hydroquinone, which is commonly used for bleaching, can also cause an allergic contact dermatitis. The clinician and patient need to be watchful of these side effects and stop the treatment when this occurs.

When medical therapies are insufficient, more aggressive treatments, such as in-office superficial chemical peels and microdermabrasion may be added to augment the results. However, special skill and care need to be exercised when using these resurfacing agents in patients with darker skin as they are more likely to develop posttreatment dyschromias.

LITERATURE REVIEW

Ablative resurfacing techniques include chemical resurfacing, mechanical resurfacing, and laser resurfacing. These modalities cause controlled skin injury to a known depth. Superficial resurfacing procedures extend from the epidermis to the papillary dermis while medium depth procedures extend to the upper reticular dermis and deep depth procedures extend to the mid reticular dermis. Healing from these procedures results in new skin growth with improved surface texture and pigmentation. Superficial chemical peels and microdermabrasion will be discussed in the chapter.

■ Superficial Chemical Peels

Chemical peels have been used for centuries since the time of ancient Egyptians, Greeks, and Romans. They used the alpha hydroxyl acids from sour milk, grape juice, and lemon extracts to improve the skin texture and color.[5] Superficial chemical peels can be accomplished via application of many agents such as Jessner's solution, salicylic acid, alpha-hydroxy acids, and trichloroacetic acid (TCA) concentrations ranging from 10%–25% (Table 5-1). They may be used to treat mild photoaging, shallow acne scars, acne, and dyschromias such as melasma and postinflammatory hyperpigmentation. The depth of the peel depends on three main factors: the amount of solution used, the pressure used to apply the peel, and the duration that the solution remains on the skin. Typically, chemical peels are performed in a monthly series with gradually increasing concentrations. Titrating the concentration to the desired effect needs to be balanced with tolerance of the chemical peel. By increasing the depth of the peel, there is an increased risk of developing dyschromia and scarring.

Alpha-hydroxy acids are naturally occurring acids such as glycolic acid from sugarcane; lactic acid from sour milk, malic acid from apples, citric acid from citric fruits, and tartaric acid from grapes.[6] It causes epidermolysis of the skin followed by desquamation. Various studies have demonstrated the efficacy and safety of using glycolic acid peels (30%–70%) in the treatment of melasma, hyperpigmentation, and acne in ethnic skin patients.[7-10] Its main side effect was temporary hyperpigmentation which occurred in approximately 5% of patients. With glycolic acid, it is important to time the treatment to know when to neutralize the acid. Neutralization occurs using either water or a 1%–5% bicarbonate solution,

TABLE 5.1 ■ Superficial Peeling Agents

Peeling Agent	Range of Concentration (%)
TCA	10–25
Jessner's solution	
Glycolic acid	20–70
Salicylic acid	10–30

TABLE 5.2 ▪ Peels Needing Neutralization

Peeling Agent
Glycolic acid

usually within 2 to 4 minutes of application. Typically, the neutralization time mark will be because of patient discomfort, mild erythema, or the specified time interval. In darker pigmented skin, neutralization should occur sooner to minimize risk of postinflammatory hyperpigmentation (Table 5.2).

Salicylic acid is a type of beta-hydroxy acid and was originally derived from the bark of the willow tree. Salicylic acid causes keratolysis of the upper, lipophilic layers of the stratum corneum. Given that salicylic acid is lipophilic, it is best used in patients with acne. In a study by Grimes, salicylic acid peels in 20% to 30% concentrations were demonstrated to be both safe and efficacious for the treatment of acne, PIH, melasma, and oily skin in Hispanic and African American patients with phototypes V and VI.[11] The patients were initially pretreated with hydroquinone 4% for 2 weeks and then a series of five peels were subsequently performed with use of hydroquinone in between treatments. Moderate to significant improvement was noted in 88% of the patients. Four in twenty-five patients experienced transitory crusting, dryness, hypopigmentation, and hyperpigmentation. A study by Lee and Kim in Asian patients also demonstrated the safety and efficacy of 30% salicylic acid peels. The main side effects noted were erythema, dryness, burning sensation, and crusting. No persistent hyperpigmentation or scarring was noted in this study[12] (Table 5.3).

A commercially available salacylic acid system is the β-lift kit. It is convenient in that it includes a pretreatment degreasing agent and a sponge applicator. It comes in 20% and 30% strengths (Figure 5.1).

TCA is also commonly used and the depth of the peel is controlled by the concentration of TCA utilized. TCA works by causing cell necrosis and a 10%–25% solution will produce a superficial peel. Benefits of using TCA are that there is no systemic absorption or toxicity and it is also self-neutralizing so does not need to be timed. Concentrations greater than 25% are considered melanotoxic and should be used with caution in skin of color. In skin phototypes IV–VI, pretreatment test patches and starting at lower concentrations are recommended. A white frost should be avoided as this increases the risk of postpeel dyschromia and scarring. The TCA peel has been used safely in ethnic skin patients with temporary side effects of erythema and postinflammatory hyperpigmentation lasting less than 3 months.[13,14]

Another superficial chemical peeling agent is Jessner's solution. It was formulated by Dr. Max Jessner in the 1960s and consists of a combination of 14 g of resorcinol, 14 g of salicylic acid, 14 g of 85%

TABLE 5.3 ▪ Self-Neutralizing Peels

Peeling Agent
TCA
Jessner's solution
Salicylic acid

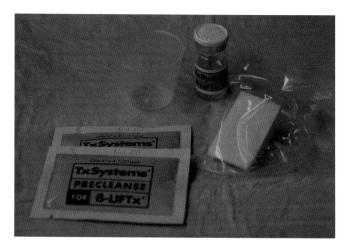

Figure 5.1 *Items provided in the commercially available salicylic acid β-lift kit.*

lactic acid, and 100 mL of 95% ethanol.[6] No individual studies to date have investigated the safety of Jessner's solution in higher skin phototypes although it is considered a superficial chemical peel. It should be used cautiously in ethnic skin patients since the resorcinol in Jessner's solution can cause depigmentation problems, particularly those of phototypes V and VI (Figure 5.2).

Clinical examination and patient history

Clinical consultation starts with addressing the patient's concerns and expectations. The physician would then gain insight on their patient's conceptions about cosmetic procedures and realistic expectations can be set at this time. The physician should address length of recovery, duration of treatment, possible side effects, and expected outcome. Patients of darker skin tones must understand their increased risk of dyschromia with any of these modalities. It is important to ensure that the patient does not have unrealistic expectations—and that multiple treatments are necessary on a monthly basis to achieve the full effect. Showing them photos of other patients prepeel, immediately postpeel, and at follow-up can help them understand the procedure. Patients who continue to entertain unrealistic expectations, appear to be emotionally unstable, or suffer from body dysmorphic disorder are poor candidates for cosmetic intervention.

In determining the type of cosmetic procedure to be performed, the patient should be asked about their priorities when undergoing a cosmetic procedure—that is, downtime vs. efficacy vs. risk of side effects. The patient can then be provided with treatment options as well as discussion of risks and benefits. Understanding both the patient's and your own threshold for risk will determine the level at which you will start and the rapidity of intensifying the treatment. As with all therapies, patient education and compliance are very important. The patient must be willing to adhere to pre- and posttreatment guidelines.

At the initial meeting to discuss options for treatment, it is also important to obtain significant history including wound healing and scarring history, ethnicity, current medications, history of herpes simplex infection, isotretinoin usage, prior cosmetic procedures, and radiation therapy. Photosensitizing drugs or oral contraceptives may be stopped after discussion with the patient and his/her physician.

TABLE 5.4 ▪ Pre-Treatment Checklist

1. History of keloids and scarring
2. History of HSV infection
3. History of radiation therapy
4. History of recent Isotretinoin therapy
5. Medication history for a photosensitizing drug

TABLE 5.5 ▪ Pre-Treatment Regimen

4% Hydroquinone
10% AHA moisturizer
Topical retinoids

If the patient has been on Isotretinoin, resurfacing treatments should be postponed for 9–12 months. If there is a history of herpes simplex, patients should receive prophylactic antivirals the day of and for 10–14 days following initiation of treatment. They should be educated about strict sun protection using at least an SPF 30 sunblock daily as well as complying with any additional topical therapies at home. The patient should also discontinue retinoids and other treatments which may compromise the epidermal barrier (i.e., waxing) 1 week prior to the peel. Male patients should not shave on the day of the peel (Table 5-4).

A careful physical examination should include evaluation of the dyschromia and amount of epidermal scarring. A hoods lamp can be useful to distinguish between epidermal and dermal pigment. Directed side lighting can also help to accentuate visual appreciation of facial scarring. Photos should be taken to help assess pre- and posttreatment results. If a patient has had radiation therapy to the area of desired treatment, the physician should carefully examine for pilosebaceous units as these are required for re-epithelialization. If there is any evidence of active infection, such as herpes or warts, treatment should be postponed until the infection has completely cleared. When it has been determined between the patient and the physician that surgical treatment would be appropriate, informed consent that the patient understands fully the benefits, risks, and limitations of the procedure is obtained.

Treatment selection

Superficial chemical peels are appealing because of their few side effects and minimal recovery time, ranging from a few days to a week. The stinging and burning associated with superficial chemical peels is mild, negating the need of a topical or local anesthetic. One of the most important factors in deciding on the type of chemical peel is the comfort and familiarity of the physician with the procedure.

Glycolic acid peels require close monitoring with neutralization of the acid at the appropriate time in order to balance the benefit from the peel with risk of hyperpigmentation and scarring. The benefit of glycolic acid peels is the ability to adjust the peel depth once it is on the patient.

Salicylic acid peels are particularly beneficial for patients with acne because of its lipophilic nature. It acts on the pilosebaceous units and is a good treatment for both open and closed comedones. Upon application of a salicylic acid peel, perifollicular frosting can be seen.

With a TCA peel, the depth of the peel can also be adjusted by the concentration of the acid as well as the number of coats applied. Because of this, it is very important not to overlap when applying the peel. When this occurs, a medium or deep depth peel may occur in the overlap zones that would lead to a higher risk of scarring and residual hypopigmentation. The ability to control the depth of the peel allows for treatment deeper than the other super-

ficial peeling agents. This is especially useful in removing dermal melanin as can be seen in melasma.

Method of treatment application

The prepeel skin regimen can include a combination of a number of agents such as hydroquinone 4%, a 10% AHA moisturizer, and a retinoid for several weeks prior to the peel. These agents should be stopped approximately a week prior to the procedure to ensure an intact epidermis. Prepeel hydroquinone helps to prevent postinflammatory hyperpigmentation by suppressing the melanocytes and blocking production of melanin. By decreasing the thickness of the stratum corneum, tretinoin increases the depth of the chemical peel. Tretinoin also works to speed epidermal heeling. Use of tretinoin and hydroquinone can be irritating for patients with sensitive skin and should be stopped or used intermittently in patients with difficulty tolerating these medications. An oral analgesic may be given prior to the procedure if the patient desires, but most patients are able to tolerate the mild stinging (Table 5.5).

Prior to performing the peel, the patient's face should be examined for retinoid dermatitis. Resurfacing of this irritated skin can lead to prolonged erythema postpeel. After a review of the risks, limitations, and benefits of the procedure, the patient can then sign the informed consent form. The patient should then cleanse his/her face with a gentle cleanser. The skin is then defatted with isopropyl alcohol or acetone wipes to allow even penetration of the peeling agent. This step allows for removal of residual oil and debris and evening of the stratum corneum. It is then complete when the wipes no longer evidence a yellow residue. The lips, corners of the eyes, and other sensitive areas can be covered with Vaseline ointment to protect them from the peeling agent. Cotton swabs should also be put in the ears and the patient advised to close their eyes or wear goggles to prevent accidental dripping of the solution into the orifices. Should any of the peeling solution accidentally drip onto the eyes, the eye should be thoroughly flushed with water at an eye wash station or with a bottle of normal saline.

The peeling agent is then applied with gauze or a sponge evenly across the face. Using gauze allows the benefit of knowing the amount of pressure applied to the skin. Depending on the chemical resurfacing agent used, a neutralizing solution may or may not be necessary. Prior to application of the chemical peel, the physician should have a predetermined pattern of application so as not to overlap or skip areas of skin. Care should be taken particularly with TCA and Jessner's peels as deeper penetration is obtained with overlapping coats. Feathering using the sponge of gauze should be done at the junction of the face and the neck to prevent demarcation lines of treated and untreated areas. Cotton-tipped applicators can also be used to spot-treat acne papules, acne scars, melasma, and other focal dyschromias and epidermal disruptions.

The patient should expect several minutes of mild stinging and burning. A hand fan or refrigerated air can be used during the peel to aid in any discomfort. The level of frosting can then be observed

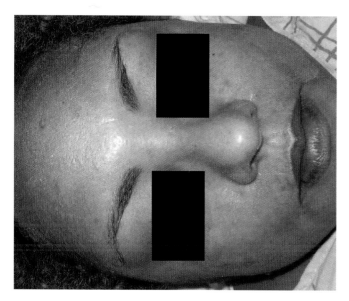

Figure 5.2 *Immediate light frosting after using a 20% salicylic acid peel.*

(Figure 5.2). Typically, in phototype IV-VI patients, minimal or no frost is desirable. A level I frost shows erythema with a mild interspersed white surface. A level II frost shows erythema with an even, but thinly white surface. A level III frost is solidly white. This frosting occurs secondary to the coagulation of epidermal and dermal proteins. Erythema with even white frost indicates that the level of the papillary dermis has been reached. The solidly white frost occurs with the peel depth has just reached the upper reticular dermis. Erythema is lost at this level because of occlusion of the blood vessels.[15]

When the peel is completed, the patient's face is draped with cool compresses of either water or 1%–5% bicarbonate (for glycolic acid peels) for symptomatic improvement of the burning. When the area is feeling better, it can then be gently cleansed with water or a gentle cleanser.

After the peel, the patient must follow strict sun protection with sunblock, hat, and avoidance measures. Use of hydroquinone post peel is also very important to prevent development of hyperpigmentation. Patients should also avoid smoking to aid in healing during the postpeel period. After several days, the patient can then resume using Tretinoin and any other pre-treatment topical medications. The patient should be instructed not to pick, peel, or manipulate the skin of the treated area. Keeping the skin well moisturized is also very important. If the patient tolerates the peel, a higher concentration may be used for subsequent peels.

Microdermabrasion

Microdermabrasion has become very popular in recent years with patients desiring rapid recovery time, lack of anesthesia, and low risk of cutaneous side effects such as scarring and dyschromia.

Microdermabrasion is similar to a superficial chemical peel in terms of its ablation depth. This mechanical ablative method utilizes a hand piece that drives aluminum oxide or salt crystals at high speeds. The crystals bombard the surface of the skin and cause graduated detachment of the stratum corneum and epidermis. The crystals and the exfoliated skin are simultaneously removed with a vacuum on the hand piece.[16]

The benefits of microdermabrasion include improvement of the appearance of solar damage, fine rhytides, and mild acne scarring. In a study of 14 patients, Shim et al.[17] demonstrated homogenization and compaction of the stratum corneum, increased epidermal thickening, and reduced melanization with more regular distribution of melanosomes after six microdermabrasion treatments. Coimbra et al.[18] also demonstrated similar results with subjective improvement in dyschromia and demonstrated increased epidermal thickening with an increase in organized collagen.

There are several theories as to what causes these histological changes. Freedman et al.[19] suggests that epidermal improvement is via stimulation of basal keratinocytes. Shpall et al.[20] think that it is the repetitive injury of the epidermis which leads to collagen stimulation. Tsai et al.[21] suggest that the physical action of the vacuum produces collagen enhancement. It is likely a combination of these factors which leads to the improvement seen in microdermabrasion.

Microdermabrasion can also be used adjunctively to aid in the absorption of other topical agents, such as retinoids, and thus improve efficacy. However, this needs to be done carefully as combining therapies also increases its potential side effects.

The risks of microdermabrasion include petechiae or purpura. This typically occurs when the vacuum suction power is too high or when the hand piece was moved too slowly across the skin. Microdermabrasion was also seen to worsen telangiectasias and facial erythema which may be temporary or permanent. Thus, patients with rosacea should be deterred from undergoing microdermabrasion. Scarring can also rarely occur if the microdermabrasion is used too aggressively and a greater depth of ablation into the papillary dermis is achieved. More conservative microdermabrasion should be utilized in patients with Fitzpatrick skin types III-VI to avoid the risk of dyschromia. Postinflammatory hyperpigmentation can largely be prevented by strict adherence to use of a broad-spectrum sunblock and sun avoidance.

Method of treatment application

Clinical examination and patient history is similar to that of chemical peels. Please see Table 5.4 and Table 5.5. After the patient's face has been cleansed and dried, the skin is then degreased with isopropyl alcohol. Goggles are then placed over the eyes to prevent corneal damage. A bottle of normal saline should be kept near the procedure area to use as an emergency eyewash should this occur.

The vacuum is then set on −8 to −15 in Hg adjusting for patient comfort. As with chemical peeling, the physician should have a predetermined pattern of application for consistency. Typically, multiple passes alternate with vertical and horizontal orientation. As the hand holding the hand piece is confidently and smoothly crossing across the skin, the other hand should hold the skin gently taut to achieve a more efficient vacuum.

The depth of ablation achieved using microdermabrasion is dependent on various factors including speed of the crystals, the rate of the movement of the hand piece, and number of passes across a given area. Deeper ablation occurs with higher velocity of the crystals, slower movement of the hand piece, and increased number of passes. Thus, microdermabrasion is able to adjust for treatment of skin with varying depths.

The forehead and chin can be treated more aggressively while the areas of thinner skin such as the periorbital region should be treated more delicately. Between each pass, a soft brush can be used to clear away the debris on the skin. The clinical endpoint is mild erythema.

After the procedure, cool water or gel may be used to soothe the skin. A broad-spectrum sunblock is then applied to the treatment area and the patient is counseled again on sun protection and avoidance. The erythema from the procedure should resolve after several hours and exfoliation is expected for the next 2 days.

For treatment of acne scarring and other focal skin lesions, multiple passes are required to reach a clinical endpoint of pinpoint bleeding. This typically requires more than 20 passes at a higher vacuum suction level (–16 to –18 in Hg). Between passes, the excess crystals are wiped away with sterile gauze. The shallow ulcerations created are then treated with antibiotic ointment and sun avoidance is again stressed.

One week after treatment, patients can resume other adjunctive skin therapies, such as topical retinoids or over-the-counter alpha or beta hydroxy products. Microdermabrasion can be used weekly or every 2 weeks, to both allow time for healing and affect improvement.

SUMMARY

In summary, both superficial chemical peels and microdermabrasion affect ablation of the epidermis to the papillary dermis. Their greatest benefit is from their minimal side effects and rapid recovery time. However, because these are superficial agents, the improvement seen is subtle and requires many repeated treatments. As there is less of an injury to the skin, risk of dyschromia or scarring is much decreased and is thus safer to use in patients of Fitzpatrick skin type III-VI. Nevertheless, counseling on this side effect is important, as is emphasis on using broad-spectrum sunblock and sun avoidance.

REFERENCES

1. The American Society for Aesthetic Plastic Surgery Statistics. http://www.surgery.org/press/statistics.php. Accessed July 14, 2008.

2. U.S. Census Bureau, 2004. U.S. interim projections by age, sex, race, and Hispanic origin. http://www.census.gov/ipc/www/usinterimproj/. Accessed July 14, 2008.

3. Halder RM, Nootheti PK. Ethnic skin disorders overview. *JAAD.* 2003;48(6):S143-S148.

4. Halder RM, Holmes YC, Bridgemen-Shah S, Kligman AM. A clinicohistopathologic study of acne vulgaris in black females. *J Invest Dermatol.* 1996;107:495A.

5. Coleman W, Lawrence N. The history of skin resurfacing. In: Coleman W, Lawrence N, eds. *Skin Resurfacing.* Philadelphia, PA: Williams and Wilkins; 1998:3-6.

6. Roberts WE. Chemical peeling in ethnic/dark skin. *Dermatol Ther.* 2004(17):196-205.

7. Wang CM, Huang CL, Hu CT, Chan HL. The effect of glycolic acid on the treatment of acne in Asian skin. *Dermatol Surg.* 1997;23(1):23-29.

8. Burns RL, Prevost-Blank PL, Lawry MA, Lawry TB, Faria DT, Fivenson DP. Glycolic acid peels for postinflammatory hyperpigmentation in black patients. A comparative study. *Dermatol Surg.* 1997;23(3):171-174.

9. Lim JT, Tham SN. Glycolic acid peels in the treatment of melasma among Asian women. *Dermatol Surg.* 1997;23(3): 177-179.

10. Javaheri SM, Handa S, Kaur I, Kumar B. Safety and efficacy of glycolic acid facial peel in Indian women with melasma. *Int J Dermatol.* 2001;40: 354-357.

11. Grimes PE. The safety and efficacy of salicylic acid chemical peels in darker racial-ethnic groups. *Dermatol Surg.* 1999: 25: 18-22.

12. Lee H, Kim I. Salicylic acid peels for the treatment of acne vulgaris in Asian patients. *Dermatol Surg.* 2003;29: 1196-1199.

13. Al-Waiz M, Al-Sharqi A. Medium-depth chemical peels in the treatment of acne scars in dark-skinned individuals. *Dermatol Surg.* 2002;28:383-387.

14. Chun E, Lee JB, Lee KH. Focal trichloroacetic acid peel method for benign pigmented lesions in dark-skinned individuals. *Dermatol Surg.* 2004;30:512-516.

15. Obagi ZE, Obagi S, Alaiti S, Stevens MB. TCA-based blue peel: a standardized procedure with depth control. *Dermatol Surg.* 1999;25:773-780.

16. Bernard RW, Beran SJ, Rusin L. Microdermabrasion in clinical practice. *Clin Plast Surg.* 2000;27(4):571-577.

17. Shim EK, Barnette D, Hughes K, Greenway HT. Microdermabrasion: a clinical and histopathologic study. *Dermatol Surg.* 2001;27(6):524-530.

18. Coimbra M, Rohrich RJ, Chao J, Brown SA. A prospective controlled assessment of microdermabrasion for damaged skin and fine rhytides. *Plast Reconstr Surg.* 2004;113(5):1438-1443.

19. Freedman BM, Rueda-Pedraza E, Waddell SP. The epidermal and dermal changes associated with microdermabrasion. *Dermatol Surg.* 2001;27(12):1031-1033.

20. Shpall R, Beddingfield FC, Watson D, Lask GP. Microdermabrasion: a review. *Facial Plast Surg.* 2004;20(1): 47-50.

21. Tsai RY, Wang CN, Chan HL. Aluminum oxide crystal microdermabrasion. *Dermatol Surg.* 1995;21:539-542.

CHAPTER 6

Epidermal and Dermal Color Improvement in Ethnic Skin: Pigment Lasers and Lights

Nicola P.Y. Chan, MB BChir, MRCP, and
Henry Hin-Lee Chan, MD, FRCP

INTRODUCTION

With the changing demographics in many parts of the world, an increasing proportion of patients who seek aesthetic services have come from a diverse ethnic background. Ethnic skin typically falls within Fitzpatrick's skin phototypes III–VI. These dark-skinned patients vary considerably in their response to sunlight, sun exposure, photodamage, and photoaging compared to the Caucasians. Therefore, it is important to be aware of the special needs of these patients with ethnic skin, and to select the most appropriate lasers and light sources in the treatment of congenital or acquired pigmentary conditions.

The cutaneous applications of lasers and light sources in dark-skinned patients differ from their use in Caucasians in several aspects. Firstly, ethnic skin tends to have more congenital and acquired pigmentary disorders. Conditions like nevus of Ota and Hori's nevus are more commonly seen in skin of color. Secondly, darker skin has larger melanocytes which produce more melanin. The melanosomes are distributed individually in keratinocytes, hence conferring significant photoprotection compared to fair skin. Aging in ethnic skin manifests 10 to 20 years later than age-matched Caucasian counterparts. Furthermore, the early signs of photoaging in dark-skinned patients commonly consist of pigmentary changes, like solar lentigines, freckles, seborrhoeic keratosis, and dermatosis papulosa nigra, rather than wrinkling as seen in Caucasians. Thirdly, the higher epidermal melanin content in ethnic skin together with the broad absorption spectrum of melanin on the electromagnetic spectrum create significant technical challenges in the use of cutaneous lasers and light sources on dark-skinned patients. The highly melanized epidermis of ethnic skin can absorb and interfere with the absorption of laser energy which is intended for another target, such as pigment within the hair follicle, a blood vessel or tattoo ink within the dermis. Hence, special considerations must be given for the selection of treatment parameters for ethnic skin in order to optimize results and to minimize unwanted side effects, such as post-inflammatory hyperpigmentation (PIH). This chapter aims to discuss the effective and safe use of lasers and light sources in the management of pigmentary conditions seen in ethnic skin. The treatment of melasma will be covered in another Chapter 15.

CLINICAL EXAMINATION AND PATIENT HISTORY

When assessing any pigmentary condition, it is paramount to make a correct clinical diagnosis before initiating treatment with lasers and light sources. For certain benign pigmented lesions, like melasma, assessment with Wood's light can help in assessing the epidermal and dermal components.

In the preoperative consultation, the patient's chief complaint, concerns and treatment expectations are addressed. These aspects should be interpreted in light of the patient's cultural background. A detailed medical history is necessary to assess for any contraindications to laser and light treatment. The use of oral retinoids within the past 6 months can increase the risk of scarring from laser treatment. Furthermore, any active infection or recent sun exposure of the treatment area, tendency for keloid and scar formation, photosensitivity, immunocompromised state, pregnancy, personal or family history of melanoma should be excluded before initiating treatment. The patient's Fitzpatrick skin type also needs to be assessed.

After a decision has been made to proceed with laser and light treatment for the pigmented lesions, the different treatment options, postoperative care, expected outcome, accepted downtime, and possible risks can be discussed with the patient. Ethnic skin has a higher risk of complications like PIH, and this should be discussed in detail preoperatively. The use of daily sun protection throughout the course of treatment as well as the avoidance of sun exposure for at least 2 weeks before laser treatment should be emphasized. Pre- and posttreatment with topical bleaching agents to lower the risk of PIH will be discussed in the following sections.

DEVICE, TREATMENT SELECTION, AND APPLICATION

▨ Solar Lentigines and Freckles

Solar lentigines and freckles are the commonest and earliest signs of photoaging in ethnic skin. Lentigines increase in number and prevalence with age. They are nonuniformly distributed and tend to vary in size and color. Histologically, the basal cell layer is hyperpigmented with an increase in the number of melanocytes. No nest formation is usually seen along the basement membrane. Epidermal rete ridges are elongated and clubbed. In contrast, freckles (or ephelides) can begin in adolescence and are more uniform in their distribution, size and color. Histologically, freckles show epidermal hypermelanosis without an increase in the number of melanocyte.

The effectiveness of Q-switched (QS) lasers in the treatment of lentigines has long been recognized. In light-skinned patients, they are often the treatment of choice for lentigines and freckles with limited complications. However, it has been shown that QS 532-nm neodymium:yttrium-aluminum-garnet (Nd:YAG) lasers, QS alexandrite laser (755 nm), and QS ruby laser (694 nm) performed on Asians carried a risk of PIH of approximately 10% to 25%.[1-3] In a study conducted by Chan et al.[4] on Oriental patients in 2000, the efficacy and complication rates of QS Nd:YAG 532 nm were

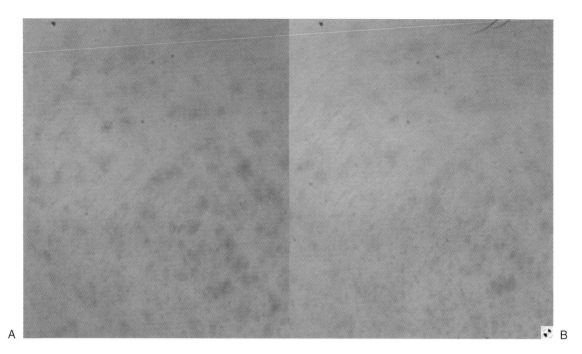

Figure 6.1 *Lentigines, (A) before and (B) after two treatments with IPL source (7–8 J/cm², 2.5 ms, 600–850 nm)*

compared with long pulsed Nd:YAG 532 nm in the treatment of facial lentigines. Although the two types of lasers had similar degree of clearing, the QS laser was associated with a greater risk of PIH. This observation is explained by the fact that QS lasers deliver short bursts (nanoseconds) of wavelength-specific energy, which causes destruction of melanin by both photothermal and photomechanical effects. The photomechanical effect also causes undesirable damage to the surrounding oxyhemoglobin, leading to inflammation of the superficial vessels and an altered activity of the melanocytes, hence resulting in PIH. Since then, a number of studies looking at the use of intense pulsed light (IPL) source and long pulsed 532-nm Nd:YAG lasers in the treatment of lentigines in dark-skinned patients have confirmed this observation.[5,6] In one study by Wang et al.[1] in 2006, QS alexandrite laser was compared against IPL for the treatment of freckles and lentigines in Chinese. It was shown that the risk of PIH was greater with QS laser. Therefore, it is now accepted that without the photomechanical effect associated with QS laser, both IPL and long pulsed laser carry a relatively lower risk of PIH when used on ethnic skin. In our practice, long pulsed 532-nm Nd:YAG is frequently employed in the removal of lentigines in Chinese patients, with an ash-gray appearance of the lesion as a clinical endpoint (2 mm spot size, 2 ms pulse duration, 6.5–8.0 J/cm² fluence without cooling or 12–14 J/cm² with cooling sapphire window). By choosing a pulse width (millisecond domain) that matches the thermal relaxation time of the epidermis (10 ms), the risk of thermal injury to the dermis is minimized.

IPL sources emit a broadband of visible light (400–1200 nm) from a noncoherent filtered flashlamp. They target pigmentation through photothermal effects. A number of studies have confirmed the efficacy and safety of IPL in the removal of lentigines and freckles in Asian skin. In 2001, Negishi et al.[5] looked at photorejuvenation with IPL in 97 Asian patients. A reduction in pigmentation in more than 90% of patients was reported after 3 to 6 treatments at

intervals of 2 to 3 weeks (cut-off filter 550 nm, 28–32 J/cm², double-pulse mode of 2.5- 4.0/4.0–5.0 ms, delay time 20.0/40.0 ms). The same group later conducted another study of IPL with an integrated contact cooling system on 73 Asian patients (cut-off filter 560 nm, 23–27 J/cm², double-pulse mode of 2.8–3.2/6.0 ms, delay time 20.0/40.0 ms).[7] Eighty percent of the patients had significant reduction in pigmentation after 3 to 5 treatments at intervals of 3 to 4 weeks. A similar study by Kawada et al.[8] showed satisfactory results of IPL in the treatment of solar lentigines and freckles in Asian patients. In all these studies, no PIH was seen. This could be explained by the photothermal effect of IPL without the photomechanical effect associated with QS lasers. Hence, IPL is advantageous in this aspect compared to QS laser in the removal of lentigines and freckles in Asian patients (Figure 6.1).

Recently, there has been an interest in the use of traditional vascular lasers in the removal of lentigines. Long-pulse pulsed dye laser (LPDL) 595-nm targets hemoglobin as well as melanin. In order to minimize the risk of bruising and subsequent PIH associated with the use of LPDL, diascopy during laser treatment has been employed. Compression of the skin surface by the flat glass window on the handpiece leads to emptying of blood vessels and therefore reduces the risks of dermal vascular damage by laser and subsequent bruising and PIH. In a study by Kono et al.,[9] the efficacy and complications of QS ruby 694-nm laser (spot size 4 mm, fluence 6–7 J/cm², pulse duration 30 ns) was compared against 595-nm LPDL delivered with compression (spot size 7 mm, fluence 10–13 J/cm², pulse duration 1.5 ms, no cryogen spray cooling) in the treatment of facial lentigines in 18 Asians. Although both lasers were shown to be effective, the LPDL with compression arm demonstrated slightly superior results with substantially less complications than the QS ruby laser. Post inflammatory hyperpigmentation was seen in 4 patients after QS ruby laser, but not in any treated with LPDL. This could be explained by the longer pulse duration

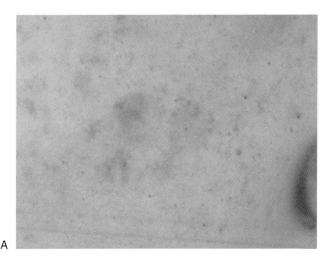

A   B

Figure 6.2 *Freckles, (A) before and (B) after with two treatments of long-pulsed 532-nm Nd:YAG laser 2-mm spot size, 12 J/cm² with contact cooling*

(milliseconds) associated with LPDL, which is more optimal for targeting the basal cell layer with minimal photomechanical effects. However, the use of long-pulse lasers in the treatment of lentigines carries the potential risk of dermal injury and scar formation because of the possible thermal diffusion from the epidermis to dermis. To prevent this, the pulse duration needs to be equal or shorter than the thermal relaxation time of the epidermal basal layer, which is in the range of 1.6 to 2.8 ms for a 20-μm thick basal layer. In the study above, 1.5 ms was used for LPDL, which yielded satisfactory clinical outcome with a lower risk of complication.

A more recent study by Kono et al.,[10] in 2007 compared the use of IPL (6 treatment sessions, fluence 27–40 J/cm², pulse duration 20 ms) to 595-nm LPDL with compression (3 treatment sessions, spot size 7 mm, fluence 9–12 J/cm² for lentigines, pulse duration 1.5 ms) in facial rejuvenation of 10 Asian patients. The improvement of lentigines was 62.3% and 81.1% for IPL and LPDL, respectively. There was no significant difference between the two devices in wrinkle reduction. No scarring or pigmentary changes were seen with either device. It was concluded that both IPL and LPDL were effective for facial skin rejuvenation in Asians, but LPDL treatment is significantly more effective for lentigines. In a further study by Kono et al.,[11] the clinical efficacy and complications of 595-nm LPDL with compression in the treatment of facial lentigines were studied in 54 Asian patients. A spot size of 7 mm was used. The mean fluence was 10.8 J/cm² (range 9–13 J/cm²), and the pulse duration was kept at 1.5 ms. Cryogen spray cooling was not used. An ash-gray color change in the lentigines without purpura was taken as the clinical endpoint. In this study, compression was achieved by a convex-type glass window, as opposed to the flat-type used in previous study, to ensure sufficient pressure for emptying blood vessels over the target area during treatment. The mean degree of clearance was 84.4% with no scarring or hypopigmentation seen. Only one patient had PIH. In view of the cumulative experience reported in the literature, it can be concluded that LPDL with compression is an effective and safe modality for treating facial lentigines in Asian patients. However, there is currently no study comparing LPDL with long pulse 532-nm Nd:YAG laser in the treatment of lentigines in ethnic skin, and further studies are warranted in this regard.

In view of the numerous devices available, an algorithm has been suggested by Chan in the treatment of lentigines and freckles in ethnic skin.[3] After discussing the advantages and disadvantages of the different treatment options with the patient, the choice of device depends on the cost-effectiveness, patient's expectation, and possible complications such as PIH. One approach is to test patients with long pulse 532-nm Nd:YAG laser, and if they respond well with no PIH, full treatment is then offered (Figure 6.2). For those who do not wish to have downtime or develop PIH at test spot, IPL is offered. IPL requires more treatment sessions to achieve the desired clinical outcome and this raises the issue of cost-effectiveness. An aggressive approach using QS lasers has the advantage of achieving significant clearing only after 1 to 2 sessions. QS lasers are also particularly effective for lightly pigmented lentigines. However, they carry a higher risk of PIH when used in ethnic skin and have a downtime of a week. Hence, their routine use in dark-skinned patient is not recommended. Recently, LPDL is an alternative treatment option which has been shown to be safe and effective in the removal of lentigines in Asians when compared to IPL and QS ruby laser (Figures 6.3, and 6.4). For patients with not only lentigines and freckles, but also melasma, seborrhoeic keratoses and Hori's macules, a combination of IPL and QS ruby laser has been shown to be safe and effective.[12] Whichever device is chosen, it is important to wear sunblock and to practice sun avoidance before and after treatment. Moreover, the use of topical bleaching agents pre-and posttreatment can help to reduce the risk of PIH.

■ Seborrhoeic Keratosis and Dermatosis Papulosa Nigra

Seborrhoeic keratoses and dermatosis papulosa nigra are common cutaneous lesions associated with photoaging in ethnic skin. No treatment is required but they can be of cosmetic concern. Removal can be achieved by scissor excision, electrodessication and laser treatment. Ablative lasers like CO_2 laser and erbium:YAG laser can be used. The chosen spot size should not exceed the diameter of the lesion so as to minimize the risk of collateral thermal damage and subsequent PIH of the surrounding skin.

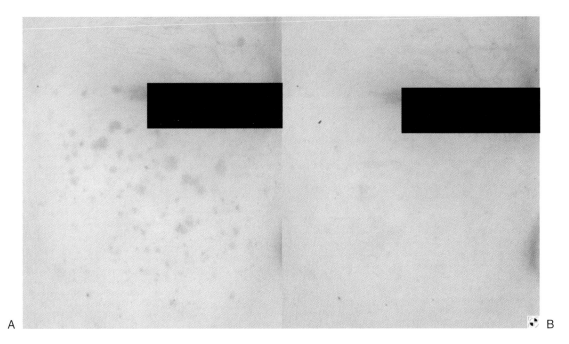

Figure 6.3 *Freckles, (A) before and (B) after single treatment with QS 532-nm Nd:YAG laser, 2-mm spot size, 0.6 J/cm²*

▧ Café Au Lait Macule

Café au lait macules (CALMs) are benign epidermal pigmented lesions that can be idiopathic or associated with neurocutaneous syndomes such as neurofibromatosis. They may increase in size with time and can be removed for cosmetic reasons. Histologically, scattered giant melanin granules are seen together with an increased melanocytic activity of the melanocytes. An increase in melanin is also present in both melanocytes and keratinocytes.

A variety of lasers have been tried on CALM with inconsistent results. Somyos et al.[13] reported good to excellent results in 15 out of 16 patients treated with 2 sessions of continuous-mode 511-nm copper vapor laser. In some cases, 510-nm pulsed dye laser and erbium:YAG laser have also been shown to be successful.[14–16] QS

Figure 6.4 *Lentigines, (A) Before and (B) after two treatments with long-pulsed 595-nm pulsed dye laser with compression 1.5 ms, 11 J/cm², 7-mm spot size*

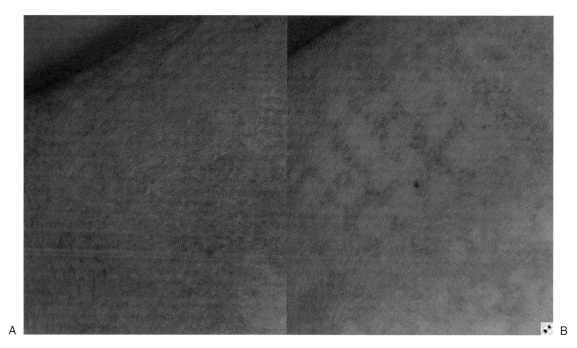

Figure 6.5 *Becker's nevus, (A) before and (B) after three treatment sessions with long-pulsed alexandrite laser 10-mm spot size, 20–25 J/cm²*

lasers yielded variable results with high recurrence rates. Paradoxical darkening has also been reported. In a study using QS 694-nm ruby laser and QS 532-nm Nd:YAG laser, it was found that the degree of clearance varied across the lesions.[17] One possible explanation was that QS lasers failed to remove the follicular melanocytic component of the CALM. Categorizing the lesion into two histological subtypes was shown not to be useful for predicting the clinical response to laser treatment.[17]

Our current approach is to use a long-pulsed pigmented laser, such as normal mode ruby laser (NMRL) or long-pulsed alexandrite laser without cooling, to remove not only the epidermal melanocytes but also the hair follicle melanocytes. In one study of 33 patients with CALM, NMRL was shown to have a lower risk of recurrence (42.4%) compared to QS ruby laser (81.8%) 3 months after a single treatment. By targeting the follicular melanocytes, long-pulse laser may help to reduce the recurrence rate.

Becker's Nevus

Becker's nevus is a pigmented hamartoma which is more common in males. It is a developmental anomaly which usually appears before 15 years of age. Clinically, a typical lesion is located over the shoulder and the back, and is characterized by changes in pigmentation, hair growth, and a slightly elevated verrucous surface. Histologically, the pigmentation is as a result of the increased melanin in the basal cells. In the past, argon and CO_2 lasers were used, which often resulted in scarring or permanent hypopigmentation. One previous study using QS ruby laser showed a post-operative increase in pigmentation after 4 weeks.[18]

Trelles et al. compared the use of erbium:YAG laser to QS 1064-nm Nd:YAG laser in 22 patients with a follow-up of 2 years.[19]

Erbium:YAG laser achieved significantly better results with complete clearance in 54% of patients after a single treatment. For QS 1064-nm Nd:YAG laser, multiple treatments were needed and only one out of eleven patients had significant clearing after three treatment sessions. Long-pulsed pigmented laser has also been employed to remove hair and pigmentation in Becker's nevus, but textural change was a possible complication.[20] In our practice, long-pulse alexandrite 755-nm laser (20–35 J/cm², 10 mm spot size, pulse duration 1.5 ms) is used to target the pigment and surrounding hair follicle (Figure 6.5). Four to eight treatment sessions are usually given with a 50% success rate. Possible adverse effects include scarring and hypopigmentation.

Nevus of Ota (Figure 6.6)

Nevus of Ota is a dermal melanocytic hamartoma characterized clinically by mottled, dusky blue and brown hyperpigmentation. The pigmentation can cause marked disfigurement and mostly affects the skin and mucous membranes innervated by the first and second branches of the trigeminal nerve. Histologically, ectopic melanocytes are present in the dermis. This condition is more common in Asians and affects approximately 0.6% of the population.[21] QS ruby 694 nm, QS alexandrite (alex) 755 nm and QS Nd:YAG 1064 nm lasers have all been used in the treatment of nevus of Ota with excellent results and minimal complications. The clinical efficacy of QS ruby laser was reported by Goldberg et al. and Geronemus in 1992.[22,23] It was later confirmed by Watanabe et al. who looked at 114 patients treated with QS ruby laser and reported a good to excellent degree of lightening after three or more treatment sessions.[24] The side effects were few, the most common being transient hyperpigmentation after the first treatment. Kono et al. reviewed 101

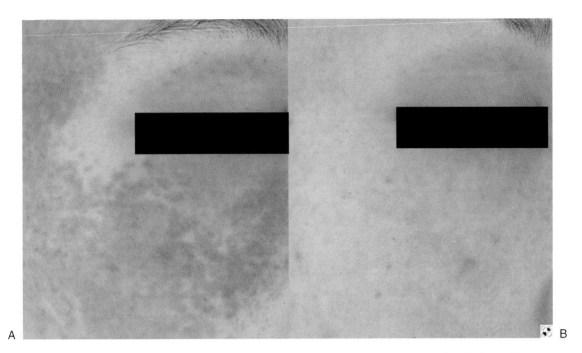

Figure 6.6 *Nevus of Ota, (A) before and (B) after five treatments with QS ruby laser (5-mm spot size, 3–4 J/cm^2)*

patients 12-months post QS ruby laser treatment, and found 56% of patients obtaining over 75% of clearance.[25] thirty-six percent of patients had complete clearance. Hypopigmentation and hyperpigmentation was seen in 17% and 6% of patients, respectively.

Chan et al. compared the use of QS alex laser with QS Nd:YAG laser in nevus of Ota, and found that most patients tolerated QS alex laser better.[26] This tolerability can be improved with pre-and posttreatment skin cooling as shown in a study of 37 nevus of Ota patients treated with QS alex laser. However, the use of contact cooling during laser treatment prevented the use of higher fluence.[27] Although QS alex is more tolerable than QS Nd:YAG laser, the latter was shown to be more effective in lightening the lesion after three or more treatment sessions.[4] In terms of complications, hypopigmentation was common, especially with QS ruby laser.[25,28] Recently, a study of 10 Asian patients with dermal pigmented lesions (three of which were nevus of Ota) showed that the use of QS alex laser delivered with compression was associated with a lower risk of purpura and dyspigmentation when compared with laser treatment without compression. The efficacy was not compromised with compression. Diascopy caused emptying of the cutaneous blood vessels and hence reduced the risk of laser injury to blood vessels.[29]

One important consideration when planning treatment is to take into account the 0.6% to 1.2% risk of recurrence, which can occur in patients after complete laser-induced clearance. This is a particularly relevant issue especially for pediatric patients. However, Kono et al.[30] showed that QS ruby laser when used for nevus of Ota in children can achieve excellent result in fewer sessions with lower complication rate than later treatment. Therefore, the pros and cons of treating nevus of Ota in childhood need to be discussed thoroughly with patients and their families before starting treatment.

▓ Acquired Bilateral Nevus of Ota-Like Macules (Abnom)/Hori's Macules (Figure 6.7)

Similar to nevus of Ota, Hori's macules are primarily dermal hyperpigmentation commonly seen in Asian patients that affects approximately 0.8% of the population. Hori's macules present as bilateral blue-gray macules typically located over the malar region in a symmetrical pattern. The lateral temples, alae nasi, eyelids, and foreheads can also be involved. Histologically, dermal melanocytes are dispersed in the papillary and middle part of the dermis. In contrast to nevus of Ota, the pigmentation of Hori's macules is acquired, has a late onset in adulthood, and does not affect the mucosa. Melasma and Hori's macules can coexist in some patients. Like nevus of Ota, QS lasers have been shown to be effective for treatment of Hori's macules.

In 1999, Kunachak et al.[31] studied a series of patients with Hori's macules treated with QS ruby laser (fluence 7–10 J/cm^2, repetition rate 1 Hz, spot size 2-4 mm). Complete clearance was seen in more than 90% of patients with no recurrence after a mean follow-up of 2.5 years. However, PIH was seen in 7% of the patients. A year later, two studies showed that QS Nd:YAG laser was also effective for Hori's macules, but the rate of PIH was between 50% to 73%.[32,33] In a retrospective analysis of 32 Chinese patients, QS alex laser (755 nm, spot size 3 mm, fluence 8 J/cm^2) was employed.[34] Eighty percent of patients achieved more than 50% clearance, while complete clearance was seen in more than 28% of patients. However, 12.5% experienced PIH, all of which resolved with topical bleaching agents. In order to increase the therapeutic efficacy of QS lasers in the treatment of Hori's macules, a group studied the use of scanned carbon dioxide (CO_2) laser for epidermal ablation followed by QS ruby laser in 13 Asian patients. The response rate

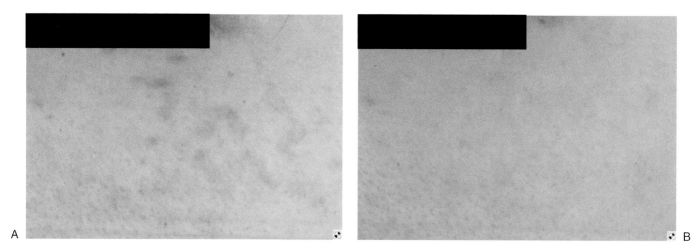

Figure 6.7 *Hori's macules, (A) before and (B) after six treatments with QS ruby laser (5-mm spot size, 3–4 J/cm²)*

was significantly higher in the combination arm compared to those treated by QS ruby laser alone. Transient hypopigmentation and erythema were seen in up to 15% of patients, but resolved at 16-month post treatment.[35]

It is the author's (H.C.) experience that Hori's macules tend to be more resistant to therapy compared to nevus of Ota. One approach is to treat these patients more frequently with repeat laser session every 4 weeks. The idea is to treat the area before epithelial repigmentation occurs. In doing so, more laser energy can reach the dermal target chromophore through a hypopigmented epidermis without the competitive absorption of epidermal melanin. For resistant cases which fail to improve after four treatment sessions, QS alex laser can be given followed immediately by QS 1064-nm Nd:YAG treatment. In this combination treatment, the fluence should be lower (4–5 J/cm² for both lasers), and the repetition rate should be reduced to no more than 3.3 Hz in order to reduce the risk of adverse effects. A similar combination approach was reported by Ee et al.[36] in 2006, which showed that QS 532-nm Nd:YAG laser followed by QS 1064-nm Nd:YAG laser is more effective in pigment clearance than QS 1064-nm Nd:YAG laser alone for Hori's macules.

Many studies have indicated a high risk of transient pigmentary disturbance when laser is used for the treatment of Hori's macules. Posttreatment PIH is common, and permanent hypopigmentation has been reported after QS ruby laser.[31] To decrease the risk of PIH, all patients should be given pre- and posttreatment topical bleaching agents. Epidermal cooling with cold air was investigated by Manuskiatti et al. as a mean of decreasing PIH after QS 1064-nm Nd:YAG treatment of Hori's macules.[37] However, epidermal cooling was associated with an increased risk of PIH after laser treatment, the reason of which is not completely clear. Finally, it should be noted IPL is not routinely recommended for the treatment of dermal pigmentary conditions, as such an approach can be associated with a high risk of scarring.

■ Congenital Melanocytic Nevus (Figure 6.8)

Melanocytic nevi are often requested by patients to be removed for cosmetic reasons. The use of laser in the removal of congenital

melanocytic nevi is controversial, since there is potentially a risk of delaying the diagnosis of melanoma. Furthermore, long-term complications, such as the increased risk of neoplastic changes, are unclear. The differences in epidemiology of melanoma in dark-skinned population compared to Caucasians suggest that the biological behaviour of melanocyte differ between these two groups. In fact, melanoma is much less common among dark-skinned patients, and they tend to be acral in location. A long-term follow-up study in Japan looking at the use of laser in the treatment of congenital melanocytic nevi showed that there was no histological evidence of malignant changes 8 years after laser treatment. Therefore, removal of melanocytic nevi with laser treatment may be more justified in dark-skinned patients compared to Caucasians, as long as there is no family history of melanoma and the lesion is not acral in location.

Different pigmented lasers have been studied in the removal of congenital melanocytic nevi. One study by Waldorf et al. looked at the use of QS ruby laser in Caucasians and found an average clearance rate of 76% after eight treatment sessions.[38] However, recurrence can be a problem. NMRL has also been used based on the principle that longer pulse duration leads to more melanocyte destruction and hence a greater extent of clearance of pigmentation.[39] A combination approach using QS ruby laser followed by NMRL was reported by Duke et al.[40] This approach intended to remove the superficial pigment first with QS ruby laser, which subsequently enhanced the penetration of NMRL. One Japanese group later reported improved clearance of pigmentation by first using NMRL to remove the epidermis, followed immediately by multiple passes of QS ruby laser.[41] In this way, the removal of epidermis allowed a greater degree of penetration by QS laser, thus enhancing the clinical efficacy.

■ Post Inflammatory Hyperpigmentation

Post inflammatory hyperpigmentation is the commonest complication of laser and light source treatment in ethnic skin. Effective prevention and treatment are therefore important. Sun protection and avoidance are necessary for at least 2 weeks before laser or IPL

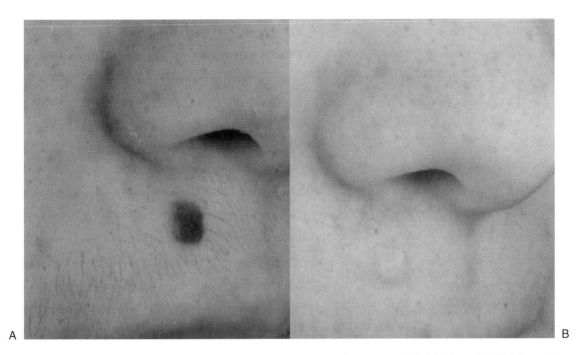

A   B

Figure 6.8 *Melanocytic nevi, (A) before and (B) after three treatments with CO_2 laser and QS 1064-nm Nd:YAG laser (3-mm spot size, 3–4 J/cm^2)*

treatment. All patients should apply titanium dioxide and zinc oxide-containing sunblock daily for 2 weeks before treatment. Application of moderate potency topical steroid immediately after laser and IPL treatment may also reduce the risk of PIH.

Pre- and posttreatment use of topical bleaching agents is important to decrease the risk of PIH. Different types of topical bleaching agents are available which contain various combinations of agents, including tretinoin, hydroquinone, steroid, alpha hydroxy acid, kojic acid, and azelaic acid. In our practice, a combination of azelaic acid, 4% hydroquinone and moderately potent steroid is given twice daily for 2 weeks pretreatment and 4 weeks posttreatment. If PIH still develops, then 5% glycolic acid is added in the morning to further reduce the hyperpigmentation. Other bleaching agents, like topical vitamin C, vitamin E, and kojic acid, can also be added depending on the degree of irritation. For cases where PIH continues to persist for longer than 6 weeks, a mild glycolic acid peel (20%–35%) alternating with microdermabrasion on a weekly basis can be offered. Phototoxic drugs, like tetracycline, can potentially increase the risk of PIH. They should be avoided for 2 weeks before any treatment, as well as in the posttreatment period.

Tattoos

Lasers can effectively remove some but not all tattoos. QS ruby, alex and 1064-nm Nd:YAG lasers can be used effectively for the removal of blue-black tattoo. Depending upon the ink composition, QS 532-nm Nd:YAG can be effective for some but not all red, yellow, orange, and purple tattoo. Tattoo darkening can occur and is thought to be related to the reduction of ferric oxide to ferrous

oxide.[42] Green tattoo can be particularly difficult to remove but QS alex can be tried.

The QS 1064-nm Nd:YAG is considered to be particularly effective in dark-skinned patients given its longer wavelength and lower risk of adverse effects.[43,44] In a Korean study, a QS alex laser was used to successfully treat 36 cases of traumatic tattoo with greater than 76% pigment removal after an average of 1.7 treatment sessions.[45] Complications such as postinflammatory hyperpigmentation can occur, but permanent side effects are seldom observed.

Despite the fact that previous study indicated the use of picosecond laser to be more effective in tattoo clearance, such device has never been commercially manufactured. More recently, tattoo ink that involves the use of microencapsulated, biodegradable and bioabsorbable dyes within colorless polymer beads have been investigated as a means to improve laser tattoo removal. Further study is necessary to confirm the efficacy of laser removal for this new type of tattoo ink.

CONCLUSION

The challenge in the use of lasers and light sources in ethnic skin is to achieve effective treatment with minimal complications. The risk of adverse effects can be minimized with the use of more conservative parameters, lower energy settings, appropriate wavelengths, and the cautious use of cooling techniques. With appropriate patient selection and physician training, laser surgery has become safer for ethnic skin. As the demand for laser and light sources treatment by dark-skinned patients continue to increase, future studies should attempt to address issues and define specific parameters for ethnic skin types.

REFERENCES

1. Wang CC, Sue YM, Yang CH, Chen CK. A comparison of Q-switched alexandrite laser and intense pulsed light for the treatment of freckles and lentigines in Asian persons: a randomized, physician-blinded, split-face comparative trial. *J Am Acad Dermatol.* 2006;54(5):804-810.

2. Murphy MJ, Huang MY. Q-switched ruby laser treatment of benign pigmented lesions in Chinese skin. *Ann Acad Med Singapore.* 1994;23(1):60-66.

3. Chan H. The use of lasers and intense pulsed light sources for the treatment of acquired pigmentary lesions in Asians. *J Cosmet Laser Ther.* 2003;5(3-4):198-200.

4. Chan HH, Fung WK, Ying SY, Kono T. An in vivo trial comparing the use of different types of 532 nm Nd:YAG lasers in the treatment of facial lentigines in Oriental patients. *Dermatol Surg.* 2000;26(8):743-749.

5. Negishi K, Tezuka Y, Kushikata N, Wakamatsu S. Photorejuvenation for Asian skin by intense pulsed light. *Dermatol Surg.* 2001;27(7):627-631.

6. Rashid T, Hussain I, Haider M, Haroon TS. Laser therapy of freckles and lentigines with quasi-continuous, frequency-doubled, Nd:YAG (532 nm) laser in Fitzpatrick skin type IV: a 24-month follow-up. *J Cosmet Laser Ther.* 2002;4(3-4):81-85.

7. Negishi K, Wakamatsu S, Kushikata N, Tezuka Y, Kotani Y, Shiba K. Full-face photorejuvenation of photodamaged skin by intense pulsed light with integrated contact cooling: initial experiences in Asian patients. *Lasers Surg Med.* 2002;30(4):298-305.

8. Kawada A, Shiraishi H, Asai M, et al. Clinical improvement of solar lentigines and ephelides with an intense pulsed light source. *Dermatol Surg.* 2002;28(6):504-508.

9. Kono T, Manstein D, Chan HH, Nozaki M, Anderson RR. Q-switched ruby versus long-pulsed dye laser delivered with compression for treatment of facial lentigines in Asians. *Lasers Surg Med.* 2006;38(2):94-97.

10. Kono T, Groff WF, Sakurai H, et al. Comparison study of intense pulsed light versus a long-pulse pulsed dye laser in the treatment of facial skin rejuvenation. *Ann Plast Surg.* 2007;59(5):479-483.

11. Kono T, Chan HH, Groff WF, et al. Long-pulse pulsed dye laser delivered with compression for treatment of facial lentigines. *Dermatol Surg.* 2007;33(8):945-950.

12. Park JM, Tsao H, Tsao S. Combined use of intense pulsed light and Q-switched ruby laser for complex dyspigmentation among Asian patients. *Lasers Surg Med.* 2008;40(2):128-133.

13. Somyos K, Boonchu K, Somsak K, Panadda L, Leopairut J. Copper vapour laser treatment of cafe-au-lait macules. *Br J Dermatol.* 1996;135(6):964-968.

14. Alora MB, Arndt KA. Treatment of a cafe-au-lait macule with the erbium: YAG laser. *J Am Acad Dermatol.* 2001;45(4):566-568.

15. Alster TS. Complete elimination of large cafe-au-lait birthmarks by the 510-nm pulsed dye laser. *Plast Reconstr Surg.* 1995;96(7):1660-1664.

16. Alster TS, Williams CM. Cafe-au-lait macule in type V skin: successful treatment with a 510 nm pulsed dye laser. *J Am Acad Dermatol.* 1995;33(6):1042-1043.

17. Grossman MC, Anderson RR, Farinelli W, Flotte TJ, Grevelink JM. Treatment of cafe au lait macules with lasers. A clinicopathologic correlation. *Arch Dermatol.* 1995;131(12):1416-1420.

18. Kopera D, Hohenleutner U, Landthaler M. Quality-switched ruby laser treatment of solar lentigines and Becker's nevus: a histopathological and immunohistochemical study. *Dermatology.* 1997;194(4):338-343.

19. Trelles MA, Allones I, Moreno-Arias GA, Velez M. Becker's naevus: a comparative study between erbium:YAG and Q-switched neodymium: YAG; clinical and histopathological findings. *Br J Dermatol.* 2005;152(2):308-313.

20. Nanni CA, Alster TS. Treatment of a Becker's nevus using a 694-nm long-pulsed ruby laser. *Dermatol Surg.* 1998;24(9):1032-1034.

21. Hidano A, Kajima H, Ikeda S, Mizutani H, Miyasato H, Niimura M. Natural history of nevus of Ota. *Arch Dermatol.* 1967;95(2):187-195.

22. Geronemus RG. Q-switched ruby laser therapy of nevus of Ota. *Arch Dermatol.* 1992;128(12):1618-1622.

23. Goldberg DJ, Nychay SG. Q-switched ruby laser treatment of nevus of Ota. *J Dermatol Surg Oncol.* 1992;18(9):817-821.

24. Watanabe S, Takahashi H. Treatment of nevus of Ota with the Q-switched ruby laser. *N Engl J Med.* 1994;331(26):1745-1750.

25. Kono T, Nozaki M, Chan HH, Mikashima Y. A retrospective study looking at the long-term complications of Q-switched ruby laser in the treatment of nevus of Ota. *Lasers Surg Med.* 2001;29(2):156-159.

26. Chan HH, King WW, Chan ES, et al. In vivo trial comparing patients' tolerance of Q-switched alexandrite (QS Alex) and Q-switched neodymium: yttrium-aluminum-garnet (QS Nd:YAG) lasers in the treatment of nevus of Ota. *Lasers Surg Med.* 1999;24(1):24-28.

27. Chan HH, Lam LK, Wong DS, Wei WI. Role of skin cooling in improving patient tolerability of Q-switched alexandrite (QS Alex) laser in nevus of Ota treatment. *Lasers Surg Med.* 2003;32(2):148-151.

28. Chan HH, Leung RS, Ying SY, et al. A retrospective analysis of complications in the treatment of nevus of Ota with the Q-switched alexandrite and Q-switched Nd:YAG lasers. *Dermatol Surg.* 2000;26(11):1000-1006.

29. Kono T, Groff WF, Chan HH, Sakurai H, Nozaki M. Comparison study of a Q-switched alexandrite laser delivered with versus without compression in the treatment of dermal pigmented lesions. *J Cosmet Laser Ther.* 2007;9(4):206-209.

30. Kono T, Chan HH, Ercocen AR, et al. Use of Q-switched ruby laser in the treatment of nevus of Ota in different age groups. *Lasers Surg Med.* 2003;32(5):391-395.

31. Kunachak S, Leelaudomlipi P, Sirikulchayanonta V. Q-Switched ruby laser therapy of acquired bilateral nevus of Ota-like macules. *Dermatol Surg.* 1999;25(12):938-941.

32. Kunachak S, Leelaudomlipi P. Q-switched Nd:YAG laser treatment for acquired bilateral nevus of Ota-like maculae: a long-term follow-up. *Lasers Surg Med.* 2000;26(4):376-379.

33. Polnikorn N, Tanrattanakorn S, Goldberg DJ. Treatment of Hori's nevus with the Q-switched Nd:YAG laser. *Dermatol Surg.* 2000;26(5):477-480.

34. Lam AY, Wong DS, Lam LK, Ho WS, Chan HH. A retrospective study on the efficacy and complications of Q-switched alexandrite laser in the treatment of acquired bilateral nevus of Ota-like macules. *Dermatol Surg.* 2001;27(11):937-941; 41-42.

35. Manuskiatti W, Sivayathorn A, Leelaudomlipi P, Fitzpatrick RE. Treatment of acquired bilateral nevus of Ota-like macules (Hori's nevus) using a combination of scanned carbon dioxide laser followed by Q-switched ruby laser. *J Am Acad Dermatol.* 2003;48(4):584-591.

36. Ee HL, Goh CL, Khoo LS, Chan ES, Ang P. Treatment of acquired bilateral nevus of Ota-like macules (Hori's nevus) with a combination of the 532 nm Q-Switched Nd:YAG laser followed by the 1064 nm Q-switched Nd:YAG is more effective: prospective study. *Dermatol Surg.* 2006;32(1):34-40.

37. Manuskiatti W, Eimpunth S, Wanitphakdeedecha R. Effect of cold air cooling on the incidence of postinflammatory hyperpigmentation after Q-switched Nd:YAG laser treatment of acquired bilateral nevus of Ota like macules. *Arch Dermatol.* 2007;143(9):1139-1143.

38. Waldorf HA, Kauvar AN, Geronemus RG. Treatment of small and medium congenital nevi with the Q-switched ruby laser. *Arch Dermatol.* 1996;132(3):301-304.

39. Imayama S, Ueda S. Long- and short-term histological observations of congenital nevi treated with the normal-mode ruby laser. *Arch Dermatol.* 1999;135(10):1211-1218.

40. Duke D, Byers HR, Sober AJ, Anderson RR, Grevelink JM. Treatment of benign and atypical nevi with the normal-mode ruby laser and the Q-switched ruby laser: clinical improvement but failure to completely eliminate nevomelanocytes. *Arch Dermatol.* 1999;135(3):290-296.

41. Kono T, Nozaki M, Chan HH, Sasaki K, Kwon SG. Combined use of normal mode and Q-switched ruby lasers in the treatment of congenital melanocytic naevi. *Br J Plast Surg.* 2001; 54(7):640-643.

42. Anderson RR, Geronemus R, Kilmer SL, Farinelli W, Fitzpatrick RE. Cosmetic tattoo ink darkening. A complication of Q-switched and pulsed-laser treatment. *Arch Dermatol.* 1993;129:1010-1014.

43. Grevelink JM, Duke D, van Leeuwen RL, Gonzalez E, DeCoste SD, Anderson RR. Laser treatment of tattoos in darkly pigmented patients: efficacy and side effects. *J Am Acad Dermatol.* 1996;34:653-656.

44. Jones A, Roddey P, Orengo I, Rosen T. The Q-switched ND:YAG laser effectively treats tattoos in darkly pigmented skin. *Dermatol Surg.* 1996;22:999-1001.

45. Chang SE, Choi JH, Moon KC, Koh JK, Sung KJ. Successful removal of traumatic tattoos in Asian skin with a Q-switched alexandrite laser. *Dermatol Surg.* 1998;24:1308-1311.

46. Ross V, Naseef G, Lin G, et al. Comparison of responses of tattoos to picosecond and nanosecond Q-switched neodymium: YAG lasers. *Arch Dermatol.* 1998;134:167-171.

CHAPTER 7

Dermal Color Improvement in Ethnic Skin: Vascular Lasers and Lights

Taro Kono, MD, PhD, and Henry Hin-Lee Chan, MD, FRCP

INTRODUCTION AND DEFINITION

Laser treatment of vascular lesions was first developed in 1960s, and the risks of scarring and texture changes were very common in the early days. In 1983, the concept of selective photothermolysis revolutionized the use of laser for the treatment of vascular lesions. Since then, pulsed dye laser (PDL) has become the gold standard in the treatment of port wine stains (PWSs). However, for technical reasons in the past, no PDL had been developed with a pulse duration longer than 1 millisecond (ms) until the late 1990s. However, complications, especially dyspigmentation such as hypopigmentation and hyperpigmentation, were common, especially in dark-skinned patients. To minimize complications caused by higher fluence in dark-skinned patients, epidermal protection by skin cooling was developed. Newer-generation PDLs provide extended pulse durations, adequate skin cooling, and higher power, leading to enhanced clinical efficacy and lower risk of complication, especially in dark-skinned patients.

Port Wine Stains

PWSs are congenital, hypervascular malformations with a dark pinkish appearance that may evolve into nodular and purple lesions later in life. For nearly two decades, PDL was the treatment of choice for PWSs. However, clearance rates vary widely and many lesions cannot be completely cleared with laser treatment. Furthermore, redarkening has been reported among patients treated with PDL 10 years after treatment.[1] Improved efficacy in PWS treatment is expected by using variable wavelengths, variable pulse durations, and higher energy fluences with selective skin cooling, and techniques such as pulse stacking.

Hemangioma

The use of PDL for the treatment of hemangioma was reported to be associated with a greater risk of complications, including pigmentary disturbance and texture change.[2] However, the fluence used was too high, and at that stage, skin cooling was not developed. More recently, extended pulsed PDL with skin cooling was found to be more suitable in the treatment hemangiomas.[3]

Facial Telangiectasia

In contrast to PWSs, facial telangiectasia responds well to 532-nm neodymium:yttrium-aluminum-garnet (Nd:YAG) laser, PDL, and intense pulsed light (IPL) source. Short-pulsed PDL (1.5 ms or less) is effective but purpura formation is very common, leading to unacceptable duration of downtime. The 532-nm or 1064-nm Nd:YAG, extended pulse PDL and IPL are recommended because of the lack of resulting purpura.

LITERATURE REVIEW/EVIDENCE-BASED SUMMARY

Wavelength

In the late 1980s, a 577-nm PDL was developed and Tan et al.[4,5] reported an in vivo study on albino pig skin that demonstrated the depth of penetration could be increased from 0.5 to 1.2 mm without affecting vascular selectivity. Verkruysse et al.[6] showed this effect by calculating the maximum depth of vascular injury versus wavelength for different amounts of blood in the dermis and for different vessel diameters. Their findings revealed that 585-nm wavelength penetrates deeper into tissue than 577-nm wavelength. However, clearance rates of PWSs treated with the 585-nm PDL varied widely and many lesions responded incompletely to therapy. Hohenleuter et al.[7] showed that the PDL failed to destroy large vessels within PWSs as partially coagulated vessels were not adequately destroyed and regeneration occurred. It has been postulated that the 585-nm wavelength failed to penetrate deep enough to reach the deep dermal vessels. When treating PWSs composed of large blood vessels, there is an inadequate amount of thermal diffusion to result in vascular injury. Kane et al.[8] proposed that the formation of a fibrous shield in the upper papillary dermis could have obstructed laser penetration in subsequent PWS treatments, thus preventing destruction of deeper dermal vessels. It is possible that resistant PWSs previously treated with a 585-nm PDL may be further improved by using lasers with longer wavelengths that penetrate to a greater depth. Although the absorption coefficient of oxyhemoglobin is 4.8 times higher at 585 nm compared to at 595 nm, Scherer et al.[9] compared the 585-nm PDL with pulsed duration of 0.45 ms and long-pulsed PDL with pulsed duration at 1.5 ms. For the long-pulsed PDL, four different wavelengths (585 nm, 12 to 15 J/cm²; 590 nm, 11–16 J/cm²; 595 nm, 11 to 18 J/cm²; 600 nm, 13–20 J/cm²) were used. They found that the long-pulsed PDL was able to treat a larger variety of vessel types in PWSs compared to the 585-nm PDL at 0.45 ms. Woo et al.[10] treated 239 patients with variable pulsed 595-nm PDL with dynamic cooling device and reported the incident of pigmentary change and scarring to be lower than expected compared with previous studies.

Fluence

Clinical end points at appropriate fluences are different for each wavelength. Patients can tolerate higher fluences when using 595 nm (7–15 J/cm²) compared to 585 nm (7–10 J/cm²) when the pulse duration (1.5 ms), spot size (7 mm), and skin cooling remain constant. For larger vessels, the reduced thermal effect as a result of reduced light absorption (secondary to the larger volume of these vessels) has to be compensated for by increasing the fluence. With very small vessels containing only a few erythrocytes (the target chromophobe), a higher fluence is also required.[11] The problem with a purely fluence-driven approach is undesirable heating of surrounding targets results in unwanted perivascular damage. This principle has been well demonstrated in PWS treatment and is especially problematic when skin cooling fails.

Pulse Duration

According to the principle of selective photothermolysis, the laser pulse durations should be equal to or less than the vessel thermal relaxation time in order to maximize laser energy deposition within the vessel and to confine thermal damage to the treated vessel. In reviewing the concept of selective photothermolysis, the mathematical model predicts that the ideal thermal relaxation time for the vessels in PWS is actually 1 to 10 ms, not 0.45 ms. Dierickx et al.[12] demonstrated that these original theoretical calculations are correct in a study that used both an animal vessel model and human PWSs. Greve and Raulin[13] reported the prospective, comparative study of 595 nm/0.5 ms versus 595 nm/20 ms PDL treatment of PWSs and found that 595 nm/0.5 ms was clearly not as effective as 595 nm/20 ms. Recently, Bernstein and Douglas[14] reported the study of a large number of PWS subjects (95 subjects) using a 585 nm/1.5 ms–pulse PDL equipped with cryogen spray cooling. They indicated that the 1.5 ms–pulse PDL was effective in improving both untreated and previously treated PWSs that had become refractory to treatment using the 0.45-ms pulse duration PDL. Asahina et al.[15] demonstrated a good correlation between clearance of PWS and the average intensity of immediate purpura observed after PDL treatment. It is worthwhile to point out that for the treatment of PWSs, regardless of the pulse duration, purpura is the appropriate end point.[16]

Spot Size

Previous studies indicated that the degree of light scattering is directional related to the spot size and that the larger the spot size, the lesser is the degree of scattering.[17,18] Large spot size can lead to greater depth of thermal injury at any given fluence. The larger beam also produces larger volumetric heat production for the same incident radiant exposure, which means that higher radiant exposure will be required to achieve the same desired end point when using smaller beam diameters. Because of deeper penetration, the larger beam diameters are more effective in reaching larger and deeper vessels.

Skin cooling

Skin cooling has increased the safety of PDL treatment. Techniques include the application of ice cubes, cold gels, aluminum rollers, and contact cooling with a sapphire window or copper plate, air-cooling, and cryogen spray cooling. Cooling devices allow the use of higher fluences, while protecting the epidermis from thermal damage. This results in better efficacy and reduce complication. Chang and Nelson[19] studied the use of a PDL (585 nm/0.45 ms) with cryogen spray cooling (PDL-CSC) for the treatment of PWS in Asian patients and compared these patients to patients who were treated with the same laser without cooling. They found that PDL-CSC

enhanced clinical efficacy and that a higher fluence could be used without an increase in complications.

CLINICAL EXAMINATION AND PATIENT HISTORY

A careful patient history and clinical examination are essential to distinguish PWS from hemangiomas and other vascular malformations. Close observation of clinical course can also be helpful. Early stage of hemangioma or salmon patch can be mistakenly diagnosed as PWSs. The patient treatment history is also important, especially among PWS patients. If he or she had been treated by traditional PDL, residual resistant vessels are relatively large or deep.

Several factors such as estrogen, corticosteroids, alcohol, chronic actinic damage, and trauma can induce telangiectasias.

The exclusion criteria included patients with active infection, patients with a personal or family history of melanoma and dysplastic nevus syndrome, immunocompromized patients, patients with photosensitivity, patients with history of keloid formation or poor wound healing, and pregnant women.

DEVICE OR TREATMENT SELECTION

When choosing an appropriate laser for treating vascular lesions (Figures 7.1 and 7.2), characteristics of wavelength have to be considered. A longer wavelength yields deeper penetration. In the treatment of PWSs and hemangiomas among dark-skinned patients, 532-nm Nd:YAG is not recommended because of its short wavelength. On the other hand, if the vessel depth of facial telangiestasia is not deep, 532-nm Nd:YAG or long-pulsed PDL can be effective. In the treatment of PWSs, PDL is the first choice (Figure 7.3). However, the risk of dyspigmentation at lip when treating PWSs is very high after PDL treatment. A 1064-nm Nd:YAG laser is recommended in the treatment of lip PWS (Figure 7.4). Alexandrite laser or 1064-nm Nd:YAG laser is recommended for the treatment of hypertrophic PWSs.

METHOD OF DEVICE OR TREATMENT APPLICATION

The pulse duration for laser treatment of vascular lesions depends on several factors, including the type of lesions, the vessel diameter, and the degree of downtime that patient can accept. For telangiectasia, purpura is often not desirable and longer pulsed duration to induce subpurpuric injury is the preferred mode of treatment. Excessive damage to proliferative hemangioma carries potential risk of complication including ulceration. Longer pulse width is therefore the preferred choice. Short duration is recommended in the treatment of PWSs and flat hemangiomas with the intention to induce purpura. Larger spot size allows deeper penetration of the laser energy (Figure 7.5). Larger spot sizes (larger than 10 cm) can be selected in the use of PDL, IPL, and 532-nm Nd:YAG laser. A smaller spot size is recommended in the use of alexandrite and 1064-nm Nd:YAG laser to reduce the risk of bulk tissue heating and therefore prevent scar formation.

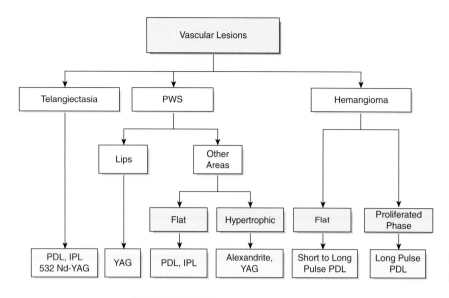

Figure 7.1 *Lasers and IPLs for vascular lesions; results may vary with each lasers and IPLs*

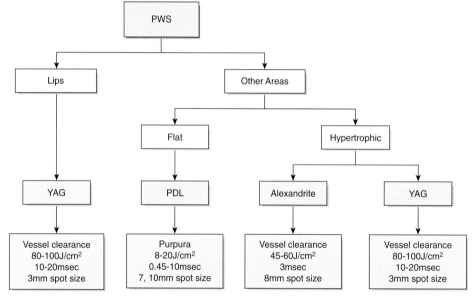

Figure 7.2 *Treatment table of PWS*

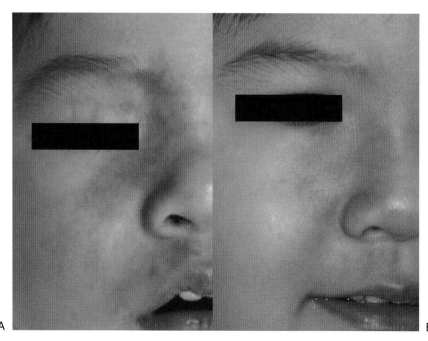

Figure 7.3 *PWS in face of a 1-year-old girl. (A) Pretreatment. (B) After four treatments with PDL (12–15 J/cm², 1.5–10 ms, 7-mm spot size, 2-3 months interval)*

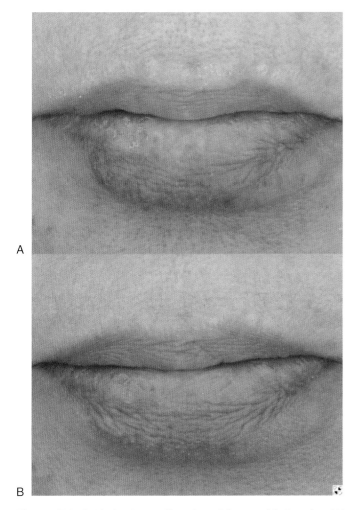

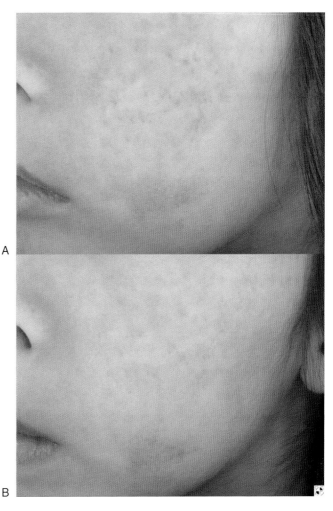

Figure 7.4 *PWS in lower lip of a 54-year-old female. (A) Pretreatment. (B) After four treatments with YAG (80–100 J/cm², 10–20 ms, 3-mm spot size, 1 month interval)*

Figure 7.5 *Traditional PDL-resistant PWS in face of a 3-year-old girl. (A) After 13 treatments with traditional PDL. (B) After two treatments with PDL (8.5–9.0 J/cm², 0.45 ms, 10-mm spot size, 3-month interval)*

Figure 7.6 *Hemangioma in hand of a 2-month-old girl. (A) Pretreatment. (B) After four treatments with PDL (11–12 J/cm², 20 ms, 7-mm spot size, 1 month interval)*

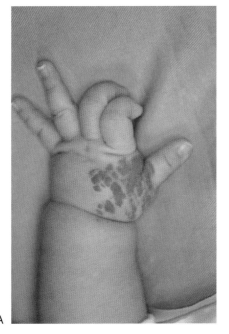

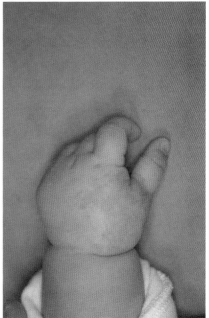

TABLE 7.1 ■ **Lasers and IPLs for Vascular Lesions; Endpoint is Different with Each Treatment Setting**

	Wavelength (nm)	Pulse duration (ms)	Endpoint	Applications
Pulsed dye	585-600	0.45-20	Purpura Vessel clearance	PWS, Hemangioma, Venous lake, Telangiectases, Cherry angioma, Venous malformation
Alexandrite	755	3-20	Purpura Vessel clearance	PWS, Venous lake, Telangiectases
Nd:YAG	1064	1-50	Vessel clearance	PWS, Venous lake, Telangiectases, Cherry angioma, Venous malformation
IPL	500-1400	1-50	Vessel clearance	PWS, Telangiectases, Cherry angioma

▓ Dose/Setting Selection

The most important thing is finding appropriate end points. Each lesion is different, and each laser/IPL device has a different end point (Table 7.1). Mild erythema or edema is the end point of IPL source; vessel clearance, for alexandrite or YAG laser; purpura, for PDL in the treatment of PWS; the maximum fluence below purpura threshold, for PDL in the treatment of hemangiomas (Figure 7.6); and vessel clearance, for PDL in the treatment of facial telangiectasias (Figure 7.7).

▓ Treatment Technique

In an attempt to enhance efficacy, the techniques of multipassing and stacking have been used in the PDL treatment of vascular lesions. However, these techniques should not been used with alexandrite laser or 1064-nm Nd:YAG laser treatment of vascular lesions. No-overlapping technique is recommended to prevent dyspigmentation and scar formation.

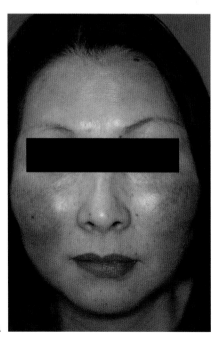
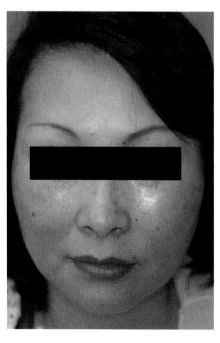

A   B

Figure 7.7 *Facial erythema and telangiectasia in face of 46-year-old female. (A) Pretreatment. (B) After two treatments with PDL (11–12 J/cm², 10 ms, 7-mm spot size, 2-month interval)*

Alternative Treatment Methods

PDL is the first choice of vascular lesions; however, there are some IPL systems that are able to emit broadband light and high fluences sufficient to heat superficial to deep vasculature. The complication rate is low, and it is also a very good option to treat telangiectasias and PWSs.

Postoperative Care

A topical antibiotic ointment may be applied for 1 week. Patients should be instructed to avoid direct sun exposure during laser treatment and for at least 3 months after the final laser treatment.

Management of Adverse Event

During the active proliferation phase, hemangiomas often show ulceration, bleeding, scarring, and infection. The most important point is to explain the possible clinical course to patients before the laser treatment. PDL treatment is also effective for ulcerated hemangiomas. On the other hand, the use of long-pulsed alexandrite laser or long-pulsed 1064-nm Nd:YAG laser must be cautious because pulse stacking and/or excessive fluence can result in ulceration.

DIRECTIONS FOR THE FUTURE AND CONCLUSIONS

PDL treatment produces reasonably good results in a limited population of PWS patients because of the ability to destroy selective dermal blood vessels. Presently, most patients are treated using similar laser parameters, with selection based on the clinical judgment of the physician. Often, these decisions are made without taking into consideration individual variations in PWS geometry or optical properties of human skin. PWS vessel diameter and depth distribution vary on an individual patient basis, and even between different areas on the same patient. Finding an appropriate PWS treatment protocol has become more complicated recently secondary to laser manufacturers introducing devices that allow the operator to vary several treatment parameters such as wavelength, pulse duration, light dosage, and skin cooling.

Future development includes the use of feedback mechanism during laser procedure to detect the individual maximum safe radiant exposure[20]; the role of topical angiogenesis inhibitor to modify the wound-healing response post laser surgery after the treatment of PWS is being also studied.[21]

REFERENCES

1. Huikeshoven M, Koster PH, de Borgie CA, Beek JF, van Gemert MJ, van der Horst CM. Redarkening of port-wine stains 10 years after pulsed-dye-laser treatment. *N Engl J Med.* 2007;356:1235-1240.

2. Batta K, Goodyear HM, Moss C, Williams HC, Hiller L, Waters R. Randomised controlled study of early pulsed dye laser treatment of uncomplicated childhood haemangiomas: results of a 1-year analysis. *Lancet.* 2002;360:521-527.

3. Kono T, Sakurai H, Groff WF, et al. Comparison study of a traditional pulsed dye laser versus a long-pulsed dye laser in the treatment of early childhood hemangiomas. *Laser Surg Med.* 2006;38:112-115.

4. Tan OT, Murray S, Kurban AK. Histologic responses of port-wine stains treated by argon, carbon dioxide, and tunable dye lasers: a preliminary report. *Arch Dermatol.* 1986;122:1016-1022.

5. Tan OT, Murray S, Kurban AK. Action spectrum of vascular specific injury using pulsed irradiation. *J Invest Dermatol.* 1989;92:868-871.

6. Verkruysse W, Pickering JW, Beek J, et al. Modeling the effect of wavelengths on the pulsed dye laser treatment of port wine stains. *Appl Opt.* 1993;132:393-398.

7. Hohenleutner U, Hilbert M, Wlotzke U, Landthaler M. Epidermal damage and limited coagulation depth with the flashlamp-pumped pulsed dye laser: a histochemical study. *J Invest Dermatol.* 1995;104:798-802.

8. Kane KS, Smoller BR, Fitzpatrick RE, Walker NP, Dover JS. Pulsed dye laser-resistant port wine stains. *Arch Dermatol.* 1996;132:839-841.

9. Scherer K, Lorenz S, Wimmershoff M, Landthaler M, Hohenleutner U. Both the flashlamp-pumped dye laser and the long-pulsed tunable dye laser can improve results in port-wine stains. *Br J Dermatol.* 2001;145:79-84.

10. Woo SH, Ahn HH, Kim SN, Kye YC. Treatment of vascular skin lesions with the variable-pulse 595 nm pulsed dye laser. *Dermatol Surg.* 2006;32:41-48.

11. Fiskerstrand EJ, Svaasand LO, Kopstad G, Ryggen K, Aase S. Photothermally induced vessel-wall necrosis after pulsed dye laser treatment: lack of response in port-wine stains with small size of deeply located vessels. *J Invest Dermatol.* 1996;107:671-675.

12. Dierickx CC, Casparian JM, Venugopalan V, Farinelli WA, Anderson RR. Thermal relaxation of port-wine stain vessels probed in vivo: the need for 1-10 millisecond laser pulse treatment. *J Invest Dermatol.* 1995;105:709-714.

13. Greve B, Raulin C. Prospective study of port wine stain treatment with dye laser: comparison of two wavelengths (585 nm vs. 595 nm) and two pulse durations (0.5 milliseconds vs. 20 milliseconds). *Lasers Surg Med.* 2004;34:168-173.

14. Bernstein EF, Douglas BB. Efficacy of the 1.5 millisecond pulse-duration, 585 nm, pulsed-dye laser for treating port-wine stains. *Lasers Surg Med.* 2005;36:341-346.

15. Asahina A, Watanabe T, Kishi A, et al. Evaluation of the treatment of port-wine stains with the 595-nm long pulsed dye laser: a large prospective study in adult Japanese patients. *J Am Acad Dermatol.* 2006;54:487-493.

16. Kono T, Sakurai H, Takeuchi M, et al. Evaluation of fluence and pulse-duration on purpuric threshold using a variable-pulse pulsed-dye laser in the treatment of port wine stains. *J Dermatol.* 2006;33:471-474.

17. Tan OT, Motemedi M, Welch AJ, Kurban AK. Spot size effects on guinea pig skin following pulsed irradiation. *J Invest Dermatol.* 1988:90;877-881.

18. Keijzer M, Pickering JW, van Gemert MJ. Laser spot size for port wine stain treatment. *Lasers Surg Med.* 1991;11:601-605.

19. Chang CJ, Nelson JS. Cryogen spray cooling and higher fluence pulsed dye laser treatment improve port-wine stain clearance while minimizing epidermal damage. *Dermatol Surg.* 1999;25:767-772.

20. Verkruysse W, Jia W, Franco W, Milner TE, Nelson JS. Infrared measurement of human skin temperature to predict the individual maximum safe radiant exposure (IMSRE). *Lasers Surg Med.* 2007;39:757-766.

21. Phung TL, Oble DA, Jia W, Benjamin LE, Mihm MC Jr. Nelson JS. Can the wound healing response of human skin be modulated after laser treatment and the effects of exposure extended? Implications on the combined use of the pulsed dye laser and a topical angiogenesis inhibitor for treatment of port wine stain birthmarks. *Lasers Surg Med.* 2008;40:1-5.

CHAPTER 8

Nonablative Dermal Resurfacing in Ethnic Skin: Laser and Intense Pulsed Light

Suneel Chilukuri, MD, and Ashish C. Bhatia, MD, FAAD

INTRODUCTION

The introduction of laser surgery resurfacing has revolutionized advanced cosmetic surgery options for all skin types over the past 25 years.[1-5] Laser resurfacing is divided into ablative and nonablative surgery. Ablative resurfacing refers to the destruction of the epidermis in an effort to improve texture, tone, and overall quality of the skin. Both the carbon dioxide (CO_2) and erbium:yttrium-aluminum-garnet (Er:YAG) lasers have proven to be extremely effective in improving photoinduced rhytides, dyschromia, and scarring in patients with Fitzpatrick I–III skin.[6] These ablative lasers have also proven to be effective in darker skin types but carry a greater risk of transient or permanent dyspigmentation.

Nonablative resurfacing refers to surgical treatment of the dermis while preserving the epidermis. A variety of lasers, including the pulsed dye lasers (PDL), Neodymium-yttrium-aluminum garnet (Nd:YAG) lasers, and the diode lasers, have been used to improve the skin tone of both fair and dark-skinned patients. In addition, intense pulsed light (IPL) and radio frequency (RF) devices have been used with varying success to rejuvenate facial skin. Herein, nonablative resurfacing techniques for darker pigmented individuals will be discussed. Preoperative, intraoperative, and postoperative considerations will be emphasized.

OVERVIEW OF LASER PRINCIPLES

Since the elucidation of the principles of selective photothermolysis in 1983,[7] laser technology in ablative and nonablative resurfacing has significantly improved. Key terms in laser medicine are given in Table 8.1. Understanding of laser properties is essential to understanding the principle of *selective photothermolysis*.

Laser light is unique in that it is monochromatic. The emitted single wavelength must be absorbed by a target to have an effect. Various *chromophores*, such as melanin, hemoglobin, and water, absorb light at different wavelengths. As the *fluence* increases, the amount of laser energy transmitted to the chromophore increases.

When the light energy is absorbed by the target, the chromophore converts the laser light energy to heat.[7] The chromophore will be destroyed if enough heat is generated at a fast enough rate. Depending on the desired outcome, different rates of energy delivery can be chosen. This rate of energy delivery must be more rapid than the rate at which heat is dissipated to the surrounding tissues by the chromophore. *Thermal relaxation time* (or dissipation of heat generated) is primarily dependent on the size of the target chromophore. In general, larger structures disseminate heat slower than smaller ones. Therefore, blood vessels (10–100 μm) will take longer to lose heat compared to the smaller melanosome (1 μm);

the vessels have a longer thermal relaxation time. Understanding the thermal relaxation time (TRT) of various chromophores allows one to adjust the pulse duration of a certain laser to achieve desired effects.

Delivering the same fluence over shorter or longer pulse durations will affect the tissue response. Delivering energy much faster than the TRT will result in destruction of the tissue, leading to rupture and purpura in the case of blood vessels, and disintegration of pigment in the case of melanin or tattoo pigment. In contrast, delivering the same fluence over a longer pulse duration results in heating of adjacent tissues without frank destruction of the chromophore. Longer pulse durations are desirable when attempting to destroy the hair bulb adjacent to a dark hair or when trying to eliminate vessels without rupturing them and causing purpura.

ABLATIVE RESURFACING

Ablative resurfacing is typically used to treat rhytides,[8,9] dyschromia,[9] and scarring.[9-11] The current technologies include high-energy pulsed and scanned carbon dioxide lasers, short-pulsed erbium:YAG lasers, variable-pulsed erbium:YAG lasers, and combined Er:YAG/CO_2 laser systems. All of these lasers target water-containing tissue to allow controlled epidermal vaporization. The adjacent thermal injury in the dermis is thought to promote collagen shrinkage and remodeling.[12,13] The clinical improvement of skin tone, color, and texture are unparalleled when compared to other resurfacing methods such as deep chemical peels, dermabrasion, and nonablative laser resurfacing.[14-18] Most studies show an average clinical improvement of rhytides and atrophic scars greater than 50%.[14-17] Unfortunately, there are inherent risks to ablative resurfacing, especially in patients with darker skin types.

The main risks with ablative laser therapy include prolonged erythema, transient and/or permanent hyperpigmentation, and delayed permanent hypopigmentation.[19-21] All patients undergoing ablative resurfacing will have some degree of edema and erythema. For this reason, it is best to wait at least a few weeks or months before judging the improvement of rhytides, since the transient edema can cause temporary improvement which can be deceiving. In some patients, prolonged erythema persists for several months rather than several weeks before partial or complete resolution.[22] Prolonged erythema is thought to be related to significantly greater thermal damage intraoperatively.

Any patient may develop transient hyperpigmentation, but this side effect is more common with darker skin types. As many as 40% of patients with Fitzpatrick skin types I–III have transient hyperpigmentation.[22,23] In contrast, 66% to 100% of patients with Fitzpatrick skin types IV–VI will develop some degree of hyperpigmentation.[24-27] While the etiology of this hyperpigmentation is not definitively known, it is presumed that the greater concentration of melanosomes in darker skin absorb more of the laser energy even

TABLE 8.1 ▪ Laser Terminology

Chromophore	The intended target of the laser light is called a *chromophore*.
Fluence	The amount of energy that is delivered to a certain surface area is called *fluence*. It is typically measured in J/cm^2.
Thermal relaxation	The conduction of heat to the surrounding tissues
TRT	The time it takes the chromophore to cool down to 50% of its peak temperature
Pulse duration	The length of time the target chromophore is exposed to the laser light
Selective photothermolysis	Using just the energy required to destroy the intended chromophore without causing damage to the surrounding tissue

at lower fluence. In addition, these melanosomes may more readily produce melanin following injury.

Permanent hypopigmentation may occur in as many as 20% of patients with Fitzpatrick skin types I and II.[15,21] The onset of this dyschromia typically occurs after 6 months following multiple pass treatment with CO_2 laser. While this hypopigmentation may be less noticeable in fair-colored individuals, this side effect may be devastating in darker individuals.

A handful of case reports and small studies reveal safe ablative laser resurfacing performed in dark skinned individuals with minimal to no long-term sequelae.[28-33] Unfortunately, in today's practice environment, few laser experts are willing to utilize these more aggressive ablation techniques on Fitzpatrick skin types IV–VI. Moreover, many patients do not want to have disruption of their normal lives for several weeks. Therefore, many practitioners wish to utilize the less destructive nonablative techniques, although cosmetic improvements are less impressive.

NONABLATIVE RESURFACING IN DARKER SKIN

Nonablative resurfacing targets dermal collagen remodeling without destruction of the epidermis. In darker skin phenotypes, nonsurface remodeling can be safely achieved with laser, light-based, or RF systems. Although melanin has an absorption spectrum ranging from 250 to 1200 nm, its absorption coefficient decreases exponentially as the wavelength of light increases.[31,33-35] Therefore, a greater amount of the energy from a 694-nm ruby laser will be absorbed by superficial melanin as compared to a 1064 Nd:YAG laser.[36] The longer wavelength of the 1064 Nd:YAG laser will penetrate deeper into the dermis.

Commonly utilized nonablative laser systems include the 1064-nm Q-switched Nd:YAG laser, 1320-nm Nd:YAG laser, 1450-nm diode laser, 1540 Er:glass laser, and the 1550-nm fractional lasers. IPL and RF systems have also been used with some success in darker pigmented individuals. Even with these less invasive systems, hyperpig-

mentation and scarring can occur. Therefore, with any of these treatments, the same preoperative, intraoperative, and postoperative precautions should be taken and procedures should be followed.

PREOPERATIVE

All patients desiring nonablative resurfacing should have a thorough preoperative consultation to assess patient expectations, attain a complete medical history, and optimize pretreatment conditions. The majority of darker pigmented individuals present for dychromia; however, some patients do present for improvement of rhytides, textural irregularities, enlarged pores, and general tissue laxity. The practitioner must address the patient's true concerns and help guide realistic expectations in order to have a successful outcome. For example, it is important to inform the patient that lessening of deep rhytides will not occur after a single treatment; rather, a series of treatments is necessary. Additionally, since many of these treatments rely on collagen remodeling, this process can take several months to manifest clinically visible results.[14,37] Moreover, there may not be photographic improvement, but only subjective improvement.[14]

A complete medical history is important when treating with any resurfacing modality. The practitioner must acquire a past surgical history, specifically regarding prior history of deep chemical peels and dermabrasion. Even with the relatively safe nonablative techniques, permanent hypopigmentation may occur in those patients who have had extensive chemical peeling and deep dermabrasion. Medical history must include inquiry regarding vitiligo and any koeberinizing conditions. Either of these preexisting medical conditions may be exacerbated with nonablative resurfacing therapies.[38] Finally, recent medications must be reviewed. No oral isotretinoin should have been used at least 1 year prior to treatment as a result of a reported higher risk of abnormal postoperative healing and scarring.[39]

Preoperative considerations include sun protection and sun avoidance, pretreatment topical tretinoin, and pretreatment hydroquinone. Although there may be no break in the epidermis, posttreatment erythema and possible posttreatment hyperpigmentation may occur even with nonablative resurfacing techniques. Therefore, the authors advocate strict sun avoidance and full-spectrum sunblock before and after treatment. Pretreatment with topical tretinoin, hydroquinone, and glycolic acid may be used. Although many use pretreatment hydroquinone, the data to support its use as such is weak. With ablative resurfacing, none of these pretreatment agents have shown to have any effect on preventing posttreatment hyperpigmentation.[27] All these agents only penetrate the epidermis which is completely removed with ablative therapy. However, these same topical treatments have proven to be effective in superficial dermabrasion and chemical peels.[40-42] Since the epidermis is similarly maintained with nonablative systems, these topical agents may be of some use in preventing and treating posttreatment hyperpigmentation.

Other preoperative treatment includes the use of an antiviral therapy. With any injury to the skin, there is an increased risk of bacterial, viral, and fungal infection. While the risk of bacterial infection is less than 1% in practice, herpetic outbreaks have been seen in up to 4% of patients treated with nonablative resurfacing. No fungal infections have been noted. Therefore, the authors routinely prescribe a low dose of valcyclovir (500 mg twice daily) to be started 3 days prior to the procedure. Variations on oral antiviral agent choice and dosing do exist, and may be chosen at the physician's discretion.

Intraoperative

There have been no reports clearly defining intraoperative technique for nonablative resurfacing for darker pigmented skin. The authors follow the similar techniques used during ablative resurfacing. While sterile intraoperative technique is not crucial in nonablative resurfacing, the authors routinely use a cleaning agent prior to starting resurfacing. During treatment, the practitioner takes care to avoid strenuous rubbing of the skin to prevent any possible mechanical damage.[43]

With laser systems, a cooling device is usually used to prevent epidermal heating and subsequent damage during treatment of the intended target, the dermis. The choice of cooling systems is important when dealing with skin of color. Typically, contact cooling systems such as sapphire lens cooling or conductive cooling are the most efficient and safe for darker skin types. Cryogen cooling can result in posttreatment hyperpigmentation of the areas. Therefore, most manufacturers of cryogen-cooled lasers recommend that the minimal cryogen duration needed to protect the epidermis be used in darker skin types. Forced air-cooling is yet another safe option in pre- and postcooling of the epidermis during a laser procedure in skin of color.

POSTOPERATIVE

Postoperative care includes a cooling fan, cool damp cloth, or ice packs to help ease any patient discomfort. A thin layer of an ointment with low sensitizing potential such as Aquaphor or petrolatum ointment is applied without an occlusive dressing. A mild cleanser, such as Aquanil, is recommended to prevent any further irritation to the skin with daily washing. Tretinoin and hydroquinone are usually stopped for 1 week following treatment to prevent further irritation to the skin. Wide-spectrum sunscreens with low incidence of allergic dermatitis, such as Solbar 50, are recommended for use on postoperative day one. Furthermore, sun avoidance is advocated. The patient is then reminded to return for another treatment; the treatment intervals vary depending on the system used.

LASER SYSTEMS

Nonablative laser and light systems target dermal tissue water by emitting light within the infrared portion of the electromagnetic spectrum (1000–1500 nm). At these wavelengths, light can attain depths of 300 to 1500 μs to cause subepidermal heating of tissues and subsequent inflammatory mediators which may cause some collagen remodeling and deposition.[44] In photodamaged skin, a band of solar elastosis exists just below the dermal–epidermal junction at a depth of 400 to 700 μm. Fortunately, infrared lasers are able to penetrate to this depth.[45]

All nonablative resurfacing devices have a cooling device protecting the epidermis from the energy of the laser. Prior to laser light emission, a cooling device may be used to increase the thermal resilience of the epidermis. In addition, parallel cooling, which is cooling applied during the pulse, may also be used to help extract heat from the surface. Finally, postpulse cooling can protect the epidermis from retrograde heating from the dermis. All these mechanisms can be used to ensure that the epidermis is protected and remains intact to allow true "subsurface" ablation.

1064-nm Q-switched Nd:YAG Laser

The first nonablative resurfacing experience was with the 1064-nm Q-switched neodymium:YAG (Nd:YAG) laser.[46] Although there is weak water absorption with this system, this laser can penetrate into the dermis and theoretically induce neocollagenesis. In addition, the nanosecond pulse duration limits thermal diffusion to surrounding structures which typically have a longer thermal relaxation time.

Goldberg and Whitworth[44] compared the effectiveness of the 1064-nm Nd:YAG laser versus CO_2 resurfacing on 11 patients with Fitzpatrick skin types I and II. At a fluence of 5.5 J/cm^2 with a 3-mm spot size, the Nd:YAG laser treatment resulted in some pinpoint bleeding. Even with this aggressive partial ablation, only three patients showed mild rhytide improvement. In all three of these patients, there was prolonged posttreatment erythema lasting 1 month or longer. In comparison, the side treated with CO_2 laser showed greater than 50% improvement in rhytides and skin texture.

Two years later, Goldberg and Metzler[47] studied true nonablative resurfacing with a low fluence 1064-nm Nd:YAG laser combined with a topical carbon solution to aid in further penetration of the light. Sixty-one patients with Fitzpatrick type I and II skin were treated with three monthly treatments at a fluence of 2.5 J/cm^2 with a 7-mm spot size. Slight improvement was seen in 97% of class I rhytides but photographic improvement was minimal. Side effects were limited to mild erythema and purpura in five patients and posttreatment hyperpigmentation in one patient.

In 2000, Newman et al.,[48] treated patients in all Fitzpatrick phototypes using the Q-switched Nd:YAG laser with a carbon-suspension solution. Four treatments at a fluence of 2.5 J/cm^2 with a 7-mm spot size and a 10 Hz repetition rate were used at 7 to 10 days intervals. While the improvement of rhytides was only 25% in all skin types, pigmentary improvement was noted in those patients with type IV–VI skin. Moreover, there were no permanent sequelae.

Based on the published studies, safe treatment with combined topical carbon suspension and the 1064-nm Nd:YAG laser may lead to some subjective improvement of mild rhytides. Dyschromia may be visibly improved as well.

980-nm Diode Laser

The 980-nm diode laser can target water, melanin, and/or hemoglobin. Low fluence and longer pulse durations more specifically target thermal heating of water. Muccini et al.[49] utilized a power range of 6 to 24 W and a 400-ms pulse duration to show in vitro tissue shrinkage similar to that of three passes with a CO_2 laser. However, only two patients of unspecified Fitzpatrick phototype were treated. Posttreatment biopsies revealed persistent moderate thickening of collagen bundles and the appearance of new elastin formation. Histologic changes were more modest than that seen with CO_2 resurfacing.

This laser system has potential use in vivo. At a fluence of 8 W and a pulse duration of 400 ms, moderate clinical changes may be observed. Further studies need to be performed to fully evaluate this laser's safety and efficacy in nonablative resurfacing in darker skin types.

1320-nm Nd:YAG Laser

The 1320-nm Nd:YAG laser (CoolTouch; ICN Pharmaceuticals, Costa Mesa, CA) was the first laser commercially developed exclusively for nonablative resurfacing through selective dermal heating. Its wavelength allows for a high scattering coefficient dispersing the thermal effect throughout the dermis at a depth of 1600 μm. Current models have a hand piece that has a thermal feed sensor that controls a cryogen spray for epidermal cooling. The dermis is heated to 60 to 65° C while the epidermis is kept at 40 to 45° C.

Various studies have been reported with both the original CoolTouch and the Cool TouchII. Menaker et al.[50] treated 10 patients in three sessions every 3 to 4 days with no statistical improvement of clinical rhytides. His group used a fluence of 32 J/cm^2 with a 5-mm spot size and series of three 300 μs pulses delivered at 100 Hz. His prototype machine did not have a thermal feedback sensor and a 20 ms cooling spray was used for epidermal protection. The researchers did not find any significant improvement in rhytides.

Kelly et al.[51] found early statistically significant improvement in all 35 patients treated with their 1320-nm Nd:YAG laser. Three treatments at 2-week intervals utilized fluences from 28 to 36 J/cm^2 with a 5-mm spot size and cryogen cooling in 20- to 40-ms spurts with a 10-ms delay. The study showed early transient improvement in rhytides, likely attributable to initial tissue edema.

Various other researchers have published similar minimal improvement with this particular laser. Goldberg[52,53] published two studies involving a total of 20 patients, of which four patients showed some visible improvement in facial rhytides and overall skin tone. These patients were treated with fluences ranging from 28 to 38 J/cm^2 with a 5-mm spot size and a 30% overlap of the pulses. The epidermal temperature was maintained at 40 to 48° C. Trelles et al.[54] and Faterni et al.[55] used similar fluences with similar results in which only 2 of 10 patients were satisfied with their final results. In all the studies, immediate mild transient erythema and edema were noted in patients with Fitzpatrick skin types I, II, and III. Two patients out of 70 (2.8%) in Kelly et al.'s[50] study and 3 of 10 patients (30%) in Menaker et al.'s[49] study developed long-term pitted scars.

Overall, these four publications indicate that there were some clinical changes that may continue to improve over 6 months or longer. This longer time period for effects to be seen may be related to long-term collagen and elastin remodeling via cytokines and inflammatory mediators rather than the immediate collagen shortening and remodeling seen with ablative laser procedures. The 1320-nm laser should be safe to use in patients with darker pigmentation, but the duration and temperature of the cooling spray may need to be adjusted to prevent cryogenic melanosome injury and permanent pitted scars. For this reason, the authors recommend using a laser which is based upon alternative cooling technologies (noncryogen based) such as contact cooling or forced air-cooling.

1450-nm Diode Laser

The 1450-nm diode laser is a low-power laser system that can penetrate the skin to a depth of 500 μm. The chromophore target, water, is heated using long 150 to 250 ms exposures versus the 1320-nm Nd:YAG which has a 20-ms macropulse. This longer pulse, with a peak power range of 16 to 20 J/cm^2, requires a sequence of pre-, intra-, and postpulse cooling spray to prevent epidermal damage.

Goldberg et al.[56] compared the 1450-nm diode laser with cryogen spray to cryogen spray alone in a split face study of 20 patients with skin types I–IV. After a single treatment with a fluence of 12 Watts and a pulse duration of 160 to 260 ms, a repetition rate of 0.5 to 1.0 Hz, and a 4-mm spot size, 10 patients showed mild improvement and three patients showed moderate improvement of class I and II rhytides after 6 months. As expected, no improvement was seen with cryogen spray alone. All patients experienced transient erythema and edema, and six patients developed small edematous papules lasting up to 7 days. One patient developed postinflammatory hyperpigmentation lasting more than 6 months.

Hardway and Ross[14] report similar moderate improvement in class I and II rhytides even with four sequential treatments using a fluence of 13 W with a 4-mm spot size. Most patients experienced general, transient erythema, but no long-term sequelae were noted.

Alster et al.[57-59] published three studies, two of which demonstrated that the 1450-nm diode laser has superior effects when compared to the 1320-nm Nd:YAG laser for perioral and periorbital rhytides and atrophic facial scars. Single pass treatment utilized the 1450-nm diode at fluences ranging from 9 to 14 J/cm^2 and a 6-mm spot size. Following three monthly treatments, clinical and histologic improvement was seen in rhytides and atrophic scars. No permanent adverse effects were reported.

The 1450-nm diode has mainly been tested on individuals with Fitzpatrick skin types I–III. There was at least one incidence of long-term posttreatment hyperpigmentation, although Goldberg et al.[55] did not indicate if this sequelae occurred in the darkest skinned test subject. When treating darker pigmented patients, the laser practitioner must monitor the effects of the cooling spray very carefully during the long pulse duration to protect the epidermis from thermal injury. Even with this precaution, ethnic patients may develop posttreatment hyperpigmentation.

1540-nm Erbium:Glass

The 1540-nm Erb:glass is similar to the aforementioned mid-infrared lasers in that its target chromophore is water. High fluences of 400 to 1200 mJ with a 5-mm spot size can lead to deep dermal penetration of 0.4 to 2 mm. Similar to the other nonablative modalities, mild-to-moderate improvement was noted for both rhytides and atrophic scars. However, a study of nine patients,[60] epidermal necrosis and scar formation was noted when using the highest fluence of 1200 mJ. Lupton et al.[61] used a weaker fluence of 10 J/cm^2 with a 3.5 ms pulse duration and a 2 Hz repetition rate with the 4-mm spot size. This resulted in no permanent sequelae. Mild-to-moderate clinical improvement of rhytides was noted at 6 months following three monthly treatments.

Of all the aforementioned laser systems, the 1540-nm wavelength is the least absorbed by epidermal melanin. Additionally, this laser is generally fired through a sapphire contact-cooling window and not with a cryogen spray mechanism. In theory, this laser system may be the most useful in darkly pigmented individuals. One must start with the lowest fluence possible to achieve transient eyrthema and then titrate up with further treatments.

IPL SYSTEM

IPL sources are flash lamp-based devices that emit light ranging from the visible spectrum of 500-nm to the infrared range up to approximately 1200 nm. These are different than the other devices discussed so far in that they are not monochromatic by design. While these devices have been typically used to treat vascular lesions and photoaging, specific filters can be used to block certain wavelengths from being emitted from the device. Limiting emission to the longer infrared wavelengths allows one to perform nonablative resurfacing rhytides with these devices in theory.

Goldberg and Cutler[62] treated thirty women (Fitzpatrick skin types I–II) with class I and II facial rhytides with mild improvement. All subjects were treated at 2-week intervals for a total of one to four treatments using a 645-nm cutoff filter, energy levels of 40 to 50 J/cm^2, with triple 7-ms pulses and 50-ms interpulse delay. Nine patients showed substantial improvement when evaluated at 6 months. The improvement in the rhytides was not as significant as that noted with ablative laser resurfacing, but photographic changes were clearly evident. While most patients had some erythema following treatment, three subjects had transient blistering after at least one treatment session. No long-term adverse effects were noted.

Other studies have shown improvement in skin pigmentation and texture, but minimal improvement in rhytides.[63,64] These studies also involved only patients with Fitzpatrick skin types I–III treated with fluences ranging from 30 to 50 J/cm^2. Recently, Kono et al.[65] compared IPL with long-pulse pulsed dye laser (LPDL) in treating rhytides and lentigines in 10 Asian patients with phototypes III and IV. While the LPDL more effectively treated the lentigines, minimal improvement of rhytides was noted with both systems. Neither laser caused any posttreatment sequelae in any of these darker patients. Further research including patients with darker skin phototypes must be performed. One of the newest advances in IPL technologies is the photopneumatic IPL systems (Figure 8.1). These are similar to traditional IPLs; however, they take advantage of a pneumatic system to stretch the skin while the light is being emitted onto the skin.

This is thought to serve three purposes. First, the negative pressure allows evaporation of moisture from the skin's surface at a lower temperature, providing evaporative cooling. Second, the stretching of the skin allows for dispersion of the epidermal pigment, effectively reducing the amount of pigment per square centimeter. This allows for more light transmission past the epidermal pigment. In addition, the vacuum exsanguinates the skin for a brief period, further reducing the absorption of the light by the superficial vascular plexus, effectively allowing more light to penetrate deeper. The chambers of these IPL heads are also covered with reflective surfaces allowing for recycling of reflected photons, which some have termed "photon recycling." These devices have recently been made available with 580-nm filters for safer use in darker skin types. Although they have clinically been proven safe and effective in darker skin types for hair removal and acne, further study on their efficacy in skin tightening is necessary.

RF SYSTEMS

Unlike laser and light systems, RF systems utilize the skin's natural resistance to the flow of ions. An electric current is applied to the skin to increase ionic energy in the skin which leads to transformation of this energy into heat. This nonselective heat can be generated within the papillary dermis and even as deep as the subcutaneous fat. Theoretically, collagen is denatured and contracts leading to some immediate results as well as further improvement occurring months following the procedure.[66,67] As with the laser-based systems, the epidermis must be protected with a cooling device to prevent the heat generated.

Because there is no light transmitted, melanocytes are relatively protected in darker skinned individuals. However, it is essential to use an appropriate surface-cooling device to prevent epidermal damage and melanocyte destruction. As with any of the laser systems, postinflammatory sequelae may follow because of the deeper inflammation. RF devices are covered in more detail in Chapter 11.

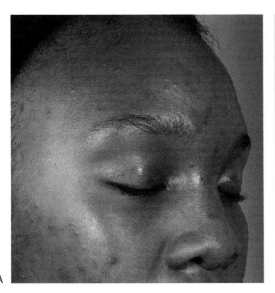 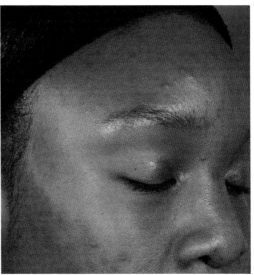

A　　　　　　　　　　　　　　　　　　　　　　　　　　　　B

Figure 8.1 *(A) Before and (B) after pictures of a Fitzpatrick skin type IV patient after one treatment with a photopneumatic IPL device. (Used with permission from Dr. Girish Munavalli, MD.)*

CONCLUSION

In comparison to ablative resurfacing, nonablative resurfacing techniques tend to be favored in the treatment of skin of color. This is primarily because of their safety in skin of color as well as the decreased risk of long-term posttreatment sequelae. These nonablative procedures also offer less downtime which is important to today's busy patient base. Unfortunately, the results are also more moderate in regards to the reduction of rhytides or improvement of skin texture. Many studies indicate that there is a decreased risk of long-term hyper- or hypopigmentation in fair-skinned individuals following nonablative resurfacing. Further research needs to be performed in those patients with Fitzpatrick skin types IV–VI, although early clinical experience seems to corroborate these findings. With the increased demand for these milder, gentler procedures, we will likely see the advent of newer technologies catering to this niche.

REFERENCES

1. Pitman S. Online spending on cosmetics increases by more than 30 per cent. http://www.cosmeticsdesign-europe.com/news/ng.asp?id=67943. Accessed May 25, 2006.

2. Smith A. Cosmetic surgery market stands firm: economic belt-tightening hasn't slowed down sales of implants, Botox or laser surgery—so far. http://www.cnnmoney.com. Accessed February 20, 2008.

3. U.S. Census Bureau. *Population Projections of the U.S. by Age, Sex, Race and Hispanic Origin: 1995—2050*. Current Population Report. Washington, DC: U.S. Government Press; 2002: 25-1130.

4. Davis M. Ethnic spending on hair, beauty, and cosmetics tops $8.4 billion says packaged facts. www.fashionwindows.com. Accessed october 17, 2006.

5. Halder RM, Grimes PE, McLaurin CI, et al. Incidence of common dermatoses in predominantly black dermatologic practice. *Cutis*. 1983;32:388-390.

6. Riggs K, Keller M, Humphreys TR. Ablative laser resurfacing: high-energy pulsed carbon dioxide and erbium:yttrium-aluminum-garnet. *Clin Dermatol*. 2007;25:462-473.

7. Anderson RR, Parrish JA. Selective photothermolysis: precise microsurgery by selective absorption of pulsed radiation. *Science*. 1983;220:524-527.

8. Fitzpatrick, RE, Goldman MP, Satur NM, et al. Pulsed carbon dioxide laser resurfacing of photo-aged facial skin. *Arch Dermatol*. 1996;132:395-402.

9. Apfelberg DB. Ultrapulse carbon dioxide laser with CPG scanner for full-face resurfacing of rhytides, photoaging, and acne scars. *Plast Reconstr Surg*. 1997;99:1817-1825.

10. Walia S, Alster TS. Prolonged clinical and histologic effects from CO_2 laser resurfacing of atrophic acne scars. *Dermatol Surg*. 1999;25:926-930.

11. Alster TS, West TB. Resurfacing of atrophic facial scars with a high-energy, pulsed carbon dioxide laser. *Dermatol Surg*. 1996;22:151-154.

12. Alster TS, Nanni CA, Williams CM. Comparison of four carbon dioxide resurfacing lasers: a clinical and histopathologic evaluation. *Dermatol Surg*. 1999;25:153-158.

13. Ross, EV, McKinlay JR, Anderson RR. Why does carbon dioxide resurfacing work? A review. *Arch Dermatol*. 1999;135:444-454.

14. Hardaway CA, Ross EV. Nonablative laser skin remodeling. *Dermatolog Clin*. 2002;20:97-111.

15. Tanzi EL, Alster TS. Side effects and complications of variable-pulsed erbium: yttrium-aluminum-garnet laser skin resurfacing: extended experience with 50 patients. *Plast Reconstr Surg*. 2003;111:1524-1529.

16. Fitzpatrick RE. Resurfacing procedures: how do you choose? *Arch Dermatol*. 2000;136:783-784.

17. Kitzmiller, WJ, Visscher M, Page DA, et al. A controlled evaluation of dermabrasion versus CO_2 laser resurfacing for the treatment of perioral wrinkles. *Plast Recontr Surg*. 2000;106:1366-1372.

18. Fitzpatrick RE, Tope WD, Goldman MP, et al. Pulsed carbon dioxide laser, trichloroacetic acid, Baker-Gordon phenol, and dermabrasion: a comparative clinical and histologic study of cutaneous resurfacing in a porcine model. *Arch Dermatol*. 1996;132:469-471.

19. Alster TS, Lupton JR. Prevention and treatment of side effects and complications of cutaneous laser skin resurfacing. *Plast Reconstr Surg*. 2002;109:308-316.

20. Alster TS, Lupton JR. Treatment of complications of laser skin resurfacing. *Arch Facial Plast Surg*. 2000;2:279-284.

21. Bernstein LJ, Kauvar ANB, Grossman MC, et al. The short- and long-term side effects of carbon dioxide laser resurfacing. *Dermatol Surg*. 1997;23:519-525.

22. Alster TS. Cutaneous resurfacing with CO_2 and Erbium:YAG lasers: preoperative, intraoperative, and postoperative considerations. *Plast Reconstr Surg*. 1999;103:619-632.

23. Nanni CA, Alster TS. Complications of carbon dioxide laser resurfacing: an evaluation of 500 patients. *Dermatol Surg*. 1998;24:315-320.

24. Sriprachya-Anunt S, Marchell NL, Fitzpatrick RE, et al. Facial resurfacing in patients with Fitzpatrick skin type IV. *Lasers Surg Med*. 2002;30:86-92.

25. Alster TS, Hirsch RJ. Single-pass CO_2 laser skin resurfacing of light and dark skin: extended experience with 52 patients. *J Cosmetic Laser Ther*. 2003;5:39-42.

26. Tanzi EL, Alster TS. Single-pass carbon dioxide versus multiplepass Er:YAG laser skin resurfacing: a comparison of postoperative wound healing and side effect rates. *Dermatol Surg*. 2003;29:80-84.

27. West TB, Alster TS. Effect of pretreatment on the incidence of hyperpigmentation following cutaneous CO_2 laser resurfacing. *Dermatol Surg*. 1999;25:15-17.

28. Sriprachya-anunt S, Marchell NL, Fitzpatrick RE, et al. Facial resurfacing in patients with Fitzpatrick skin type IV. *Lasers Surg Med*. 2002;30:86-92.

29. Battle EF Jr., Hobbs LM. Laser therapy on darker ethnic skin. *Dermatol Clin*. 2003;21:713-723.

30. Bhatt N, Alster TS. Laser surgery in dark skin. *Dermatol Surg.* 2008;34:184-194.

31. Kim JW, Lee JO. Skin resurfacing with laser in Asians. *Aesth Plast Surg.* 1997;21:115-117.

32. Ko NY, Ahn HH, Kim SN, Kye YC. Analysis of erythema after Er:YAG laser skin resurfacing. *Dermatol Surg.* 2007;33:1322-1327.

33. Ruiz-Espara J, Lupton JR. Laser resurfacing of darkly pigmented patients. *Dermatol Clin.* 2002;20:113-121.

34. Tanzi EL, Alster TS. Cutaneous laser surgery in darker skin phototypes. *Cutis.* 2004;73:21-30.

35. Baba T, Narumi H, Hanada K, et al. Successful treatment of dark-colored epidermal nevus with ruby laser. *J Dermatol.* 1995;22:567-570.

36. Macedo O, Alster TS. Laser treatment of darker skin tones: a practical approach. *Dermatol Ther.* 2000;13:114-126.

37. Bhatia AC, Dover JS, Arndt KA, Stewart B, Alam M. Patient satisfaction and reported long-term therapeutic efficacy associated with 1320 nm Nd:YAG laser treatment of acne scarring and photoaging. *Dermatol Surg.* 2006;32:346-352.

38. Fulton JE. Complications of laser resurfacing: methods of prevention and management. *Dermatol Surg.* 1998;24:91-99.

39. Roenigk HH. Dermabrasion: state of the art. *J Dermatol Surg Oncol.* 1985;11:306-314.

40. Alster TS. Combined laser resurfacing and tretinoin treatment for facial rhytides. *Cosmet Dermatol.* 1997;10:39-42.

41. Alster TS, Lupton JR. Pre-treatment of skin for laser resurfacing: is it necessary? *Cosmet Dermatol.* 2000;3:21-24.

42. Lowe NE, Lask G, Griffin ME. Laser skin resurfacing: pre and posttreatment guidelines. *J Dermatol Surg.* 1995;21:1017-1019.

43. David L, Ruiz-Esparaza J. Fast healing after laser resurfacing. The minimal mechanical trauma technique. *Dermatol Surg.* 1997;23:359-361.

44. Alster TS, Lupton JR. Are all infrared lasers equally effective in skin rejuvenation. *Sem Cutan Med Surg.* 2002;21:274-279.

45. Ross EV, Sajben FB, Hsia J, et al. Nonablative skin remodeling: selective dermal heating with a midinfrared laser and contact cooling combination. *Lasers Surg Med.* 2000;26:186-195.

46. Goldberg DJ, Whitworth J. Laser skin resurfacing with the Q-switched Nd:YAG laser. *Dermatol Surg.* 1997;23:903-906.

47. Goldberg DJ, Metzler C. skin resurfacing utilizing a low-fluence Nd:YAG laser. *J Cut Laser Ther.* 1999;1:23-27.

48. Newman J, Lord J, McDaniel D. Non-ablative laser therapy in skin types I-IV: clinical evaluation of facial treatment using QS 1064 nm Nd:YAG laser combined with carbon suspension lotion. *Lasers Surg Med Suppl.* 2000;12:70.

49. Muccini J, O'Donnell F, Fuller T, et al. Laser treatement of solar elastosis with epithelial preservation. *Lasers Surg Med.* 1998;23:121-127.

50. Menaker GM, Wrone DA, Williams RM, et al. Treatment of facial rhytides with a nonablative laser: a clinical and histologic study. *Dermaotl Surg.* 1999;25:440-444.

51. Kelly KM, Nelson S, Lask GP, et al. Cryogen spray cooling in combination with nonablative laser treatment of facial rhytides. *Arch Dermatol.* 1999;135:691-694.

52. Goldberg DJ. Nonablative subsurface remodeling: clinical and histologic evaluation of a 1320 nm Nd:YAG laser. *J Cutan Laser Ther.* 1999;1:153-157.

53. Goldberg DJ. Full-face nonablative dermal remodeling with a 1320 nm Nd:YAG laser. *Dermatol Surg.* 2000;26:915-918.

54. Trelles MA, Allones I, Luna R. Facial rejuvenation with a nonablative 1320 nm Nd:YAG laser: a preliminary clinical and histologic evaluation. *Dermatol Surg.* 2001;27:111-116.

55. Fatemi A, Weiss MA, Weiss RA. Short-term histologic effects of nonablative resurfacing: results with a dynamically cooled millisecond-domain 1320 nm Nd:YAG laser. *Dermatol Surg.* 2002;28:172-176.

56. Goldberg DJ, Rogachefsky AS, Silapuni S. Non-ablative laser treatement of facial rhytides: a comparison of 1450-nm diode laser treatment with dynamic cooling as opposed to treatment with dynamic cooling alone. *Lasers Surg Med.* 2002;30:89-81.

57. Tanzi EL, Williams CM, Alster TS. Treatment of facial rhytides with a nonablative 1450-nm diode laser: a controlled clinical and histologic study. *Dermatol Surg.* 2003;29:124-128.

58. Alster TS, Tanzi El. Treatment of transverse neck lines with a 1450 nm diode laser. *Lasers Surg Med.* 2002;14:33.

59. Tanzi EL, Alster TS. Comparison of a 1450 nm diode laser and a 1320-nm Nd:YAG laser in the treatment of atrophic facial scars: a prospective clinical and histologic study. *Dermatol Surg.* 2004;30:152-157.

60. Ross EV, Sajben FP, Hsia J, et al. Nonablative skin remodeling: selective dermal heating with a mid-inrared laser and contact cooling combination. *Lasers Surg Med.* 2000;26:186-195.

61. Lupton JR, Williams CM, Alster TS. Nonablative laser skin resurfacing using a 1540 nm erbium glass laser: a clinical and histologic analysis. *Dermatol Surg.* 2002;28:833-835.

62. Goldberg DJ, Cutler KB. Nonablative treatment of rhytides with intense pulsed light. *Lasers Surg Med.* 2000;26:196-200.

63. Bitter PH. Non-invasive rejuvenation of photodamaged skin using serial, full face intense pulsed light treatments. *Dermatol Surg.* 2000;26:835-843.

64. Weiss RA, Weiss MA, Beasley KL. Rejuvenation of photoaged skin: 5 years experience with intense pulsed light of the face, neck, and chest. *Dermatol Surg.* 2002;28:1115-1119.

65. Kono T, Groff WF, Sakurai H, et al. Comparison study of intense pulsed light versus a long-pulse pulsed dye laser in the treatment of facial skin rejuvenation. *Ann Plast Surg.* 2007;59:479-483.

66. Fitzpatrick R, Geronemus R, Goldberg D, et al. Multicenter study of non-invasive radiofrequency for periorbital tissue tightening. *Lasers Surg Med.* 2003;33:232-234.

67. Alster TS, Tanzi EL. Improvement of neck and cheek laxity with a non-ablative radiofrequency device: a lifting experience. *Dermatol Surg.* 2004;30:503-507.

CHAPTER 9

Ablative Dermal Resurfacing in Ethnic Skin: Laser, Deep Peels, and Dermabrasion

Tina Bhutani, MD, and Sonia R. Batra, MD, MSc, MPH

INTRODUCTION

Historically, people in many societies have searched for methods to restore youthful appearance and rejuvenate aging skin. Stories recount the efforts of ancient Chinese emperors and Spanish explorers to seek mythical substances and supernatural powers thought to have the ability to reverse the aging process. During the Dark Ages, European alchemists spent endless hours investigating magical methods for prolonging life and restoring youthful beauty. These beliefs have become rooted in modern-day society, as people continue to seek assistance for facial skin rejuvenation from healthcare professionals all over the world. In fact, because of the unbounded interest in this field and the aging population, more options now exist than ever before for reversing cutaneous changes caused by long-term exposure to sunlight. More recently, the spectrum of skin issues for which these methods have been utilized has expanded past the treatment of photoaging to include many skin problems more common in youth such as pigmentary disorders and acne scarring.

The population of the United States is not only aging, but also becoming more ethnically diverse. Data from the 2000 census revealed that 31% of the U.S. population is of ethnic background, and this statistic is expected to reach 50% within just a few years.[1] Although, Caucasian skin is more prone to ultraviolet light injury, ethnic skin also exhibits characteristic changes of photoaging. In 2003, racial and ethnic minorities accounted for 20% of all cosmetic procedures, and dermatologists and cosmetic surgeons likely will see an increasing influx of patients with darker skin types seeking rejuvenation treatment for aging skin and other cutaneous problems.[2] Hence, it is imperative to understand the differences in techniques, results and side effects in using these procedures on ethnic skin as compared to lighter colored skin types.

In this chapter, we will discuss these considerations in the context of ablative skin resurfacing, which can be accomplished using lasers, chemical peels, and microdermabrasion. Techniques and possible adverse reactions for these modalities in the treatment of ethnic and darker skin types will be considered.

ETHNIC SKIN—DEFINITION

Skin color in different ethnic groups varies dramatically from dark to light, as exemplified by central African and northern Scandinavian individuals, respectively, despite the fact that the density of melanocytes in the skin of these two skin types is identical. Numerous investigators have studied the biological basis of human skin color variation over the years. The intrinsic coloration is determined by the amount and type of melanin in the skin. However, an equally important determinant of skin color is the variation in the quantity, packaging, and distribution of epidermal melanin within keratinocytes of different ethnic groups. It is well documented that the melanosomes within keratinocytes of dark skin are distributed individually in the cytosol, predominantly over the nucleus, whereas the melanosomes within keratinocytes of light skin are clustered together in membrane-limited groups of two to eight melanosomes, also in the cytosol predominantly over the nucleus (Figure 9.1). Studies have also demonstrated that there is a progressive variation in melanosome size with ethnicity, African skin having the largest melanosomes, European skin the smallest melanosomes, and the melanosomes in Indian, Mexican, and Chinese skin being intermediate in size. Hence, skin color is not determined by the number of melanosomes but rather by relative size and localization within the cell.[3]

Because of the marked variability in skin color across the globe, Fitzpatrick[4] in 1988 developed a standardized method to classify skin types according to color and reaction to sun exposure (Table 9.1). Skin types range from I to VI, with ethnic skin usually classified in the spectrum between types IV-VI.[4] Since melanin is thought to have photoprotective effects, darker skinned individuals are less prone to the direct damage of ultraviolet light and are able to maintain a naturally youthful appearance later into life. In fact, studies have shown that approximately three to four times more UVA light reaches the upper dermis of Caucasians when compared to blacks.[5] Consequently, long-term exposure to differing intensities of light produce varied changes between these two groups. While lighter skinned individuals are more likely to present with deep-seated wrinkles, darker colored patients are usually seen with finer wrinkles, mottled hyperpigmentation, and unique skin lesions such as dermatosis papulosa nigra and actinic lentigines (Figure 9.2). Therefore, it is important to understand the common manifestations of photoaging in ethnic skin in order to provide the best treatment options. As will be discussed later, it is critical to determine a patient's skin type before deciding on a procedure since results and adverse effects will differ accordingly.

CLINICAL EXAMINATION AND PATIENT HISTORY

Proper patient selection and assessment of each individual's skin type is crucial prior to determining if an ablative procedure is indicated. The preoperative consultation is important in identifying at-risk patients who are best avoided or who necessitate an extra-cautious approach, as well as selecting patients who are ideal candidates for an ablative procedure. It is imperative to identify the key goals of the patient, such as an improvement in color or texture, expected time frame or number of procedures, and patient tolerance for recovery or "down" time postoperatively. The physician should explore whether a patient may tolerate more down time or

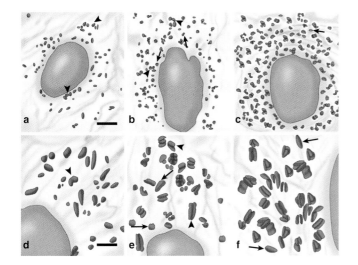

Figure 9.1 *Melanosome distribution in dark versus light skin. Melanosomes in dark skin from an African American (A,D) are predominantly distributed individually, with a few as membrane-bound clusters (arrowheads) throughout the cytoplasm of epidermal keratinocytes. Melanosomes in light skin from a Caucasian (C,F) are distributed as membrane-bound clusters with a few as individuals (arrows). Melanosomes in Asian skin (B,E) showed a combination of individual (arrows) and clustered (arrowheads) distribution pattern intermediate between the African American and Caucasian skin. Melanosomes in all types of skin frequently aggregated apically over the nucleus. (A-C) Low magnification; (D-F) higher magnification. Bars: (A-C) 5.2 μm; (D-F) 2.0 μm.*

TABLE 9.1 ▪ Fitzpatrick Skin Types

Skin type	Color	Skin characteristics
I	White	Always burns, never tans
II	White	Usually burns, tans less than average
III	White	Sometimes mild burn, tans about average
IV	White	Rarely burns, tans more than average
V	Brown	Rarely burns, tans profusely
VI	Black	Never burns, deeply pigmented

tions, anticipated results, and limitations as well as the potential risks of the procedure. A thorough history should include other medical conditions, past surgeries and complications (including a history of excessive scarring or keloid formation), past resurfacing modalities, and a detailed list of medications. Chronic medical illnesses, prior radiation, chemical or thermal burns, and medication known to delay wound healing may all play a role in predisposing to scarring. A history of abnormal scar formation or pigmentary alterations after prior procedures should influence a more conservative therapeutic approach.[6]

The preprocedure consultation is an opportunity to not only identify and discuss therapeutic options for the patient's chief complaint, but to understand whether the patient's expectations of the procedure, postoperative period, and results are realistic. It is essential that the patient's goals and expectations are reasonable prior to selecting the patient for a procedure, as this has a strong correlation with postoperative patient satisfaction. The patient must fully understand the potential benefits, limitations, and risks, and an informed consent must be signed prior to performing the procedure.

multiple treatments/interventions (such as use of topical bleaching cream) in order to achieve the primary goal.

At the time of the initial consultation, the dermatologist must evaluate the patient for relative contraindications; discuss the indications for the procedure; and assess the patient's goals, expecta-

Figure 9.2 *Differences in manifestations of photoaging in light versus ethnic skin. (A) Signs of photoaging in a lighter skinned individual including fine lines, coarse wrinkles, and loss of skin elasticity. (B) Typical photoaging changes in East and Southeast Asians include actinic lentigines; flat, pigmented seborrheic keratoses; and mottled hyperpigmentation. In addition, sun-induced melasma is also more common in this group than whites (not pictured here)*

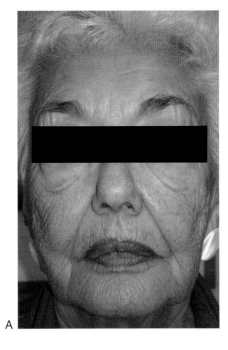

A

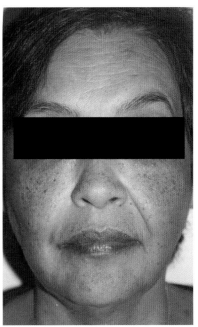

E

Moreover, to achieve a successful procedural outcome, a physician's understanding of cultural differences and preferences among ethnic patients is equally as important as the technical proficiency in the procedures to be performed. Cultural preferences can be understood through open discussion with the patient and knowledge of the manner in which cultural variations can affect communication. For example, Asian cultures place great importance on physical beauty to the extent that some believe that prospects for personal success in life are related to one's physical traits. In addition, many Asian patients have great respect for authority, which may limit communication with the physician since the patient may assume that the physician will understand and do what the patient desires. Questioning authority is considered disrespectful in some cultures as well. Consequently, the doctor should encourage the patient to verbalize concerns and expectations in order to achieve the greatest patient satisfaction ultimately.[7] Care must also be taken to make the patient feel comfortable in the clinical setting and to provide continuous support through the postprocedural period and beyond.

DEVICE OR TREATMENT SELECTION

As noted above, the patient's goals and severity of condition will guide the therapeutic plan. All ablative options discussed in this chapter can address photoaging, pigmentary disturbance, acne, and scarring in ethnic patients. In general, laser skin resurfacing (LSR) provides the greatest depth of ablation and is an excellent option for severe acne scarring or photoaging. However, the potential improvement in texture afforded by this technique must be weighed against the greater potential for pigmentary alteration and/or scarring in ethnic skin types. A greater depth of ablation will usually require increased recovery time, which must also be made clear to the patient. Figure 9.3 depicts the spectrum of ablative modalities in terms of aggressiveness.

An alternate, more conservative, approach in ethnic patients is to choose a less aggressive modality, such as chemical peels, and for the patient to undergo a series of treatments. This is particularly

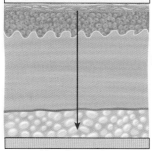

Commonly Used Ablative Modalities for Facial Skin Resurfacing

Least Aggressive

Microdermabrasion
Superficial Chemical Peel
Medium-Depth Chemical Peel
Deep Chemical Peel
ER:YAG Lasers
Combination CO_2/ER:YAG
CO_2 Lasers

Most Aggressive
(Greatest Depth of Ablation)

Figure 9.3 *Spectrum of ablative modalities (least to most aggressive)*

true of microdermabrasion, which affords the best results with regular therapy sessions.[8] In any ablative modality, strict sun protection must be emphasized to the patient postoperatively to minimize the risk of pigmentary alteration.

METHOD OF DEVICE OR TREATMENT APPLICATION

Laser Resurfacing

The word "laser" is an acronym, which stands for light amplification by the *stimulated emission of radiation*. Laser light has unique properties that allow it to be used therapeutically. Consequently, the popularity of laser procedures has skyrocketed in the past decade as the indications for use and types of lasers available continue to multiply. Laser light is monochromatic (single wavelength), coherent (in phase, both in time and space), and collimated (light waves are parallel). These properties make possible the generation and delivery of high fluence (energy per area), which can interact with the skin. Additionally, the monochromaticity of laser light is essential for selective targeting of structures in the skin, which preferentially absorb light of that wavelength. Commonly targeted chromophores in the skin, which each have their own unique absorption spectrum for laser light, include water, hemoglobin, and melanin.[9]

In the mid-1980s, Anderson and Parrish[10] revolutionized the therapeutic use of lasers with the development of the theory of selective photothermolysis; by using ultrashort pulses of high energy laser light rather than a continuous beam, collateral thermal damage could be minimized. Pulse duration is considered optimal if it is shorter than the target chromophore's relaxation time, defined as the time required for the targeted site to cool to one-half of its peak temperature immediately after laser irradiation.[10] In addition, the majority of cutaneous lasers are now used with systems to cool the epidermis to prevent collateral damage to epidermal structures from laser light intended to target deeper structures.

Carbon dioxide lasers

LSR with the carbon dioxide (CO_2) laser remains the gold standard for clinical and histologic improvement in severely photodamaged and scarred facial skin. In fact, it was the development of high-energy pulsed CO_2 systems in the early 1990s that revolutionized aesthetic laser surgery and ushered in a new decade of rapidly evolving laser technology.[9] Producing a wavelength of 10,600 nm, the CO_2 laser penetrates approximately 30 um into the skin by the absorption and vaporization of water containing tissues.[11] Energy densities of approximately 5 J/cm^2 must be applied in order to achieve tissue ablation.[12] With each subsequent laser pass, vaporization of very thin (20–30 um) layers of skin occurs, leaving a small amount of residual thermal necrosis.[13] With each subsequent laser pass, further tissue ablation occurs, but because the area of residual thermal necrosis increases (effectively reducing the amount of tissue water and hence the targeted chromophore), the amount of ablation with each pass diminishes until a peak of approximately 100 um is reached.[14] Delivering more than three to four passes or use of excessive energy densities significantly increases the risk of excessive thermal injury and subsequent scarring.

Dose/setting selection In ethnic patients, more conservative laser settings and fewer passes may decrease the risk of scarring and/or pigmentary change. With an Ultrapulse (Lumenis, Inc., Santa Clara, CA), the CPG scanner is used primarily and a 3 mm collimated spot for feathering or small areas. Overlap should be 10% or less. The authors prefer a pattern shape of 2 (parallelogram), pattern size 9, density 5250 mJ per pulse fluence, 50 W power, and repeat rate 1.5/s. The fluence and power may be decreased at the periphery of treatment to blend with surrounding skin and to minimize the risk of scarring.

Treatment technique Postinflammatory hyperpigmentation is a common postoperative side effect in patients with phototypes IV to VI.[15] For at least 6 weeks preoperatively, patients may use topical tretinoin in the highest tolerable concentration. If a patient is retinoid intolerant, an alpha-hydroxy acid may be substituted. Concomitantly, topical lightening agents, such as hydroquinone, soy extract, kojic acid, or azelaic acid can be used. Patients should also be counseled to avoid being tanned prior to the procedure and to minimize postoperative sun exposure.

All patients receive prophylactic antibiotics starting the day before resurfacing and continuing for 1 week. Dicloxacillin 500 mg twice daily, or in penicillin allergic patients levofloxacin 750 mg daily are common choices. Prophylactic antiviral therapy with valacyclovir 500 mg twice daily is also begun 2 days preoperatively and continued for 10 days after resurfacing.[16]

Vaporization of epidermal and dermal tissue causes significant pain, and adequate anesthesia must be achieved. This can be accomplished by a combination of topical anesthesia, local infiltration, and regional nerve blocks. Oral sedatives and analgesics may be used adjunctively.

The patient should wash his or her face thoroughly with a gentle cleanser and thereafter an antiseptic may be used to prep the skin. Scalp hair may be wrapped with moist towels and Surgilube (Fougera) applied to eyebrows and scalp margins. Corneal shields may be inserted to protect the eyes.[15]

The first pass is performed using a CPG with spots placed next to one another with no more than 10% overlap. After the first pass, desiccated proteinaceous debris can be removed by wiping with saline-moistened gauze. Some authors believe that a single pass that leaves the char in place to act as a biologic dressing may minimize the risk of pigmentary change and scarring.[17] Increased passes may be used for areas of deeper wrinkling or scarring. In ethnic or darker skin types, no more than three to four passes should be performed as this greatly increases the risk of scarring.

Postoperative care Following LSR, either open or closed wound care techniques may be employed. Most open wound care regimens consist of frequent soaks with cool compresses of 0.25% acetic acid, normal saline, or cool tap water lasting 10 to 20 minutes every 2 to 4 hours, followed by gentle wiping of the skin. Cold compresses are immediately followed by the application of a bland emollient ointment. Popular ointments include Catrix®-10 (Lescarden) and Aquaphor® Healing Ointment (Beiersdorf AG). The frequency of soaks and ointment application decreases as re-epithelialization progresses and is tapered off when re-epithelialization is complete.

Studies indicate that closed wound care regimens utilizing occlusive dressings for 48 to 72 hours postoperatively may hasten re-epithelialization and reduce crusting, discomfort, erythema, and swelling.[18] Dressings employed after resurfacing include the composite foam Flexzan® (Dow Hickam Pharmaceuticals), the hydrogel product 2 nd Skin® (Bionet), the plastic mesh N-terface® (Winfield Laboratories), and the polymer film Silon-TSR® (Bio Med Sciences). Occlusive dressings are applied for 2 to 3 days, postoperatively. Longer applications increase the risk of infection with subsequent scarring. The authors employ the Silon-TSR®, a silicone dressing with a polytetrafluorethylene inner polymer network.

Immediately after resurfacing, the face is blotted dry and the dressing is applied. Openings are cut for the eyelids, nose, and central lips, and a smaller patch of dressing is applied to cover the nasal bridge. Gauze 4×4 dressings are applied over the mask to absorb exudates and are held in place by tube gauze. Patients are seen on the first postoperative day and the gauze is removed. The resurfaced area is inspected through the transparent mask, and accumulated exudate or crust is removed from uncovered areas with saline. Patients are instructed to begin ice-water soaks through the mask for 20-minutes periods at 2 to 4 hours intervals while awake. Patients return again at the third postoperative day and the dressing is removed. Patients continue soaks at 3 to 4 hours intervals followed by application of Aquaphor® healing ointment.

In both open and closed wound care regimens, by 7 to 10 days after the procedure, soaks are replaced with gentle cleansing, and patients switch to the application of a moisturizer-sunscreen.[19]

Management of adverse events As noted above, prophylactic antibiotics and antivirals should be begun preoperatively, and any sign of infection should be treated aggressively as it may result in scarring. Over 80% of patients note pain in the immediate postoperative period.[20] This can be minimized by intraoperative use of supplemental local anesthesia as well as systemic pain medication. After LSR, ice packs, cold compresses, and acetaminophen help to alleviate pain. Approximately 85% of patients require pain medications for the first 3 days postoperatively and those not relieved by acetaminophen often benefit from acetaminophen with codeine phosphate or acetaminophen with hydrocodone bitartrate.

Pruritus often occurs during re-epithelialization and typically lasts approximately 10 days. Pruritus can often be relieved by cool compresses and emollients, although over half of patients require oral antihistamines. In more severe cases of severe pruritus, medium-to-high potency topical steroids may be required. Control of pruritus is essential since excoriation may result in scarring. Erythema typically occurs for up to several months after LSR. Erythema can be camouflaged with make-up containing green foundation. As noted above, particularly in ethnic patients, sun protection and avoidance should be encouraged during the entire period of post-LSR erythema to minimize postinflammatory hyperpigmentation. Edema develops in the first 48 hours after LSR. The severity can be controlled with ice packs and head elevation at night. In cases where marked edema develops during or immediately after the procedure, oral corticosteroids may be necessary.

Erbium: yttrium-aluminum-garnet laser
The short pulsed Er:YAG laser was developed in the mid-1990s in an attempt to replicate the results of the CO_2 laser while minimizing the side effect profile. The emitted wavelength of 2940 nm has a higher affinity for water and is therefore absorbed 12 to 18 times

TABLE 9.2 ▪ **Side Effects and Complications of Ablative LSR***

Side effects	Mild complications	Moderate complications	Severe complications
Transient erythema	Prolonged erythema	Pigmentary change	Hypertrophic scar
Localized edema	Milia	Infections (bacterial, fungal, viral)	Ectropion
Pruritus	Acne		
	Contact dermatitis		

*In general, side effects and complications following Er:YAG lasers are similar but less severe and more transient when compared with those experienced after CO_2 laser resurfacing

more efficiently by superficial cutaneous tissues and approximately 2 to 5 μm of ablation occurs per pass with very narrow zones of thermal necrosis.[21] Clinically, this translates into a shorter postoperative healing time with a lower risk of posttreatment erythema and risk for hyperpigmentation than CO_2 lasers. However, multiple passes with the laser are necessary to ablate a similar depth as one pass of the CO_2 laser, making the procedure potentially slower than CO_2 resurfacing. Also, because the Er:YAG effects are photomechanical rather than photothermal (like the CO_2), intraoperative hemostasis is often difficult to achieve.[15,22]

Several studies have documented the effectiveness of the Er:YAG laser in the treatment of mild to moderate rhytids, photodamage, and atrophic scars, with the use of multiple passes, high fluences, and/or multiple sessions yielding improved clinical outcomes. The Er:YAG has also been proven to be a good option for treatment of patients with darker skin types because of its lower risk of pigmentary alteration[23] and has even been used to treat melasma.[24]

Dose/setting selection With the Er:YAG, approximately 4 μm of tissues is vaporized per J/cm^2 of energy applied.[21] Therefore, a fluence of 5 J/cm^2 will ablate the epidermis in four passes. Settings can be adjusted depending on the depth of ablation desired. A repetition rate of 1 to 10 Hz and spot sizes of 3 to 7 mm can be selected with most Er:YAG lasers.

Treatment technique Patient preparation and anesthesia are performed similarly to the CO_2 laser. After the first pass, proteinaceous material may be wiped with moistened gauze; however, after ablation of the epidermis, wiping is not necessary. The treated area is covered with moderately overlapping spots. The surgeon must keep track of the number of passes performed to minimize the risk of scarring and pigmentary alteration.

If using a long-pulsed Er:YAG laser, the effect is similar to that of a CO_2, and initial passes may be performed to induce collagen tightening and coagulation of small dermal vessels. Thereafter, the short-pulsed mode may be used for ablation and to remove thermal damage. This technique is similar to combination CO_2/Er:YAG resurfacing, in which the CO_2 is used first, followed by one to two passes of an Er:YAG.[16]

Postoperative care Wound care is performed similarly to that following CO_2 resurfacing.

Management of adverse effects Side effects and complications are varied and greatly influenced by postoperative care, patient selection, and operator skill. In general, the side effect profile after Er:YAG

laser resurfacing is similar but less severe and more transient when compared with those experienced after CO_2 laser resurfacing (Table 9.2). For example, postoperative erythema lasting an average of 4.5 months, is an expected occurrence in all CO_2 laser treated patients and is a normal consequence of the wound healing process. Erythema after short-pulsed Er:YAG resurfacing is comparably transient of 2 to 4 weeks duration.[25] In addition, time to re-epithelialization averages 8.5 days with multipass CO_2 laser resurfacing compared with 5.5 days after Er:YAG resurfacing.[15]

Hyperpigmentation is a relatively common side effect typically seen 3 to 6 weeks after the procedure. After CO_2 resurfacing, the reported incidence is 5% in the perioribital area and 17% to 83% in other facial sites, with an even greater incidence in patients with darker skin tones.[26] Hyperpigmentation also occurs after Er:YAG laser resurfacing. However, when compared with multipass CO_2 laser, hyperpigmentation caused by dual pass Er:YAG resolves 6 weeks earlier.[27] Hyperpigmentation typically fades spontaneously but dissipates more rapidly with application of any of a variety of glycolic, azelaic, or retinoic acid creams, light glycolic acid peels, and/or hydroquinone compounds. Hypopigmentation can also be seen after delayed onset ($\geq$6 months postprocedure), and is more often long standing and is very difficult to treat. Fortunately, it is seen far less frequently than is hyperpigmentation.[28]

A potentially more serious complication of laser LSR is infection—viral, bacterial, or fungal. Even with appropriate antiviral prophylaxis, herpes infection (usually reactivation of latent virus) occurs in 2% to 7% of patients postoperatively. In addition, patients must be followed closely in the postoperative period and placed on appropriate antibiotics if bacterial or fungal infection is suspected. As noted above, if infections are left undiagnosed or untreated, systemic infections or even scarring can result.[29]

Scarring has also been attributed to the use of aggressive laser parameters and/or overlapping or stacking of laser pulses, which leads to excessive residual thermal necrosis of tissue. In addition, it is best to avoid resurfacing of the neck and chest because of the scarcity of pilosebaceous units in these regions with resultant slow re-epithelialization and potential for scarring.

▪ Considerations for Ethnic Skin

The most common complication in dark skinned patients after laser surgery is postinflammatory hyperpigmentation, as mentioned above. Although this is transient in nature, it can last for several months and therefore is poorly tolerated by most patients. Recent advances in skin cooling, longer laser wavelength, and shorter

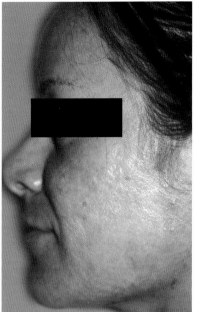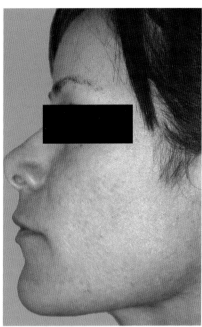

Figure 9.4 *Pre- and postablative laser resurfacing (combination CO_2/Er:YAG) in a Hispanic patient with acne scarring and preexisting hypopigmentation from a prior laser procedure* A ___ B

pulse durations have improved treatment outcomes; however, this still remains an important issue.

Because of the higher risk of postoperative complication and less deep wrinkling in dark skinned patients, nonablative technologies are currently first-line therapy.[30] However, when ablation is required for deep-seated damage, it has been suggested that the combination approach in which three passes of CO_2 laser are followed immediately by one pass of Er:YAG laser, be adopted (Figure 9.4). This combination has been associated with reduced erythema and hyperpigmentation. More recently, long-pulsed Er:YAG lasers have been used with the aim of achieving better hemostasis and some degree of collagen contraction. Jeong et al.[33] studied the use of such a system among skin types III and IV patients with pitted acne scars. They found an excellent response in 93% of patients, but erythema lasting more than 3 months was seen in 54%. Patients should be warned that several treatments may be necessary to achieve a significant degree of improvement, but there will be less downtime and lower risk of hyperpigmentation. Single pass CO_2 laser resurfacing has also recently been shown to be effective in the treatment of acne scar and wrinkle reduction in dark skinned patients with a reduction in severity and duration of laser associated complications.

In addition, just as in all other patients, sun avoidance and sun protection prior to surgery are encouraged in order to reduce the risk of postinflammatory hyperpigmentation. It is not uncommon for patients to misunderstand the meaning of sun avoidance, and only avoid sun bathing. Therefore, it is important to emphasize to all patients that they should apply sunblock (preferentially containing titanium dioxide and zinc oxide) for 2 weeks daily before and 6 weeks after laser surgery, whether or not they engage in outdoor activities. UV light-protected clothing and a broad-rimmed hat are also useful.

Recent studies have also shown that application of a moderate potency topical steroid immediately after laser surgery may also reduce the risk of hyperpigmentation. The use of topical bleaching agents before and after surgery such as combinations of tretinoin, hydroquinone, topical steroid, AHA, kojic acid, and azelaic acid has been advocated. A sample regimen is to give all patients a combination of 0.025% tretinoin cream mixed with 4% hydroquinone and a moderate potency steroid twice daily preoperatively and then postoperatively for another 4 weeks. If postinflammatory hyperpigmentation develops despite the use of such agents, the addition of 5% glycolic acid in the morning may further reduce pigmentation. Depending on the degree of irritation, other bleaching agents are then added including vitamin C, vitamin E, and kojic acid. If hyperpigmentaion persists, a mild glycolic acid peel may be performed approximately 6 to 8 weeks after surgery.[31] The use of microdermabrasion may also be effective as an adjunctive means to improve superficial pigmentation.

Newer Technology—Fractional Lasers and Plasma Skin Regeneration

While ablative skin resurfacing with CO_2 and Er:YAG lasers has proven highly effective in reversing the signs of facial photoaging and atrophic scars, the associated lifestyle hindrance and potential complications are often unacceptable to patients. In recent years, focus has shifted to nonablative technologies that deliver either laser, light-based, or radio frequency energies to the skin without alteration of the epidermal surface. Although effective for collagen contraction and popular for a low side effect profile and minimal recovery period, the use of nonablative lasers for more severe photodamage has revealed inconsistent results with no epidermal resurfacing effects and modest clinical results at best.

Fractional lasers attempt to bridge this gap between ablative and nonablative laser modalities, and are now being used in many centers to treat the epidermal and dermal effects of skin aging. By targeting water as a chromophore, the 1550 nm erbium fiber laser

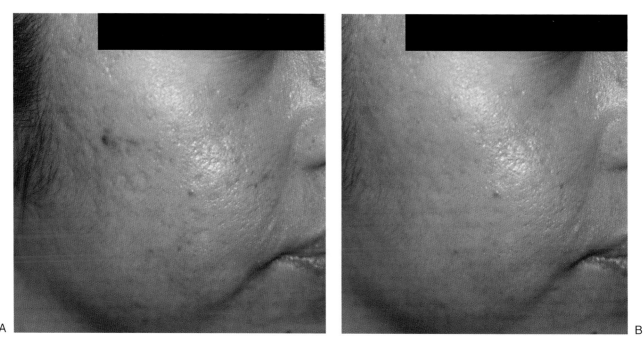

Figure 9.5 *Pre- and postseries of four fractional resurfacing treatments in a phototype IV patient with acne scarring*

induces a dense array of microscopic, columnar thermal zones of tissue injury that do not perforate or impair the function of the epidermis. In addition, for every microthermal zone the laser targets and treats intensively, it leaves the surrounding tissue unaffected and intact. This "fractional" treatment allows the skin to heal much faster than if the entire area were treated at once. The skin remodeling that ensues can be used to treat, with less downtime, epidermal pigmentation, melasma, and rhytides, as well as textural abnormalites that include acne related and surgical scars[32] (Figure 9.5).

A newer modality uses energy delivered from plasma rather than light or radio frequency. In a pilot study evaluating the use of a single full facial treatment at high energy (3–4 J), Kilmer, et al.[34] demonstrated a mean improvement in overall facial rejuvenation of 50% by 1 month.

Although these technologies have shown promising results in many large scale studies, none thus far have focused on the effects in darker skin complexions. Early data has shown that postinflammatory hyperpigmentation is less common with these modalities. Consequently, further large-scale studies examining their use in the treatment of photoaging in darker skinned patients is necessary. In the meantime, great care must be taken with these modalities in Fitzpatrick skin types IV-VI as to avoid possible side effects.

Chemical Peels

The first chemical peels date back to the Egyptians who used the lactic acid in sour milk baths, various chemicals, and sandpaper in order to attain a smoother skin surface. In the Middle Ages, old wine with tartaric acid as its active ingredient was used for the same purpose. Modern-day chemical peeling originally was promoted by dermatologists, such as P.G. Unna, who first described the properties of salicylic acid, resorcinol, phenol, and trichloroacetic acid (TCA). In the 1960s, Baker and Gordon developed a deep peeling agent that contained alpha hydroxy acids, which was able to smooth deeper furrows, especially around the mouth. From the 1980s to the present, many different types of peels, each for a specific range of problems have been developed.[35]

The chemical peel works by producing a controlled partial thickness injury to the skin. Following the insult, a wound healing process ensues that can regenerate epidermis from surrounding epithelium and adnexal structures, decrease solar elastosis, and replace and reorient the new dermal connective tissue. The result is an improved clinical appearance of the skin, with fewer rhytides and decreased pigmentary dyschromia.[36]

Chemical peels are categorized into superficial, medium depth, and deep types of wounding depending on the level of penetration, destruction, and inflammation (Table 9.3). Although deep peels are usually indicated for patients requesting ablative resurfacing, they are usually not recommended for ethnic skin because of the increased risk of hyperpigmentation following the procedure.[37] Therefore, in this chapter, we will focus on only superficial and medium-depth peels that have been found to be safe and effective in all skin types.

Agents for chemical peeling

Many agents are available for chemical peeling today. New agents are being researched, and older agents are being used in different combinations and formulations to create new ways of peeling. As a result of the wide range of options, it is important to recognize the strengths of each solution, so that better recommendations can be offered to patients.

Glycolic acid is an alpha hydroxy acid (AHA), which belongs in a class of naturally occurring compounds derived from food sources such as sugar cane and fruits. Glycolic acid peels can

TABLE 9.3 ■ **Chemical Peels Organized by Depth**

Peel depth	Depth of penetration	Indications
Superficial	Superficial exfoliation Epidermal necrosis	Melasma, epidermal Postinflammatory hyperpigmentation Acne vulgaris Pseudofolliculitis barbae Mottled dyschromia (ethnic skin)
Medium	Papillary dermal necrosis	Mild to moderate photoaging Actinic keratoses Melasma, dermal Atrophic acne scars, moderate Pigmentary dyschromias
Deep	Reticular dermal necrosis	Severe photodamage

range in concentration from 20% to 70% and are generally performed every 3 to 4 weeks for a total of four to six treatments. These peels are indicated in the treatment of melasma, postinflammatory hyperpigmentation, mild photoaging, and acne. In addition, glycolic acid peels are usually well tolerated in all skin types and colors.

Salicylic acid is a beta hyrdoxy acid and is also a naturally occurring substance which can be found in the bark of the willow tree. Peels range in concentration from 20% to 30% and are performed every 3 to 4 weeks for a total of three to five treatments. Salicylic acid peels are indicated in the treatment of acne vulgaris, melasma, postinflammatory hyperpigmentation, rough and oily skin with enlarged pores, and mild to moderate photodamaged skin.

Jessner's peel is a solution that combines resorcinol, salicylic acid, 85% lactic acid, and 95% ethanol. These peels are indicated in the treatment of inflammatory and comedonal acne and melasma, as well as hyperkeratotic skin disorders. This peel was developed in order to lower the concentration of any one agent and to enhance the keratolytic activity. However, the limitation of Jessner's solution is the storage requirement of a dark bottle to prevent photo-oxidation.

Finally, TCA produces superficial peeling when used in strengths from 10% to 35%. At these strengths, TCA is indicated for the treatment of fine rhytids, actinic damage, mild epidermal dyschromia, reduction of superficial keratoses, scars, and comedone formation. Treatment intervals between applications are generally within 7 to 28 days. Unlike the other peels, the solution is self-neutralizing, and does not require water or bicarbonate solution to terminate the peeling action. Therefore, TCA is often considered the gold standard of chemical peeling agents. It is a stable agent (shelf life greater than 6 months) that is not light sensitive and requires no refrigeration. Often, the skin is primed with other peeling agents (glycolic acid, Jessner's solution) or solid CO_2 which can allow for penetration of lower and safer concentrations of TCA that is deeper and more evenly distributed. The end result is more uniform peeling with fewer complications.[38]

Treatment technique After thorough cleansing and degreasing of the skin, the chemical agent is applied sequentially to six aesthetic units: forehead, perioral region, right cheek, left cheek, nose, and periorbital region. After mixing, the solution should be kept in a glass bowl or basin with a broad bottom so the solution can be gently agitated without danger of spilling or splashing. One to two cotton tip applicators are used to stir the solution and to apply it to the skin. The patient's eyes should be kept closed throughout the procedure. The applicator tip is stroked quickly and with moderate pressure over the cosmetic unit while watching for a whitening frost that appears within 10 seconds. Frosting with different wounding agents is variable in rate and appearance and depends on the pre-existing degree of photodamage, the choice of applicator used, and adequacy of defatting. This segment is then considered "painted." After each segment is evenly frosted, dry, cold compresses and fanned air are used to help minimize the burning sensation. Also, ice packs can be used to symptomatically cool the skin. Depending on the agent used and the concentration, the amount of time the agent is left on the skin varies, generally between 2 to 4 minutes. Neutralization of the agent is used with either water or sodium bicarbonate.[39]

Postoperative care After the procedure, as noted above, all patients who undergo any type of resurfacing must adhere to strict sun avoidance and sun-protective measures. In addition, patients should be counseled not to smoke, as smoking impairs the healing process. Patients may resume their prepeel rejuvenation regimen after compete re-epithelialization has occurred. Typically, the recovery time postpeel is minimal.[40]

Management of adverse events Complications and risks of superficial and medium-depth peels are fewer with the advent of the combination peel but still exist. The most common complication following a chemical peel is hyperpigmentation, and the most common factor responsible is early sun exposure.[41] Patients are routinely instructed to avoid significant sun exposure in the weeks leading up to and following the procedure and to wear a broad-spectrum sunscreen with UVA/UVB block. Pretreatment with retinoic acid and hydroquinone can reduce the risk of postinflammatory hyperpigmentation, but those with darker skin types and/or those being treated for pigment problems are at greater risk and may not be affected by pretreatment. If it arises, postpeel pigmentation can be managed with retinoic acid, hydroquinone products, midpotency topical steroids, and follow-up peels (approximately 3-6 months later) until a lightening effect is

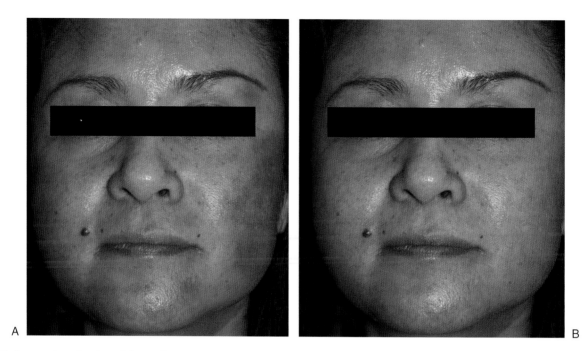

A   B

Figure 9.6 *Pre- and postseries of three glycolic peels in an Asian patient with pigment dyschromia*

achieved. Postpeel hypopigmentation is less frequently a problem and treatment options are few and less reliable. Although previously thought only to occur with deep chemical peels, hypopigmentation has been reported with 20% and 35% TCA peels.[42] In darker skin types, this potentially permanent side effect can be devastating.

Hypertrophic scarring is a rare but disastrous complication of chemical peels. Those at increased risk include patients who have recently undergone facial plastic surgery and patients who have taken isoretinoin (Accutane) within 1 year.[42] Special care in not allowing the agent to drip or be drawn into unwanted areas is of critical importance. Maintaining a container with water and 10% sodium bicarbonate close at hand to neutralize glycolic acid and TCA, respectively, can tighten the physician's control over chemical that contacts the skin. Conditions that predispose to delayed healing as described in section "Clinical Examination and Patient History" may also be responsible for the development of hypertrophic scarring in certain patients. The areas most vulnerable to disfigurement are the jaw line, skin overlying the zygomatic arch, and the perioral perimeter. Treatment options include massage, compression bandages, topical or intralesional steroids, and silicone gel sheeting as soon as the potential for scarring is suspected.[43]

Herpes simplex reactivation is a risk of any skin resurfacing procedure and therefore, patients are routinely prophylaxed with antiviral medication. Less serious but more common side effects also include milia, acne flares, and cyst formation following a chemical peel. Bland emollients are necessary to prevent such side effects, protect the newly laid epithelium, and promote wound healing. Lastly, persistent erythema beyond the accepted 60 days may indicate an incipient scar, contact dermatitis, or infection, and warrants careful proactive management in most cases.[44]

Considerations for ethnic skin When considering the use of chemical peels in ethnic skin, it is critical to identify the patient's Fitzpatrick skin type as well as determine the patient's ethnicity prior to selecting a peeling agent. Indications for chemical peeling in darker skin include, acne vulgaris, PIH, melasma, scarring, photodamage, and pseudofolliculitis barbae. However, the primary indication for chemical peeling in skin types III-VI is for pigment dyschromias (Figure 9.6).

In darker skinned patients, specific properties of the peeling agents must be considered to choose the most appropriate agent to address the patient's dermatological needs. For example, glycolic acid and salicylic acid peels are excellent tools to treat acne in skin of color. In addition, salicylic acid in ethanol is appropriate for ethnic skinned patients with melasma or PIH, whereas glycolic acid is less favorable in the darkest patients because it may actually induce PIH in skin types V and VI. TCA at low concentrations of 10% to 25% also works well to treat acne scarring in skin of color, and when used in combination with 70% glycolic acid gel, it also rejuvenates uneven, mottled skin pigmentation. Jessner's solution may create depigmentation in patients with skin types V and VI but may be successful for spot peeling for PIH in ethnic skin. In addition, TCA 25% and salicylic acid are also important tools for spot peeling.[40]

Regardless of the peeling agent chosen, treatment should proceed judiciously in darker skinned patients. Treatments should first be attempted at low concentrations and dry times to decrease the risks of adverse side effects. Multiple treatments of low intensity may outweigh the benefits of deeper and more severe peels. As noted for other ablative modalities, it is critical to start a prepeel regimen that includes the morning application of sunscreen with UVA/UVB protection and an SPF of at least 30, a moisturizer containing alpha hydroxy acid as well as an evening combination including retinoid, hydroquinone, kojic acid, or azelaic acid and possibly a low potency steroid. Following the peel, patients must also be followed closely with frequent follow-up in order to assess signs of hyperpigmentation or scarring early on in the process.[45]

▨ Microdermabrasion

With more than two dozen products by different manufacturers on the market, microdermabrasion has gained significant popularity in Europe, Australia, and the United States since its development in Italy in 1985. The various machine types can be divided into the higher power physician's model and the lower power aesthetician's model. The physician's model is capable of creating pressures up to 70 mm Hg, affecting deeper layers of the skin and requiring the supervision of a physician.[46] The technique of microdermabrasion relies on two basic functions: (1) superficially abrading the skin with fine, sharp crystals (aluminum oxide, salt, or sodium bicarbonate) via positive or negative flowing pressure, and (2) a vacuum closed loop suction device to remove the crystals, along with dead skin, oil, and surface debris.[47]

In brief, microcrystals are deposited on the skin via short, rapid strokes of the hand piece. A tube contained within the hand piece of the machine simultaneously aspirates the crystals and skin debris. Particle flow rate and vacuum pressure determine the volume of particles impacting the skin. Skin depth of the microdermabrasion procedure is determined by the strength of the flow of crystals, speed of movement of the hand piece, and the number of passes per anatomic site. Slow movement of the hand piece and a higher number of passes increase the depth of microdermabrasion.[48]

As an alternative to laser resurfacing and chemical peels, microdermabrasion is indicated for similar skin issues but with the limitation of having relatively superficial results. Described as "skin polishing", this procedure can be used for atrophic acne scars, mild facial rhytids, melasma, and for improvement in skin texture and appearance. It can be used to prime the skin for superficial chemical peels by stripping the stratum corneum to ensure even more absorption. Therefore, a less potent peeling method can be used to obtain similar results to deep peeling with fewer side effects.[46] There is substantial patient satisfaction with microdermabrasion. In most circumstances, the patient has minimal discomfort, there is no down time, and the patient perceives immediate improvement in tone, texture, and pigmentation.[48]

Treatment technique The technique of microdermabrasion is noninvasive and quite simple. Prior to treatment, the area is cleansed and allowed to dry completely. Vacuum level and crystal pressure maybe determined by testing an area of nonfacial skin, but patient tolerance can also dictate an adjustment in power setting. The first pass is performed by allowing gentle suction of the skin into the hand piece as it is made to glide along the skin surface. The surface area being treated is stretched taut by the clinician's free hand to avoid excess suction in any one area, which can cause an abrasion or pinpoint bleeding. A second pass is made at a right angle to the first, and if more passes are required, they should continue to follow this alternating pattern to avoid streaking. Reducing the level of suction and or number of passes maybe necessary around the eyes and other delicate areas of the face. The intensity of the treatment, as determined by the number of passes

and level of suction, is chosen based on the condition being treated. When the treatment is completed, the residual crystals should be gently brushed off the skin in the direction away from the eyes so as to prevent eye irritation. The skin can then be rinsed with tepid water and a moisturizer with adequate sunscreen applied. Some practitioners advocate the use of a mask when performing microdermabrasion to minimize the risk of inhalation of any airborne particles.[40]

Periprocedural care Patients are instructed to avoid keratolytic agents, including retinoids, alpha-hydroxy acids, and benzoyl peroxides 3 days before and 3 days following the treatment. Patients are also asked to avoid waxing, electrolysis, and laser hair removal 1 week before treatment and are often given prophylaxis for HSV infection as is standard with other resurfacing methods.

Management of adverse events Overall, the treatment is considered a safe, noninvasive procedure with few reported side effects. It is safe in all Fitzpatrick skin types; however, complications can occur with this procedure. These include postinflammatory hyperpigmentation and streaking from intense pressure of the hand piece. Petechiae and purpura are also complications of aggressive treatment.[48] Additionally, even though adhesive ocular shields should be worn during the procedure, ocular complications can occur if aluminum crystals enter the eye. These include eye irritation, chemosis, photophobia, and punctuate keratitis.[49] In contrast, if sodium chloride enters the eye, immediate, thorough rinsing dissolves the particles and usually alleviates ocular symptoms.

The subject of cross contamination with microdermabrasion equipment has also recently been reported. Shelton found bloody material on the hand piece after performing microdermabrasion on a patient with acne scarring, indicating that it is not sufficient to sterilize the distal cap of the hand piece or to use disposable caps. Therefore, it was suggested that the hand piece itself must be sterilized to prevent the transmission of infectious particles to a subsequent patient receiving microdermabrasion.[50]

Considerations in ethnic skin With predictably superficial results, microdermabrasion has been safely performed on all skin types. The concerns for hyperpigmentation that may hinder many ethnic patients from elective resurfacing procedures are greatly reduced in microdermabrasion, and if present, are extremely short lived. Poor candidates include only those who have been on isoretinoin within the last year, those with cutaneous malignancies, recent herpes outbreaks, warts involving the treatment area, flared rosacea, draining acne vulgaris, unstable diabetes, and autoimmune disorders.

CONCLUSION

Multiple ablative modalities, including LSR, chemical peels, and microdermabrasion can be used to address cosmetic concerns in ethnic patients. Common goals include improvement of photodamage and rhytids, pigmentary dyschromia including postinflammatory hyperpigmentation and melasma, and acne scarring. Treatment of these patients must be pursued cautiously and with specific precautions against scarring and pigmentary alteration. In addition, treatment of patients with ethnic skin may be challenging because cultural preferences and expectations may differ from the physician's own views of a successful procedure. With the increasing number of ethnic patients who will request ablative procedures in the future, it is critical to learn about these differing expectations as well as refine the techniques to be used in this patient population.

ACKNOWLEDGMENTS

The authors thank Ava T. Shamban, MD, for sharing clinical photographs, and Isabella Toma, for helping with figure preparation.

REFERENCES

1. 2000 U.S. Census Bureau Government Data. Available at http://www.census.gov/popest/race.html. Accessed March 2007.

2. American Society for Aesthetic Plastic Surgery. Survey Data. 2005. Available at http://www.surgery.org/press/news-release.php?iid=325. Accessed March 2007.

3. Thong HY, Lee SH, Sun CC, Boissy RE. The patterns of melanosome distribution in keratinocytes of human skin as one determining factor of skin colour. *Br J Dermatol*. 2003; 149(3):498-505.

4. Fitzpatrick TB. The validity and practicality of sun-reactive skin types I through VI. *Arch Dermatol*. 1998;124(6):869-871.

5. Pathak MA. The role of natural photoprotective agents in human skin. In: Fitzpatrick TB, Pathak MA, eds. *Sunlight and Man*. Tokyo: University of Tokyo Press; 1974.

6. Rubenstein R, Roenik HH, Stegman SJ, Hanke CW. Atypical keloids after dermabrasion of patients taking isoretinoin. *J Am Acad Dermatol*. 1986;15:280-285.

7. McCurdy JA. Facial surgery in asian patients. In: Matory WE, ed. *Ethnic Considerations in Facial Aesthetic Surgery*. Philadelphia, PA: Lippincott-Raven; 1998:263-284.

8. Jackson BA. Cosmetic considerations and non-laser cosmetic procedures in ethnic skin. *Dermatol Clin*. 2003;21:703-712.

9. Tanzi EL, Lupton JR, Alster TS. Review of lasers in dermatology: four decades of progress. *J Am Acad Dermatol*. 2003;4:1-32.

10. Anderson RR, Parrish JA. Selective photothermolysis: precise microsurgery by selective absorption of pulsed radiation. *Science*. 1983;220:524-527.

11. Lanzafame RJ, Naim JO, Rogers DW, et al. Comparisons of continuous-wave, chop-wave, and super pulsed laser wounds. *Laser Surg Med*. 1988;8:119-124.

12. Alster TS, Garg S. Treatment of facial rhyties with a high energy pulsed carbon dioxide laser. *Plast Reconstr Surg*. 1996;98: 791-794.

13. Alster TS, Kauvar ANB, Geronemus RG. Histology of high-energy pulsed CO_2 laser resurfacing. *Semin Cutan Med Surg*. 1996;15:189-193.

14. Fitzpatrick RE, Smith SR, Sriprachya-anunt S. Depth of vaporization and the effect of pulse stacking with a high energy, pulsed carbon dioxide laser. *J Am Acad Dermatol*. 1999;40:615-622.

15. Alster TS. Cutaneous resurfacing with CO_2 and Erbium: YAG lasers: preoperative, intraoperative, and postoperative considerations. *Plast Reconstr Surg*. 1999;103:619-632.

16. Hruza GJ, Fitpatrick RE, Arndt KA, Dover JS. Lasers in skin resurfacing. In: Kaminer MK, Dover JS, Arndt KA, eds. *Atlas of Cosmetic Surgery*. Philadelphia, PA: WB Saunders; 2002: 328-350.

17. Ruiz-Esparza J. Barba Gomez JM. Long-term effects of one general pass laser resurfacing: a look at dermal tightening and skin quality. *Dermatol Surg*. 1999;25:169-173.

18. Batra RS, Ort RJ, Jacob C, Hobbs L, Arndt KA, Dover JS. Evaluation of silicone occlusive dressing after laser skin resurfacing. *Arch Dermatol*. 2001;137:1317-1321.

19. Batra RS. Ablative laser resurfacing—postoperative care. *Skin Therapy Lett*. 2004;9:6-9.

20. Lowe NJ, Lask G, Griffin ME. Laser skin resurfacing: pre and post treatment guidelines. *Dermatol Surg*. 1995;21:1017-1019.

21. Kaufman R, Hibst R. Pulsed erbium: YAG laser ablation in cutaneous surgery. *Lasers Surg Med*. 1996;19:324-330.

22. Walsh JT Jr, Deutsch TF. Erbium: YAG laser ablation of tissue measurement of ablation rates. *Lasers Surg Med*. 1989;24: 81-86.

23. Polnikorn N, Goldberg DT, Suwachinda A, et al. Erbium: YAG laser resurfacing in asians. *Dermatol Surg*. 1998;24:1303-1307.

24. Manaloto RMP, Alster TS. Erbium: YAG laser resurfacing for refractory melasma. *Dermatol Surg*. 1999;25:121-123.

25. Alster TS. Clinical and histologic evaluation of six Erbium: YAG lasers for cutaneous resurfacing. *Lasers Surg Med*. 1999;24: 87-92.

26. Alster TS, Lupton JR. Prevention and treatment of side effects and complications of cutaneous laser resurfacing. *Plast Reconstr Surg*. 2002;109:308-316.

27. Alster TS, Lupton JR. Erbium:YAG laser for cutaneous laser resurfacing. *Dermatol Clin*. 2001;19:453-466.

28. Alster TS, Doshi S. Laser skin resurfacing. In: Burgess CM, ed. *Cosmetic Dermatology*. Berlin, Germany: Springer; 2005:111-126.

29. Alster TS, Nann CA. Famciclovir prophylaxis of herpes simplex virus reactivations after laser skin resurfacing. *Dermatol Surg*. 1999;25(3):242-246.

30. Munavalli GS, Weiss RA, Halder RM. Photoaging and nonablative photorejuvenation in ethnic skin. *Dermatol Surg*. 2005;31: 1250-1261.

31. Chan HL, Kono T. Laser treatment in ethnic skin. In: Goldberg D, ed. *Procedures in Cosmetic Dermatology Series: Lasers and Lights,* vol. 2. Philadelphia, PA: WB Saunders Co; 2005:89-101.

32. Rahman Z, Alam M, Dover JS. Fractional laser treatment of pigmentation and texture improvement. *Skin Therapy Lett*. 2006;11(9):7-11.

33. Jeong JT, Kye YC. Resurfacing of pitted facial acne scars with a long pulsed Erbium: YAG laser. *Dermatol Surg*. 2001;27 (2):107-110.

34. Kilmer S, Fitzpatrick R, Bernstein E, Brown D. Long-term follow-up on the use of plasma skin regeneration (PSR) in full facial rejuvenation procedures. *Lasers Surg Med*. 2005;36 (Suppl 17):22.

35. Brody HJ, Monheit GD, Resnik SS, Alt TH. A history of chemical peeling. *Dermatol Surg.* 2000;26:405-409.

36. Brody H. History and classification of chemical peels. In: Patterson AN, ed. *Chemical Peeling*, 1st ed. St. Louis, MO: Mosby; 1992:7-22.

37. Grimes PE. The safety and efficacy of salicylic acid chemical peels in darker racial ethnic groups. *Dermatol Surg.* 1999;25: 18-22.

38. Roberts WE. Chemical peeling in ethnic/dark skin. *Dermatol Ther.* 2004;17:196-205.

39. Brody HJ. Skin resurfacing: chemical peels. In: Freedberg IM, Eisen AZ, Wolf K, eds. *Fitzpatrick's Dermatology in General Medicine*, 6th ed. New York: McGraw-Hill; 2003:2530-2535.

40. Bourelly PE, Lotsikas-Baggill AJ. Chemoexfoliation and superficial skin resurfacing. In: Burgess CM, ed. *Cosmetic Dermatology*. Berlin, Germany: Springer; 2005:53-83.

41. Mendelsohn JE. Update on chemical peels. *Otolaryngol Clin North Am.* 2002;35(1):55-72.

42. Resnik SS, Resnik BJ. Complications of chemical peeling. *Dermatol Clin.* 1995;13(2):309-312.

43. Gold MH. A controlled clinical trial of topical silicone gel sheeting in the treatment of hypertrophic scarring and keloids. *J Am Acad Dermatol.* 1994;30:506-507.

44. Monheit GD, Chastain MA. Chemical peels. *Facial Plast Surg Clin North Am.* 2001;9(2):239-255.

45. Monheit GD, Zeitouni NC. Skin resurfacing for photoaging: laser resurfacing versus chemical peeling. *Cosmet Dermatol.* 1997;10(4):11-22.

46. Koch RJ, Hanasono M. Microdermabrasion. *Facial Plast Surg Clin North Am.* 2001;9(3):377-382.

47. Tan M, Spencer J, et al. The evaluation of aluminum oxide crystal microdermabrasion. *Dermatol Surg.* 2001;27: 943-949.

48. Grimes PE. Microdermabrasion. *Dermatol Surg.* 2005;31: 1160-1165.

49. Morgenstern KE, Foster J. Advances in cosmetic oculoplastic surgery. *Curr Opin Ophthalmol.* 2002;13:324-330.

50. Shelton RM. Prevention of cross-contamination when using microdermabrasion equipment. *Cutis.* 2003;72:266-268.

CHAPTER 10

Hair Removal in Ethnic Skin: Laser, Lights, and Medical and Mechanical Epilation

Roopal V. Kundu, MD

INTRODUCTION

Many men and women elect to remove unwanted body and facial hair for cosmetic, cultural, social, or medical reasons. There are two main medical causes for excessive hair: hirsutism and hypertrichosis. Hirsutism is characterized by an androgen-dependent hair pattern with excessive and increased body and facial terminal hair distributed in a male pattern.[1] It can be idiopathic or genetic in origin; however there are medical conditions that can cause hirsutism (Table 10.1).

Hypertrichosis is a condition of excessive hair that is not influenced by androgens.[2] It can be an adverse effect of drug administration such as cyclosporine, minoxidil, or phenytoin (Table 10.2) or an underlying medical condition such as porphyria cutanea tarda, thyroid disorders, or malnutrition/anorexia. Primary hypertrichosis has been classified based on the age of onset (congenital or acquired) and the extent of distribution (localized or generalized forms).[2]

A medical investigation to elicit the cause of excessive hair should be conducted prior to or in conjunction with treating the unwanted hair. There are several medical conditions associated with hirsutism (Table 10.1). Patients who may have any underlying medical condition leading to hirsutism may also suffer from seborrhea, acne, androgenetic alopecia, irregular menses, or virilization.[1] Rapid onset of hirsutism or other signs of androgen excess should prompt a hormonal evaluation, including levels of free and bioavailable testosterone and dehydroepiandrosterone-sulfate (DHEA-S), to rule out the presence of an androgen-secreting tumor. When underlying disease is suspected, it is advisable to work in conjunction with the primary care physician and/or a specialist if indicated (i.e., gynecologist and/or endocrinologist for polycystic ovary syndrome).

In people of color, there are other medical indications for hair removal, including but not limited to pseudofolliculitis barbae (PFB) (Figure 10.1), acne keloidalis nuchae (AKN) (Figure 10.2), and dissecting cellulites (Figure 10.3). Finally, facial or body hair in excess of the cultural norm can be very distressing to some patients and is more commonly seen in some ethnic subgroups, such as South Asians.

The current available treatment methods for masking and removal of excessive hair include bleaching, trimming, waxing, physical and chemical depilatories, electrolysis, intense pulsed light (IPL) therapy, and laser hair reduction (Table 10.3). Each method has its own advantages and limitations. This chapter will further discuss the different methods for hair removal paying particular attention to the nuances of treatment in people of color.

TEMPORARY HAIR MASKING

▨ Bleaching

Bleaching is an inexpensive method used to disguise unwanted hair. It is quick, easy, and painless process that removes natural hair pigment partially or totally, lightening the hair to a yellowish hue.[3] The active ingredient is hydrogen peroxide, which softens and oxidizes the hair. Bleaching can last up to 4 weeks. Common sites for bleaching include the upper lip, beard area, and arms. Multiple commercial bleaches are available. It is strongly advisable to apply the bleach to a test site to assess for contact dermatitis. The disadvantages of this method include skin irritation, temporary skin discoloration, and pruritus. Furthermore, this method is problematic in people of color because of the prominence of the yellow-toned bleached hair when viewed against the skin of a more darkly pigmented person.

▨ Trimming

Trimming of the hair is a recommended option for persons with either localized or diffuse hypertrichosis or hirsutism, and especially for those prone to PFB, AKN, and dyschromia. Close trimming can also be an effective alternative to shaving while patients are undergoing a laser hair reduction treatment protocol. Trimming involved areas will make the hair less noticeable and will not alter the innate patterns of hair regrowth. The main limitations to this technique are the length of time involved to trim large areas of excessive hair and the lack of a smooth, hair-free surface after trimming is complete.

TEMPORARY HAIR REMOVAL

▨ Physical Depilation and Epilation

Physical depilation includes shaving or any one of the multiple forms of epilation.[4] Epilation involves the removal of the entire hair shaft and comprises the most effective group of methods for temporarily removing hair. Epilation involves tweezing or plucking, waxing, threading, abrasives, sugaring, and the use of mechanical devices.[4] For this method to be effective, treated hairs should be long enough to be grasped by the device used, typically several millimeters in length at minimum. Repetitive epilation leads to wounding of the hair follicle and may result in permanent matrix damage, with the end result possibly being finer or thinner hairs.

▨ Shaving

Shaving is the most frequently used method to temporarily remove unwanted hair. It is fast, easy, painless, effective, and inexpensive. The main limitation is that the results are temporary, lasting from

TABLE 10.1 ▪ Medical Conditions Associated with Hirsutism

Polycystic ovary syndrome
Congenital adrenal hyperplasia
Androgen-secreting neoplasms
Cushing's syndrome
HAIR-AN syndrome (hyperandrogenism, insulin resistance, and acanthosis nigricans)

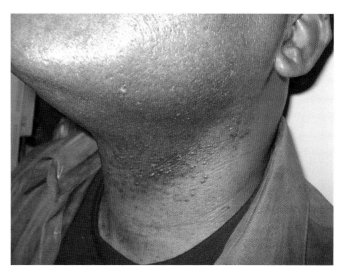

Figure 10.1 *PFB with postinflammatory hyperpigmentation in an African American male. Perifollicular hyperpigmented and erythematous papules on the cheek and neck*

only 1 to 3 days, and require a continual commitment to maintain a hair-free appearance. In persons of color, further limitations occur in those patients who are prone to folliculitis and PFB that can eventually lead to postinflammatory hyperpigmentation, dyschromia, and/or scarring. Shaving is performed on wet skin with a razor blade. Shaving cream or other lubricants are often used to decrease trauma to the skin in the form of nicks, cuts, and folliculitis and is advocated for darker skinned patients. Shaving is typically done against the grain of the hair growth in order to achieve a close, smooth shave. Again, in those patients prone to PFB, alternative shaving instructions are often advised including shaving in the direction of hair growth and shaving less frequently if possible. Since dry or electric shaves are not as close as wet shaves, a dry electric razor is often recommended to treat patients with PFB.

Contrary to popular belief, shaving does not affect the width or rate of regrowth of individual hairs,[5] but the hairs as they grow out are thicker and coarser, without the finer tapered end of unshaven hair. As a result, daily shaving must often be undertaken or the cosmetic result is worsened. Certain areas of excessive hair, such as the legs, may be amenable to daily shaving. Males also have the option of shaving excess hair on the beard and mustache regions, but this may be unacceptable psychologically for women. Often women of color who begin to shave excess facial hair develop PFB that only leads to more frustration with the addition of dyschromia, acneiform papules, and scarring to the baseline problem of excessive hair.

▪ Tweezing or Plucking

Tweezing is an effective temporary hair removal method, but it is a slow, tedious, and painful process. It is best used for removing an occasional coarse hair or small group of hairs such as on the eyebrows, chin, or periareola. Plucking often leads to a longer-lasting

TABLE 10.2 ▪ Medications Associated with Excessive Hair

Acetazolamide
Cyclosporine
Diazoxide
Glucocorticosteroids
Hormonal therapy
Immunosuppressives
L-thyroxine
Minoxidil
Penicillamine
Phenytoin
Psoralens (trimethylpsoralen, methoxypsoralen)
Streptomycin

result than shaving as hair is pulled from the hair shaft as in waxing. However, this temporary method often only tears off anagen hair bulbs in varying break patterns allowing for regrowth of the hair follicles. Complete removal of the follicular bulb including both the matrix epithelium and papilla rarely occurs.[6] For persons of color, plucking may be a feasible option for very localized areas of increased hair growth but too demanding for diffuse hair growth. Adverse reactions are common in this patient population and include hyperpigmentation, folliculitis, scarring, ingrown hairs, and distorted follicles.[7] The results of this form of depilation can last up to 4 weeks, but is particularly transient in these patients with hypertrichosis, leading to rapid hair regrowth within a week or two.

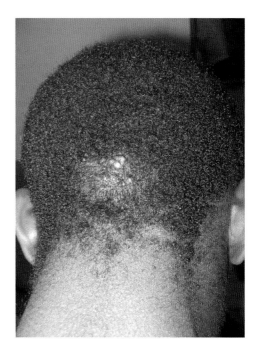

Figure 10.2 *AKN in an African male. Firm, flesh-colored to hyperpigmented papules over the posterior scalp and neck*

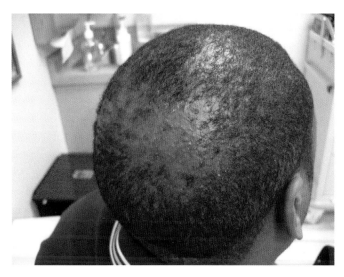

Figure 10.3 *Dissecting cellulitis in an African American male. Residual large patches of scar and alopecia after the inflammatory active phase of disease*

Waxing and Sugaring

Wax epilation is a painful process for the removal of either fine vellus hair or terminal hair. Waxing methods are used with cold, warm, or hot wax. After the hairs become embedded into the hardened wax, it is quickly stripped off against the direction of hair growth. If the hair root is successfully extracted, a soft regrowth typically occurs within 3 to 5 weeks. All areas of the body, excluding genital regions, can be treated with waxing methods. Waxing causes greater discomfort and is more expensive than shaving. Other possible adverse effects include skin irritation and folliculitis.[8] Another drawback of this epilating technique includes the requirement for the hair to be a minimum length of 2 to 3 mm to be grasped by the wax. Therefore, no other hair removal methods may be used for several days prior to waxing.[9] It is often recommended that patients using systemic retinoids, such as isotretinoin or soriatane, avoid waxing until treatment has been discontinued for at least 6 months to 1 year to avoid tearing of the skin and scarring. This is particularly prudent advice in patients of color that may be genetically predisposed to hypertrophic scarring and/or keloid formation. Waxing should also be avoided on skin being treated with topical retinoids, along with skin that is irritated or inflamed.

Sugaring is an alternative to waxing that has been in use for thousands of years, commonly in the Middle East. Sugaring paste is prepared by heating sugar, lemon juice, and water. The paste is then applied to the skin and quickly stripped away,[10] ideally entirely removing the hair from the hair shaft. This is a common at-home alternative is used in many Middle Eastern and Southeast Asian communities and in those people who are sensitive to wax. Premade sugar wax kits may also be purchased from manufacturers. The risk and benefits are similar to those of waxing.

Threading

Threading is a popular hair removal technique used in Arabic countries and India. It involves the use of a long, twisted loop of thread that is rotated rapidly across the base of the visible hair shaft. The twisted string first entraps the hairs and then they are pulled or broken off. Side effects are similar to plucking. It is becoming a more popular technique here in the United States, especially for eyebrow shaping and definition. The advantages to this method include less cutaneous irritation, lower cost, and shorter treatment time. The limitations of this method are pain during the procedure, risk of folliculitis, and transient local cutaneous reactions such as pruritus, erythema, edema, and dyspigmentation.[11]

Abrasives

Abrasives, such as pumice stones and devices made of fine sandpaper, physically rub the hair away from the skin surface. This method is irritating and uncomfortable. In darker skinned persons, it can lead to a secondary problem of irritant dermatitis and postinflammatory hyper- or hypopigmentation (Figure 10.4).

Chemical Depilation

Chemical depilatories contain sulfides, enzymatic depilatory agents, and/or thioglycolates. They break down hair by cleaving its cysteine linkages and disrupting sulfide bonds of hair keratin[12] and cause minimal damage to the underlying skin. Sulfides are quick, easy, and effective, but the generated hydrogen sulfide releases an unpleasant odor and can often irritate the skin. Enzymatic depilatory agents do not have the offensive odor and are nonirritating, but they are not as effective.

Most commercially available chemical depilatories, as a result, consist of thioglycolates (sodium or calcium). Thioglycolates are less odiferous and less irritating, but require a longer time to act than the sulfide-based depilatories. They can be used in more

TABLE 10.3 ■ Hair Removal Treatment Modalities

Temporary masking	Temporary reduction	Temporary removal	Permanent reduction	Permanent removal
Bleaching	Vaniqa®	Abrasives	Laser	Electrolysis
Trimming	(eflornithine HCL 13.9%)	Depilatories	Diode	Galvanic
		Plucking	Long-pulse ruby	Thermolysis
		Shaving	Alexandrite	Blend
		Sugaring	Long-pulse	
		Tweezing	Nd:YAG	
		Waxing	IPL	

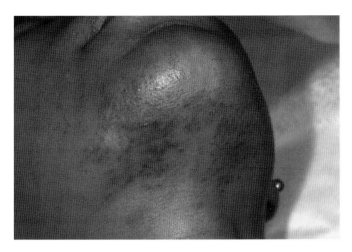

Figure 10.4 *Hirsutism and irritant dermatitis from an abrasive used for hair removal with postinflammatory hyperpigmentation in an African female. Hyperpigmented papules coalescing into plaques with increased terminal hair over the chin and neck*

sensitive areas, such as the face, and work best on fine vellus hair of at least moderate length. These agents should not be used on eyebrows, near mucous membranes, or on broken skin. They are available as gels, creams, lotions, aerosols, or roll-ons.

The use of chemical depilatories is limited as a result of several disadvantages: (1) suitable for small areas only, (2) association with a risk of allergic contact dermatitis, (3) messy application, (4) unpleasant odor, (5) relatively expensive, especially if treating larger areas, and most importantly (6) localized cutaneous irritation which is a well-known and common potential adverse reaction, especially if applied for longer than indicated.[13] Other side effects include burns, folliculitis, ingrown hairs, and allergic contact dermatitis to either the thioglycolate or fragrances. Therefore, it is advisable to apply the chemical depilatory to a test site first, closely adhere to the manufacturer's instructions particularly the recommended time limitations, wash the treated area thoroughly after application is complete, and follow with the use of a moisturizer.

Temporary Hair Reduction

A novel method for retarding excessive hair growth (not removing hair) is Vaniqa® (eflornithine hydrochloride 13.9%) cream, which irreversibly inhibits ornithine decarboxylase, an enzyme present in hair follicles that is important in hair growth.[14] When this enzyme is blocked by the medication, metabolic activity in the hair follicle decreases, and hairs grow in more slowly. Twice daily application reduced excessive, unwanted facial hair compared with vehicle treatment.[14] Side effects have been limited to local irritation, characterized by burning, stinging, and/or tingling.[15] Improvement is typically seen after 4 to 8 weeks of treatment. After stopping treatment, hair growth approaches pretreatment levels within 8 weeks. Since Vaniqa® does not remove hair, it should be used in conjunction with other epilation methods. It has recently been shown to lead to a more rapid and complete reduction of unwanted facial hair in women for up to 6 months when used in combination with laser hair reduction.[16] Long-term follow-up studies have not been

conducted to date. Vaniqa® is classified as pregnancy category C and should not be used during pregnancy.

Permanent Hair Removal

Permanent hair removal methods include electrolysis, also called electrology. Electrolysis, a permanent hair removal technique, can be accomplished by 1 of the 3 following methods: galvanic, thermolysis, or blend.[7] For all methods, multiple treatment sessions are required in order to achieve a clinically significant result.

Proper technique is critical for the successful use of electrolysis: accurate needle insertion, appropriate intensities and durations of current. Correct needle insertion is more difficult in people of color who have curved hair follicles, which is commonly seen in African and African American persons. Since many of these procedures are not performed in physician offices, it is imperative to advise patients of their potential side effects: scarring (both atrophic and keloidal), postinflammatory hypopigmentation or hyperpigmentation, pain, and local cutaneous infections.

The main disadvantage of electrolysis is the associated pain. Although preapplication of ice packs or topical anesthetics, such as a eutectic mixture of 2.5% lidocaine and 2.5% prilocaine hydrochloride (EMLA®) or 4% topical lidocaine (LMX®) may decrease discomfort, electrolysis is often poorly tolerated. Other adverse effects include transient postinflammatory erythema and whealing, bruising, swelling, and, in darker-skinned patients, postinflammatory hyperpigmentation.[7]

Galvanic Electrolysis

In galvanic electrolysis, a direct electric current is delivered to the hair follicle through an inserted needle. The current produces sodium hydroxide (lye), a caustic agent that destroys the hairbulb and dermal papilla.[17] This modality is the most effective, but the slowest, sometimes requiring a minute or more for each hair with repeated insertion into the follicle.

Thermolysis

In thermolysis, a high-frequency alternating current produces heat in the follicular tissue causing destruction of the hair bulb.[17] This method is quick, requiring only a few seconds per hair, but not as effective in thick hairs or in highly curved hair follicles, such as in African American hair.

Blend

The blend method combines galvanic electrolysis and thermolysis, and is the most efficient electrolysis technique.[7] The best result occurs if the area is shaved several days before epilation so that only anagen hairs are epilated. Permanent hair removal can occur only if the needle is inserted deep into the follicle, enabling the current to travel to the germinative bulb.[18] Hair is not an electrical conductor and cannot transmit an electrical current to the hair bulb. Therefore, the commercially promoted home electric tweezer method does not produce permanent hair removal.[7] These devices more likely represent a temporary hair removal method, similar to waxing or plucking.

Permanent Hair Reduction

Laser therapy (alexandrite, diode, neodymium:YAG, and ruby lasers) and IPL therapy are the newest available permanent hair removal systems.[19] Laser technology was developed to efficiently remove unwanted facial and body hair over large areas of skin with as few complications as possible. Although this treatment modality is considerably more expensive than electrolysis, it is faster and arguably less painful. Darker skin types are more difficult to treat, but can still be treated. Electrolysis remains the only proven method for permanent hair removal; however laser-assisted hair reduction is quickly becoming the treatment of choice. Studies have shown that this method can lead to permanent removal of some hairs along with markedly delayed growth of others.

These techniques remove unwanted hair through the principle of selective photothermolysis[20] of melanin-rich structures, allowing light energy absorption primarily in hair follicles and minimal absorption by surrounding tissues. When melanin in the hair follicle absorbs the laser light energy, the hair follicle is heated and destroyed, preventing its ability to produce new hair while leaving other skin structures unharmed. This hair removal system is most successful for dark, coarse hair, with decreased efficacy for fine vellus hair, and little to no efficacy for white or gray hair. Treatments result in significant clearance of excess hair, with the neck, chin, and lip as common requested areas of treatment.

Laser therapy in pigmented skin poses several challenges because of the constant competing chromophore of melanin. The key components of treating skin of color are laser and laser setting choice. There are multiple laser and light sources currently available for the treatment of unwanted hair: IPL, long-pulsed ruby, alexandrite, diode, and long-pulse Nd:YAG.[21] The optimal wavelength, pulse duration, and fluence to provide both safe and permanent long-term hair reduction are under continual investigation. However, the ideal patient for laser-assisted hair reduction has light skin and dark hair leading to this patient profile most commonly chosen for laser studies. Since darker-skinned patients have more competing melanin in the surrounding structures, they are prone to experience more side effects. To date, in darker skinned patients, particular Fitzpatrick skin phototype V and VI, the longer wavelength lasers, in particular the long-pulse Nd:YAG is the laser of choice.[22]

Expected Benefits

The average number of laser treatments needed to achieve a significant reduction of excess hair is between five and six treatments performed in 1- to 3-month intervals. The number of treatments needed to obtain the best results for different anatomic sites is unknown. However, anecdotal evidence reveals that certain areas may require more treatments such as the axilla, bikini area, and beard area in men. Maintenance treatments ranging from every 6 months to 1 year are typically needed to maintain hair reduction. Expected outcomes can be summarized as fewer hairs, thinner hairs, slower regrowing hairs, and lighter hairs.

An average of 20% to 25% hair loss can be expected with each treatment, with a goal for long-term hair reduction of approximately 70% to 80%. It should be stressed to all patients that the removal of all hair is unlikely.

Patient Interviews

In order to achieve optimal success, a thorough patient history should be obtained. Discussion of patient expectations, previous hair removal strategies, dermatological history, local infections, history of scarring, medications, recent sun exposure, hobbies or habits which might interfere with treatment, and assessment of the etiology of excessive hair should be performed.

A discussion of previously used hair removal strategies, including types, effectiveness, and side effects, can help set the stage for patient expectations and outcomes. Patients with dermatological diseases such as vitiligo and psoriasis should be warned of the risk of koebnerization following laser surgery. Thus far, this is primarily a theoretical risk and clinically rarely seen. Patients with active cutaneous infections should not be treated. Patients with a history of recurrent staphylococcal and herpes simplex infections can be started on appropriate prophylaxis to diminish the likelihood of an outbreak. Patients with a history of hypertrophic scarring or keloids can be treated, but should be done so conservatively to minimize risk of burn or blister formation. It is advisable to wait a minimum of 6 to 12 months after completion of an isotretinoin course before undergoing cosmetic hair removal treatment. Recently tanned patients should delay cosmetic laser hair reduction treatment as a result of the increased risk of dyschromia from the recently stimulated and activated melanocytes. Patients with underlying etiologies for excessive hair (i.e., medication use or hormonal stimulation) should be advised that hair removal may not be as effective.[23]

Pretreatment Counseling

Pretreatment instructions for patients include refraining from any epilating hair removal techniques for a minimum of 1 to 2 weeks prior to treatment. Trimming is the ideal alternative during this time period, although shaving and bleaching are acceptable alternatives.

For all patients, especially those of skin of color, pretreatment with broad-spectrum sunscreen and/or sun avoidance is recommended for at least 2 weeks prior to laser treatment. In addition, a bleaching cream containing hydroquinone, may also be considered for those prone to postinflammatory hyperpigmentation.

The patient should be instructed to shave or trim the area to be treated the day of or day before laser treatment. A depilatory cream can also be used instead if care is taken not to irritate the skin.

Day of Treatment

The area to be treated should be clean and free of make-up. Laser hair removal is not a painless procedure. Most patients experience some discomfort during and immediately after treatment. A topical anesthetic can be used 1 to 2 hours prior to treatment to reduce these effects. Preapplication of topical anesthetics, such as a eutectic mixture of 2.5% lidocaine and 2.5% prilocaine hydrochloride (EMLA®) or 4% lidocaine (LMX®) may be applied.[24] Careful instruction to avoid overuse of topical anesthetics over large body surface areas is imperative to avoid risk of lidocaine toxicity.

Treatment Strategy

The long-pulse Nd:YAG has proven to be the best laser choice for darker pigmented skins[22,25] Other devices including the diode laser[26] using long pulse durations[27] and long-pulsed alexandrite[28] have also been effective. IPL can also be used for hair removal in various skin types (I to V) but often requires more treatment sessions and has a higher risk of dyspigmentation in the darkest skinned patients.[29] Therefore, it is advisable to become familiar with a long-pulse Nd:YAG laser device in order to treat all darker-skinned patients. There are multiple laser devices available and the individual manufacturer's instructions should be carefully reviewed. There is relatively reduced melanin absorption at these higher wavelengths which necessitates the need for higher fluences in order to adequately damage hair. However, the poorer melanin absorption at this wavelength coupled with epidermal cooling device makes the long pulsed Nd:YAG a safer laser treatment for darker skin types. The important targets for permanent hair follicle destruction are the follicular stem cells located in the hair bulge, near the attachment of the arrector pili muscle, approximately 1.5 mm below the epidermis. Therefore, the use of long pulse width 1064 nm Nd:YAG laser in darker skin types is further supported because it can penetrate deeper into the dermis to ideally reach the whole length of the hair follicle and is expected to produce sufficient follicular injury for a more persistent hair reduction. This can be done with less epidermal damage in patients with darker skin types compared to shorter wavelength laser and light systems.[29]

A treatment grid can be applied in order to provide an outline of the area to be treated. In the absence of a grid, careful attention must be paid to prevent double treatment and skipped areas.

Ideal treatment parameters must be individualized for each patient. For further epidermal protection in darker skinned patients, utilizing longer pulse durations (minimum 30 ms) and optimal cooling is recommended. Laser units equipped with cooling tip devices are best, especially those with embedded sapphire cooling plates (Figure 10.5). Although some devices have cryogen spray incorporated, this may lead to further dyschromia in darker-skinned patient and should be used cautiously. With or without a cooling device, a thick layer of cooled gel should be applied before delivery of the

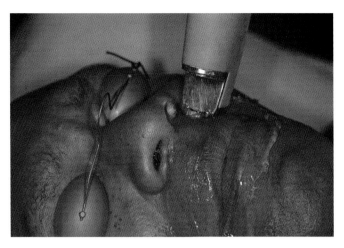

Figure 10.6 *Laser treatment. Firm pressure should be applied during the laser hair reduction treatment.*

laser pulse. Prior to pulse delivery, the hand piece is pressed firmly against the skin and special attention should be paid to adequately precool every treatment site, including the first pulse administered (Figure 10.6). The hand piece should be wiped clean periodically to remove debris. Between patients, disinfection of the hand piece is mandatory.

With most lasers available for laser hair reduction in darker skinned patients, performing test sites at inconspicuous areas is crucial. The maximum fluence tolerated is determined by the epidermal pigmentation. The treatment fluence is carefully increased while the skin is observed for signs of acute epidermal injury, such as whitening, blistering, or ablation. Slightly overlapping (approximately 10% overlap vertically and horizontally) laser pulses should be delivered with a predetermined spot size. It is recommended that the largest spot size and the highest tolerable, safe fluence are used to obtain best results.

The ideal immediate response is vaporization of the hair shaft with no other apparent effect. After a few minutes, perifollicular edema and erythema may appear and should last no more than a few hours (Figure 10.7). If this is pronounced or there is sign of epidermal damage, the fluence should be reduced.

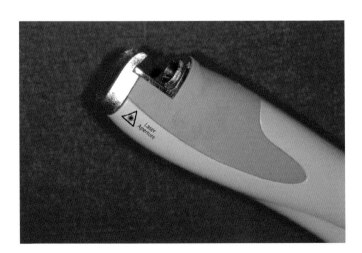

Figure 10.5 *Laser hand piece. A cooling plate that is a fixed part of the laser hand piece is recommended*

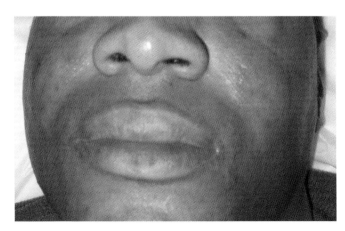

Figure 10.7 *Posttreatment erythema. Erythema and perifollicular edema over the beard area in a skin phototype IV mixed ethnicity male*

▨ PostTreatment Counseling

Patients can cleanse with cool water to remove gel and cool the skin. Ice packs reduce postoperative pain and minimize edema. Analgesics are not typically required. Prophylactic courses of antivirals should be completed when indicated. Topical antibiotic ointment should be applied twice daily if any epidermal injury occurred. Any trauma (i.e., picking or scratching) should be avoided, especially for those patients with PFB or preexisting dyschromia. Direct sun exposure should be avoided and sunblock used daily for a minimum of 2 weeks posttreatment. Routine skin care and make-up regimen may be resumed the day following treatment unless blistering or crusting develops. The damaged hair is often shed during the first weeks after treatments. Patients should be reminded that this is not a sign of hair regrowth.

Retreatment typically occurs in 1 to 3 months and can be performed as soon as regrowth appears, which follows the natural hair cycle and varies by anatomic location (Figure 10.8).

▨ Side Effects, Complications, and Special Considerations

Patient education in the form of benefits, risks, treatment procedure, realistic expectations, time course and importance of long-term follow-up are critical for a successful patient–physician relationship.

With particular regards to skin of color, patients should be advised that there is an inherent increased risk of scarring, dyspigmentation, and failure of response especially if appropriate fluences cannot be safely reached. In addition, recent reports indicate the rare induction of hair growth after laser hair removal.[30,31] This was found to occur in young female patients with skin types III-IV of Mediterranean ancestry who were undergoing treatment for fine vellus hairs on the cheeks and neck. Laser-induced hypertrichosis typically occurred in adjacent nontreated zones and was effectively treated with further laser treatments. Although the mechanism is not understood for this side effect, patients should be advised of the possibility prior to treatments, especially those requesting treatment of fine vellus hairs on the face and neck.

Transient pigmentary changes are one of the most common side effects in darker skin types or when patients have had a recent tan. Permanent pigmentary changes are less common and can be prevented if the ideal patient and treatment fluences are chosen. Scarring is rare except in cases of overaggressive treatment or postoperative infection. Other side effects include posttreatment erythema, edema, blisters, and crusting.

Sun protection and avoidance of tanning should be advised strongly before, during, and after the treatment series.

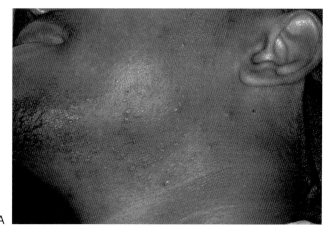

A

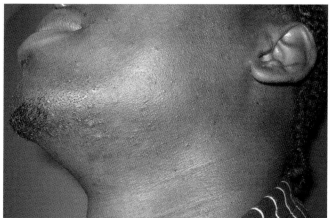

B

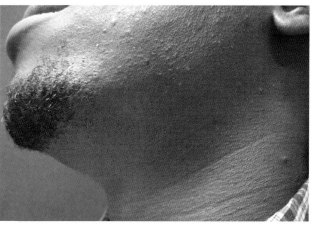

C

Figure 10.8 *PFB. A Fitzpatrick skin phototype V patient (A) prior to laser hair reduction, (B) 1 month after one treatment with long-pulse Nd:YAG (30 J, 30 ms, 1 Hz, 10-mm spot size), and (C) 4 months after three monthly treatments with long-pulse Nd:YAG*

Regardless of skin phototype, patients should not be treated within the orbital rim to avoid risk of ocular injury.[32] Proper eye protection must be worn by the patient and operating personnel at all times.

SUMMARY

Temporary and permanent methods of hair removal and reduction are an important component in the management of patients with unwanted hair. No one method is ideal for all patients. A medical investigation for underlying problems should always be conducted. Other factors including size and location of treatment area, cost of treatment, and expertise of the technician must be considered when choosing a method for hair removal.

REFERENCES

1. Essah PA, Wickham EP III, Nunley JR, et al. Dermatology of androgen-related disorders. *Clin Dermatol.* 2006;24:289.

2. Wendelin DS, Pope DN, Mallory SB. Hypertrichosis. *J Am Acad Dermatol.* 2003;48:161.

3. Wagner RF Jr. Physical methods for the management of hirsutism. *Cutis.* 1990;45:319.

4. Ramos-e-Silva M, de Castro MC, Carneiro LV Jr. Hair removal. *Clin Dermatol.* 2001;19:437.

5. Lynfield YL, Macwilliams P. Shaving and hair growth. *J Invest Dermatol.* 1970;55:170.

6. Bassukas ID, Hornstein OP. Effects of plucking on the anatomy of the anagen hair bulb. A light microscopic study. *Arch Dermatol Res.* 1989;281:188.

7. Richards RN, Meharg GE. Electrolysis: observations from 13 years and 140,000 hours of experience. *J Am Acad Dermatol.* 33:6621995

8. Richards RN, Uy M, Meharg G. Temporary hair removal in patients with hirsutism: a clinical study. *Cutis.* 1990;45:199.

9. Olsen EA. Methods of hair removal. *J Am Acad Dermatol.* 1999;40:143.

10. Tannir D, Leshin B. Sugaring: an ancient method of hair removal. *Dermatol Surg.* 2001;27:309.

11. Scott MJ Jr, Scott MJ III, Scott AM. Epilation. *Cutis.* 1990; 46:216.

12. Klein AW, Rish DC. Depilatory and shaving products. *Clin Dermatol.* 1988;6:68.

13. Vashi RA, Mancini AJ, Paller AS. Primary generalized and localized hypertrichosis in children. *Arch Dermatol.* 2001; 137:877.

14. Balfour JA, McClellan K. Topical eflornithine. *Am J Clin Dermatol.* 2001;2:197.

15. Hickman JG, Huber F, Palmisano M. Human dermal safety studies with eflornithine HCl 13.9% cream (Vaniqa), a novel treatment for excessive facial hair. *Curr Med Res Opin.* 2001;16:235.

16. Hamzavi I, Tan E, Shapiro J, et al. A randomized bilateral vehicle-controlled study of eflornithine cream combined with laser treatment versus laser treatment alone for facial hirsutism in women. *J Am Acad Dermatol.* 2007;57:54.

17. Kligman AM, Peters L. Histologic changes of human hair follicles after electrolysis: a comparison of two methods. *Cutis.* 1984;34:169.

18. Verdich J. A critical evaluation of a method for treatment of facial hypertrichosis in women. *Dermatologica.* 1984;168:87.

19. Haedersdal M, Gotzsche PC. Laser and photoepilation for unwanted hair growth. *Cochrane Database Syst Rev.* 2006: CD004684.

20. Anderson RR, Parrish JA. Selective photothermolysis: precise microsurgery by selective absorption of pulsed radiation. *Science.* 1983;220:524.

21. Goldberg DJ. Laser- and light-based hair removal: an update. *Expert Rev Med Devices.* 2007;4:253.

22. Lanigan SW. Incidence of side effects after laser hair removal. *J Am Acad Dermatol.* 2003;49:882.

23. McGill DJ, Hutchison C, McKenzie E, et al. Laser hair removal in women with polycystic ovary syndrome. *J Plast Reconstr Aesthet Surg.* 2007;60:426.

24. Guardiano RA, Norwood CW. Direct comparison of EMLA® versus lidocaine for pain control in Nd:YAG 1064 nm laser hair removal. *Dermatol Surg.* 2005;31:396.

25. Alster TS, Bryan H, Williams CM. Long-pulsed Nd: YAG laser-assisted hair removal in pigmented skin: a clinical and histological evaluation. *Arch Dermatol.* 2001;137:885.

26. Battle EF Jr, Hobbs LM. Laser-assisted hair removal for darker skin types. *Dermatol Ther.* 2004;17:177.

27. Greppi I. Diode laser hair removal of the black patient. *Lasers Surg Med.* 2001;28:150.

28. Garcia C, Alamoudi H, Nakib M, et al. Alexandrite laser hair removal is safe for Fitzpatrick skin types IV-VI. *Dermatol Surg.* 2000;26:130.

29. Goh CL. Comparative study on a single treatment response to long pulse Nd: YAG lasers and intense pulse light therapy for hair removal on skin type IV to VI—Is longer wavelengths lasers preferred over shorter wavelengths lights for assisted hair removal. *J Dermatolog Treat.* 2003;14:243.

30. Kontoes P, Vlachos S, Konstantinos M, et al. Hair induction after laser-assisted hair removal and its treatment. *J Am Acad Dermatol.* 2006;54:64.

31. Lolis MS, Marmur ES. Paradoxical effects of hair removal systems: a review. *J Cosmet Dermatol.* 2006;5:274.

32. Halkiadakis I, Skouriotis S, Stefanaki C, et al. Iris atrophy and posterior synechiae as a complication of eyebrow laser epilation. *J Am Acad Dermatol.* 2007;57:S4.

CHAPTER 11

Liposuction in Ethnic Skin

Murad Alam, MD

INTRODUCTION, DEFINITION, AND HISTORY

Liposuction, also referred to as "liposculpture," is a form of surgical "body contouring" that aims to reduce focal subcutaneous, suprafascial fat accumulation at various sites by transcutaneous vacuum-assisted extraction of fat particles through small punctures in the skin.

Liposuction was introduced to medicine in 1976 by Fischer, an otolaryngologist who pioneered the use of the hollow cannula. In France, Illouz and Fournier refined the process of liposuction, and their contributions included the "wet technique," or injection of hypotonic saline and hyaluronic acid prior to fat removal (Illouz)[1] and the criss-cross motion of cannulas for smooth contouring and syringe removal (Fournier).[2,3]

While the first liposuction in the United States was performed in 1982, a sea change occurred in 1987 with Jeffrey Klein's report that liposuction with local anesthesia alone could be safe and effective. The advent of so-called tumescent liposuction eliminated the need for pain control through general anesthesia or conscious sedation. Additionally, since tumescent anesthesia entailed intralesional infusion of an extremely dilute anesthetic solution of lidocaine with epinephrine (Table 11.1), the resulting vasoconstriction markedly reduced intraoperative blood loss, one of the major causes of complications during nontumescent liposuction. This refined procedure enjoyed growing popularity and authoritative reviews of tens of thousands of cases confirmed the safety of the procedure. Ostad et al.[4] demonstrated that a total dose of at least 55 mg/kg of body weight was not associated with any lidocaine toxicity.

In recent years, there have been concerns raised by some that liposuction may not be as safe as believed and this has led to a move to restrict liposuction to physicians licensed to perform this procedure in hospital operating rooms. However, these fears have not been borne out and tumescent liposuction continues to enjoy an unparalleled safety record when performed according to accepted protocols. Paradoxically, reports of mortality associated with liposuction have been exclusively associated with liposuction performed under general anesthesia or conscious sedation by nondermatologists.

In an era of minimally invasive, extremely safe, low-downtime cosmetic procedures, liposuction remains a timely and appropriate procedure. Unlike some minimally invasive procedures, however, liposuction is associated not with mild efficacy, but rather with dramatic cosmetic improvement. Up to several liters of fat aspirate can be removed in a single procedure. The cost-benefit tradeoff associated with liposuction is thus exceptionally favorable.

LITERATURE REVIEW/EVIDENCE-BASED SUMMARY

Since the cosmetic efficacy of liposuction is both clinically obvious and difficult to measure by objective techniques, few high-quality studies on clinical efficacy and persistence are available. In general, appropriate patient selection is associated with maximal efficacy. Efficacy appears to be diminished when liposuction is performed on obese patients; patients with significant excess or thin skin; patients with little or no excess fat; and older adults or deconditioned patients.

The largest body of studies pertains to establishing parameters for safe liposuction, and for assessing the benefits of these in protecting patients. The safety of tumescent liposuction was already well accepted in 1995, when Hanke et al.[5] reviewed 15336 cases of liposuction performed by members of the American Society for Dermatologic Surgery. They found only minor complications, and no reports of death, pulmonary or fat embolism, hypovolemic shock, perforation of the peritoneum or thorax, or thrombophlebitis. In 1996, Ostad et al.[4] demonstrated on a cohort of 60 patients that a mean lidocaine dose of 55 mg/kg was not associated with lidocaine toxicity, whether assessed by subjective signs or plasma lidocaine levels (Table 11.2).

The low risk of liposuction under tumescent anesthesia was verified by a review of malpractice claims. Based on Physicians Insurance Association of America malpractice data from 1995 to 1997,[6] hospital-based liposuction was more than three times as likely to culminate in malpractice settlements, as was office-based liposuction. Fewer than 1% of liposuction claims settlements were found to be against dermatologists.

In 1999, a widely read article in the New England Journal of Medicine reported a series of so-called tumescent liposuction-related deaths more than a 5-year period in New York.[7] Notably, all four of the reported deaths were associated with so-called liposuction under general anesthesia or conscious sedation, and one was in a patient with severe coexisting morbidities and multiple interacting medications. As such, this case series did not provide any information regarding the safety of true tumescent liposuction technique under local anesthesia alone as pioneered and perfected by dermatologists.

Following the sensational and poorly understood report from the New England Journal of Medicine, the dermatologic surgery community embarked on additional studies to assess the safety of true tumescent liposuction and to try to allay the concerns of patients and policymakers. In 2000, Florida mandated all adverse events occurring in physician's offices be reported and Coldiron et al.[8] undertook a review of all such reports from 2000 to 2004. Among these, there were seven complications and five deaths associated with the use of intravenous sedation or general anesthesia, and liposuction and/or abdominoplasty under general anesthesia or intravenous sedation were the surgical procedures most commonly associated with complication and death. However, there were no adverse events associated with the use of dilute local (tumescent) anesthesia alone.

A study initiated by the Accreditation Association for Ambulatory Health Care Institute for Quality Improvement prospectively collected data from 688 patients undergoing tumescent liposuction at 39 centers between February 2001 and August 2002.[9] Patients were followed for 6 months after surgery to track any delayed

TABLE 11.1 ■ Recipe for Commonly Used Tumescent Anesthesia Concentrations*

Ingredient	Quantity	Final Concentration or pH
Normal saline (0.9%)	1 L	—
Lidocaine 2% (select one)	50 mL	0.1%
	37.5 mL	0.075%
	25 mL	0.05%
Epinephrine (1:1000)	1 mL	0.1%
Sodium bicarbonate (8.45%)	12.5 mL	pH 7.4
Triamcinolone acetonide (optional)	10 mg	—

*Different values for lidocaine dosage are *alternatives*. Only *one* of these quantities should be infused in any given bag of saline.

adverse events. Minor complications were found to occur at a rate of 0.57% and the major complication rate of 0.14% was accounted for single patient, who required hospitalization.

A mail survey of 517 dermatologic surgeons who were members of the American Society for Dermatologic Surgery in August 2001 elicited retrospective information on numbers of patients receiving liposuction, the operative setting, and associated complications for the period 1994 to 2000.[10] The overall response rate was 89%, of which 78% had performed liposuction procedures during the interval of interest. Based on a total of 66570 reported cases, the overall serious adverse event rate was 0.68 per 1000 cases. Complication rates were higher when intramuscular or intravenous sedation was used, as versus no or oral sedation. No deaths were reported. Detailed information was obtained for each reported complication.

Experienced physicians have adapted liposuction to their practices and minor differences in technique abound. However, certain studies clarify elements of technique that are now widely accepted. Many of these are described in the American Society for Dermatologic Surgery's recently updated guidelines of care for tumescent liposuction.

Recent papers suggest the utility of other technique modifications. Kaplan and Moy's[11] double-blind randomized crossover study in 1996 demonstrated that upon infusion into subcutaneous fat, local anesthetic warmed to 40°C elicited reduced pain com-

pared to room temperature anesthetic solution. Similar work by Yang et al.[12] in 2006 confirmed these results and also indicated a similar pain reduction benefit for neutral tumescent anesthesia with sodium bicarbonate added compared to nonneutralized solution.

While tumescent liposuction is most often performed with syringe suction or a mechanical aspirator, other approaches have met with variable success. Ultrasound-assisted liposuction, which was purported to be an improvement over standard mechanical suction, was one of the earliest such variations and has not been widely adopted by U.S. dermatologists. Lawrence and Cox (2000)[13] performed a randomized control trial comparing efficacy and safety of liposuction with such high-intensity continuous wave ultrasound to a placebo control of extremely low-intensity ultrasound and found no benefit of the therapeutic high-intensity ultrasound. More recently, power-assisted liposuction has been compared with traditional liposuction,[14-16] with the former found to be associated with briefer procedure times, less intraoperative and postoperative pain, diminished surgeon fatigue, increased rate of fat aspiration per minute, and reduced recovery time with lower incidence of ecchymoses and edema. Laser-assisted lipolysis is a very new technique in which an Nd:YAG or similar laser probe is introduced into the subcutis and used to melt fat.[17,18] Laser lipolysis may be effective for treatment of small pockets of fat or in combination with traditional suction liposuction for larger volume procedures.

The metabolic effects of tumescent technique and of liposuction continue to be studied. High-pressure injection of anesthetic solution does not appear to increase plasma levels or metabolic rate.[19] On the other hand, introduction of dilute epinephrine slows redistribution of lidocaine into the systemic circulation and delays the peak plasma concentration of lidocaine by more than 7 hours. This effect may be partly responsible for the exceptional safety of tumescent anesthesia. Specifically, the delay in absorption may permit some lidocaine to be preemptively removed from the subcutis by liposuction; moreover, the gradual rise to peak plasma levels may enable the development of systemic tolerance to high lidocaine plasma levels. Interestingly, when tumescent anesthesia is injected into the head and neck, some of this benefit may be lost.[20] Peak plasma lidocaine concentration after neck injection occurs in approximately 6 hours, compared to 12 hours after thigh injection.

CLINICAL EXAMINATION AND PATIENT HISTORY

Prior to liposuction, the following must be assessed: the patient's medical suitability for safe liposuction, the likelihood that the cosmetic deficit of concern will be addressed by the procedure envisioned, and the patient's mental state and expectations of the surgery.

Liposuction under tumescent anesthesia can be safely accomplished in most patients (Table 11.3), but there are some contraindications to treatment. Pregnancy is an absolute contraindication, and history and pregnancy tests should be obtained before surgery on women of childbearing age. Other relative contraindications include significant concurrent illness, including systemic immunosuppression, significant cardiovascular or neurovascular illness, bleeding disorders, hepatic disease, and wound healing

TABLE 11.2 ■ Recommended Maximum Total Tumescent Anesthesia Volumes (55 mg/kg Total Dose)

Body Weight		0.1% Solution (L)	0.075% Solution (L)
In kg	In lb		
40	88	2.2	2.9
50	110	2.7	3.7
60	132	3.3	4.4
70	154	3.8	5.1
80	176	4.4	5.9
90	198	4.9	6.6

TABLE 11.3 ■ **Patient Selection Criteria for Liposuction***

Category	Specific criterion
Medical fitness	Not pregnant or seeking to be pregnant
	Good general health
	Medications do not interact with tumescent anesthesia
	Absence of serious bleeding disorders or abnormalities
	Liver function within normal limits
	Immune status consistent with low risk of infection
Medical indication	Patient not obese
	Focal areas of fat excess
	Either satisfactory "snap test" OR patient amenable to postoperative skin excess or subsequent skin resection
	Targeted fat is not visceral fat
Emotional readiness	Reasonable expectations
	Patient accepts that perfect symmetry is not attainable
	Patient accepts that not all fat can or should be removed
	Patient accepts risks of mild, and rarely serious, adverse events.

*Contraindications are rarely absolute, and must be assessed in the context of the patient's overall welfare and safety.

diatheses. Numerous prior surgeries to the target site, such as multiple abdominal surgeries in a patient desiring abdominal liposuction or currently placed catheters or gastrointestinal devices, may also be contraindications, or at least strongly suggestive of a need to reduce the scope and intensity of any liposuction. Many but not all surgeons may request a preoperative complete blood count with differential and a comprehensive chemistry panel to confirm good general health. Coagulation parameters, hepatitis panels, liver function tests, and HIV tests may also be obtained.

Regarding the cosmetic deficit of interest, it is important that it be not only amenable to correction by liposuction, but also of salience to the patient. This distinction can be easily overlooked by an enthusiastic physician who is a novice at cosmetic dermatology. If there is an objectively obvious cosmetic deficit, such as bulging hips in an otherwise healthy, normal weight, and young person with good skin tone, a patient may be an excellent candidate for liposuction, but if the patient does not perceive this deficit as problematic, even the most technically skilled procedure will not meet with the patient's approval. As cosmetic procedures are inherently optional and designed to please and not save the patient, it is imperative to focus on correcting problems that the patient considers major and to relegate areas of secondary interest to subordinate status.

While liposuction is a safe procedure, there are associated risks and downtime that should be communicated to the patient. The procedure can last from an hour to several hours, and requires lidocaine and epinephrine injections followed by puncture inci-

sions to permit entry of cannulas. As such, the area undergoing liposuction will eventually display several small dot-like atrophic scars, which may be hypo- or hyperpigmented. Immediately after liposuction, significant swelling will result, with copious watery and serosanguinous drainage for at least 1 day. Widespread bruising to the treated site is inevitable, and may resolve gradually in 1 to 3 weeks. In the immediate aftermath of a liposuction procedure, reduction in apparent contour or girth is not evident and the area may even seem thicker or fuller. Only after several weeks will the contour improve, as fluid is resorbed, edema diminishes, and the subcutis contracts and readheres to the fascial layer. The evening following a liposuction procedure, patients should have a friend or family member staying with them or at least checking to make sure that they are doing well. Finally, patients who are unwilling to wear a support and compression garment to the treated site for several weeks after the procedure should be advised that this reluctance will diminish the efficacy of the procedure. It is often useful to provide patients contemplating a liposuction procedure with written material about liposuction, as well as a consent form. These documents should also encourage patients to preoperatively avoid unnecessary anticoagulants, such as alcohol, certain herbal medications, vitamin E, and self-prescribed nonsteroidal anti-inflammatory drugs. Patients who are unwilling to prepare appropriately for the liposuction procedure, or who cannot accede undergoing some of the key steps, should be dissuaded from continuing. In some cases, other procedures may be suggested as an alternative option.

GENERAL TREATMENT APPROACH

■ Dose Setting/Selection

Liposuction is performed similarly at various body sites. Concentrated (0.1%) tumescent fluid may be used at more sensitive body sites, and dilute fluid (0.05%-0.075%) at less sensitive sites. Total dose of lidocaine is usually adjusted in accordance with patient body weight to conform to a level of 55 mg/kg. Patients with skin of color may be more prone to hyperpigment or develop hypertrophic scars at puncture sites where cannulas are inserted. This risk is not mitigated by reducing the overall dose of lidocaine but may be addressed by minimizing the number of entry sites, concealing these in skin folds or other anatomic areas, and reducing skin trauma during liposuction to avoid spreading or tearing of skin apertures. Men may have more fibrous subdermal fat and also more total suprafascial fat thickness; this may require more aggressive infusion of anesthetic solution to prevent discomfort during suctioning, and also more aggressive suctioning during removal.

■ Treatment Technique (Table 11.4)

Prior to treatment, a detailed patient consultation should be conducted, as described above. At this point, it is appropriate to provide prescriptions for preoperative, intraoperative, and postoperative medications (Table 11.5). Drugs may include oral antibiotics, which are usually started several days or at least an hour before surgery; sedatives or analgesics to be used intraoperatively; and posttreatment pain medications.

TABLE 11.4 ■ **Major Procedural Steps in Tumescent Liposuction**

Obtain consent and prepare patient
    Review consent form and answer questions
    Provide patient with opportunity to decline procedure
    Mark patient skin, and have patient review examine markings in mirror
    Provide oral sedation, if any
Sterile prep and drape
Infuse tumescent solution
    Anesthetize and perforate entry sites
    Infuse tumescent solution 1 to 2 cm beyond feathering borders at multiple levels
    Reposition patient and repeat infusion from other entry sites
Aspirate fat
    Optional re-prep and drape
    Remove fat via criss-cross technique
    Observe and avoid danger zones
    Periodically pinch and palpate skin to ensure even and complete suctioning
    Usually, one side is suctioned, then the other; the process is repeated as needed
Prepare patient for discharge
    Clean patient skin, and apply dressings to entry sites
    Apply compression garments
    Review postoperative instructions
    Schedule follow-up appointment

Preoperative photographs, often front and side views, are obtained. Informed consent is obtained, and if so desired, the patient is premedicated with sedatives or analgesics, often oral diazepam. After discussion with the patient, and appreciation of which exact areas the patient is concerned about and which are feasible to treat, the sites to be treated are marked. A medium tip black permanent marker (e.g., Sharpie) can be used to demarcate areas that require active suctioning; areas that require light suctioning, or feathering or blending with the surrounding areas; and areas that should not be suctioned (Figure 11.1). Markers are also used to pinpoint entry sites, which are usually symmetrically placed on both sides of the body, and in such a manner as to enable easy suctioning, triangulation during suctioning, and optimal concealment of such sites after the procedure.

Thereafter, the patient is sterilely prepped and draped, and placed in a supine or prone position. A short, fine (e.g., 30-gauge, 0.5-in) needle attached to a small (e.g., 3 mL) syringe containing 0.1% to 2% lidocaine solution is then used to raise blebs at the sites of cannula entry. A no. 11 blade or other similar device (e.g., 1.5- to 2-mm punch biopsy instrument) is then used to make at each potential entry location a shallow stab incision 3 to 4 mm in length that is oriented along the relaxed skin tension lines. A spinal needle or blunt-tipped infusion cannula is inserted and infusion of tumescent fluid is begun. The fluid flows from the peristaltic pump, passive pressure cuff or large syringe into the subcutis.

To protect underlying structures, the insertion of the infusion cannula is initially vertical but then angled laterally as it is advanced. The cannula is advanced and retracted with full motions that ensure that the tip disgorging anesthetic covers the maximum radius and hence provides anesthetic to the largest possible area. Movement of the cannula should be gradual to allow adequate filling at each site. When the cannula is near withdrawn, it can then be redirected in a slightly different direction; in this manner, a round area around the cannula is infused. Redirection of the cannula should only be performed when the cannula is pulled back, because intrastroke redirection puts stress on the entry site, with the attendant risk of friction trauma, and also causes tenting and dimpling of the skin that may result in subsequent uneven suctioning. Several layers of fat including immediately subdermal, mid-fat, and deeper fat should all be infused since each of these will ultimately be suctioned. Rates of tumescent fluid delivery vary, but very high flow speeds may be antithetical to even and complete anesthesia, patient comfort, and conservation of anesthetic fluid. Common infusion rates are less than 100 mL/min with higher rates

TABLE 11.5 ■ **Oral Medications Frequently Used in Conjunction with Tumescent Liposuction**

Medication category	Specific types	Indication	When dosed
Antibiotics	Broad spectrum (cephalosporins, other)	Infection prevention	Starting before procedure and usually for several days
Sedatives	Benzodiazepines (diazepam, lorazepam, and other)	Intraoperative sedation, muscle relaxation	Immediately before procedure
Analgesics (if necessary)	Mild narcotics	Pain control	After surgery, usually for a brief course
Antinausea agents (if necessary)	Nonsteroidal agents (prochlorperazine, ondansetron)	Nausea reduction	After surgery, if patient experiences significant nausea
Vitamins	C, K, and multivitamins	Stress tolerance	Preoperatively (less commonly) recommended by a minority of surgeons

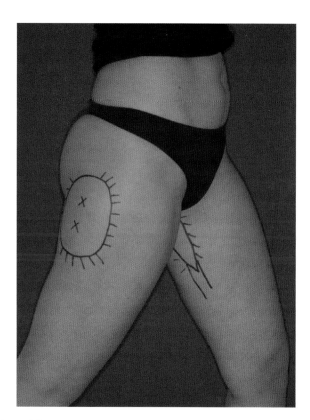

Figure 11.1 *Marking of areas of excess fat should be done before infusion of tumescent fluid, which can distort anatomy. Notations should be used to distinguish between dense fat pockets, smaller areas of fat removal, and regions at the periphery that require light feathering only. Discussion with the patient can increase the likelihood that areas of particular aesthetic concern are targeted*

tolerable, if the patient is relatively more sedated. A small degree of burning sensation is to be expected immediately upon starting infusion at a particular site, and this quickly diminishes. Especially when treating a larger area, it is important not to prematurely deplete the total allowable supply of tumescent fluid. After the fat has been infused adequately from one entry site, this cycle is repeated from the other sites. Horizontal and vertical criss-crossing of cannula paths from multiple sites is recommended to avoid missing areas that may then be painful during suctioning.

Delay required between infusion and suction varies according to anatomic site, and ranges from 15 to 45 minutes. Vasoconstriction may occur in as little as 15 minutes, but 30 to 45 minutes may be necessary for complete anesthesia, which enables precise and painstaking suctioning. Visible white blanch at the area to be treated is a good clinical indicator of adequacy of anesthesia.

If bilateral liposuction is being performed, fat removal commences on the side anesthetized first. Fat is removed from both areas of significant accumulation and from the edges of such areas. Feathering refers to the process of conservative fat removal from peripheral areas to create a smooth contour with the surrounding skin and prevent a precipitious drop-off at the edge of the fat pocket of interest. As with infiltration, full back and forth cannula movements are needed to ensure even fat removal and to avoid over suctioning at any one site. Continual manipulation of the

skin and subcutis is necessary to ensure that appropriate amounts of fat are being removed. Tactile feedback is provided by pinching, pressing, and moving the skin with the hand not holding the suction cannula. In this manner, the surgeon ensures that the area is evenly defatted and that focal, asymmetric minipockets of fat do not elude treatment. Compressing the skin with the nondominant hand also helps to guide the cannula to various depths, helping to remove not only mid-fat, but also superficial and deep fat. For instance, if the skin and subcutis are pinched and then the cannula is used to push through the superficial pinched fat, fat just below the dermis may be gently removed; similarly, if a cannula is moved laterally below a handful of pinched skin, this may be preferentially target deeper fat. Triangulation is a key concept in cannula movement. To ensure smooth, even decrease in the fat layer, localized fat deposits are suctioned from two or three sites located approximately 120 degrees apart. If triangulation is not performed, there is a risk of over suctioning in one or more grooves, thus creating an uneven topography of hills and valleys. Larger bore cannulas are used early in liposuction of a particular anatomic area. At this point, anesthetic effect is at its peak, and the larger cannulas slide through the fat comfortably. As the volume of fat is decreased and much of the tumescent fluid is removed by suction, smaller bore cannulas come into use. Fine diameter cannulas cause less trauma and hence less discomfort, and they are also more effective for removing lesser amounts of residual fat without causing overlying textural abnormalities.

During the liposuction process, the surgeon needs to be aware of the evolving character of the liposuction aspirate. A pale yellow aspirate is ideal, but a degree of serosanguinous fluid is usually inevitably elicited as the procedure continues. Frank blood is a sign of caution and the aspiration cannula should be repositioned. Vigorous suctioning accompanied by very little fat removal indicates that, a particular area or depth may have been fully suctioned. Lower or higher cannula elevation may result in further fat mobilization. Dimpling or worsened cellulite can be avoided by aiming the cannula holes downward. As the dermis on the trunk can be thick, the surgeon should understand that the first 0.5 to 1 in. that are pinched may be skin rather than subcutis. Suctioning should be discontinued at a point when sufficient fat remains to ensure a smooth postoperative contour.

ALTERNATIVE TREATMENT METHODS

Technique in liposuction is frequently anatomic site specific (Table 11.6) and distribution of fat can be gender specific. Effective, speedy, and safe suctioning of different body areas requires minor and sometimes major adjustments.

◼ Neck and Jowls

The neck and jowls are perhaps the body region most commonly treated with liposuction. Neck youthfulness can be measured by the cervicomental angle, which is the intersection of the vertical anterior facial plane and the submental plane. In young patients, ideal cervicomental angles are approximately 80 to 95 degrees. Another important parameter is the submental-cervical angle; ideally relatively sharp, which is defined by the submental plane and

TABLE 11.6 ▪ Anatomic Areas Most Commonly Treated by Liposuction (in descending order)

Men	Women
Flanks/"love handles"	Abdomen
Abdomen	Outer thighs
Neck/jowls	Hip/waist
Breast	Neck/jowls

the anterior border of the neck. As fat accumulates in the submental area and the skin becomes more lax, normal aging results in descent of the cervical point, the junction between the submental area of the face and the neck. Under the neck, skin is the thin bilateral platysma muscle, the local continuation of the superficial muscular aponeurotic system (SMAS), which may need to be resuspended in the aging neck. Subplatysmal fat that lies below the platysma may contribute to the appearance of a thickened anterior neck. Lateral jowl fat pads are accentuated as gravitational descent results in ptosis of the jowls. Depending on its position, the hyoid bone, a floating point within the anterior neck muscles that is important in swallowing, can make the anterior neck appear more or less full.

The optimal neck liposuction patient is a woman with excess submental fat. Lateral neck profile in such often mildly obese patients can be improved by liposuction alone. Elevation of the cervicomental point results in a better cervicomental angle. Jowls are treated more sparingly to avoid oversuction and consequent indentations.

Contraction of the skin can improve the overall outcomes of liposuction. Such contraction occurs as the dermis readheres to the underlying fascia postoperatively. Thinner patients with limited submental fat and excess skin may benefit from a concurrent skin resection procedure, such as a rhytidectomy. Effects of skin removal may be enhanced by platysmaplasty, a procedure in which the platysma is tightened by suture plication. Such a procedure can reduce platysmal bands, which may become evident once submental fat is removed. Subplatysmal fat can be removed by careful liposuction in patients with significant deep fat accumulation. Notably, an anteriorly displaced hyoid bone can complicate neck liposuction and reduce the enhancement associated with this procedure.

In the standard approach to neck liposuction, the patient is positioned with the neck hyperextended. Reduction of the anterior neck fat is commenced from one submental and two infralobular incisions. Jowls may be approached also from two infrajowl incisions. These three to five incisions may be suctioned by machine suction or by syringe suction, with syringe suction alone often practical for less fatty necks.

Postliposuction, a pressure dressing and a compression garment resembling a chin strap is worn by the patient day and night for several days. Thereafter, this garment may be worn at night only.

Adverse events after neck liposuction include edema, swelling, and bruising, which are seen in most cases. Jowl swelling may remit more slowly than neck swelling and may be evident over a week later. Hematoma can occur, and is more common after platysmaplasty. Risk of seroma formation may be reduced by extended use of compression. In some cases of large volume liposuction, a skin-fold may emerge proximal to the submental incision;

this may eventually involute or be treated with intralesional steroid injection. A potentially serious complication of neck and jowl liposuction is injury to the marginal mandibular nerve. Liposuction cannulas do not usually sever the nerve but may traumatize or stretch it, leading to temporary paresis of the ipsilateral lip depressors. Resolution within a few weeks to a month is routine.

▪ Back and Abdomen

The torso is among the more common sites for liposuction, which can provide dramatic improvement of body contour in this area. Female and male body habitus differences require similarly diverse approaches to removal of fat. Ideal shape in women is an hourglass figure, with the minimal width at the hips contingent on the structure of the iliac crest. A "V" shape is more appropriate in men, in whom the chest tapers to the flatter hips. In both men and women, the ideal upper and lower abdomens, as well as the back, have little subcutaneous fat.

Stable pretreatment weight, and an ongoing diet and exercise regimen, are crucial preconditions for liposuction of the trunk. Personal trainers and nutritionists may be helpful consultants for those who have been unable to achieve physical fitness on their own. Resistant areas that persist despite attempts at modification by diet and exercise are optimal targets for liposuction. For instance, a patient in good physical shape and at near-optimal weight may have a lower abdominal bulge that no amount of exercise and only extreme weight loss can address. Focal treatment of this localized adiposity would be an indication for liposuction. Overall truncal obesity is not an indication for liposuction. Most patients undergoing truncal liposuction will be within 10 to 25 lb of ideal body weight, and will have good skin tone that will allow the skin to contract postoperatively.

While body contour may be abnormal, it may not be susceptible to improvement by liposuction. Skeletal abnormality like scoliosis or kyphosis must be excluded. Tactile assessment of the proposed treatment area with the "pinch test" will reveal the degree of subcutaneous adiposity. Intra-abdominal (i.e., "beer belly") and visceral fat is not amenable to liposuction. Such deep, sequestered fat may be relatively more copious in the male lower abdomen.

Silhouette in clothing is improved after truncal liposuction. Patients who are seeking this improvement will often be pleased with the results. Small corrections in patients with minor contour abnormalities may also improve appearance in more revealing clothing or bathing suits.

Truncal liposuction has the same anesthesia-associated risk as liposuction at other sites, but the greater volume of infused tumescent fluid potentially increases cumulative risk. Strictures on maximum total dose of lidocaine should be observed. If the area to undergo treatment would require more than the body weight-specific total dose, the liposuction must be divided into two or more procedures performed on different days.

Prior history of abdominal surgery must be elicited before abdominal liposuction. Scars and appliances will need to be avoided, or the areas around them treated exceptionally gently. Umbilical, ventral, and inguinal hernias should be noted on physical examination. Again, cautions should be observed intraoperatively, or the liposuction should be truncated or avoided. Severe laxity or redundancy of abdominal skin suggests that skin retraction after liposuction will be incomplete. Patients with such skin should be advised that skin resection or abdominoplasty may be necessary to treat excess skin, if removal of this is desired.

Within the trunk, there are several cosmetic units that may be separately approached. Women may be concerned about localized areas of the upper lateral mid-back. These so-called "bra bulges" are usually amenable to liposuction. At the hips, a double-bulge commonly observed in women can look unattractive in clothes. Suctioning the hips alone to reduce both these protrusions and blend them better can be highly cosmetically effective. Both men and women frequently request reduction of the abdomen. Assuming the fat collection is not subrectus and hence, unreachable by liposuction; liposuction is often effective at reducing even relatively large accumulations. "Spare tire"—type circumferential fat coalescing into "love handles" at the lateral flanks is commonly seen in the lower abdomen of men. Liposuction of the lower abdomen and flanks is often effective at correcting this. In women, fat is frequently distributed in both the upper and lower abdomen. While the fat accumulation in the lower area may be greater than that in the upper abdomen, adequate suctioning of both areas precedes good final contour. Temptation to concentrate on the lower abdomen can result in the under suctioned upper abdomen pushing down on the lower and causing the umbilicus to be elongated horizontally like an inverted crescent or an unhappy mouth.

Technically, a single supraumbilical entry site may be best for abdominal liposuction. Horizontal motion of the aspiration cannula at this site can create a well-defined, cosmetically elegant midline sulcus between the upper and lower abdomen. This approach also permits use of fine cannulas to completely suction around the umbilicus. "Doughnut" like residual fat around the umbilicus is important to avoid by adequate suctioning, and smaller cannulas can remove more of this fat while minimizing pain at this very sensitive area.

Debulking of a large abdomen may require either large bore, aggressive cannulas, or powered liposuction equipment. Transitioning to smaller cannulas after much of the fat has been removed permits even and smooth fat reduction. Scarpa's fascia divides the fat compartment, with some suctionable fat lying below this. For optimal removal of abdominal fat, gentle mobilization and removal of fat below Scarpa's fascia is necessary. This should be done with great care to avoid injury to underlying muscle.

Given that, abdominal and truncal liposuctions tend to be relatively extensive procedures compared to liposuction at other sites, several days of postoperative recovery may be required. Abdominal binders and garments should be worn to allow smooth contour emergence as swelling and bruising diminishes (Figure 11.2). Pain control may require medication adjustment. Postoperative nausea may need to be treated with drugs. Occasional hematomas and seromas should be monitored for self-resolution or drained if they are larger. Asymmetry or dimpling can occur, and usually at least 6 to 12 months are allowed to elapse before a touch-up procedure is considered. Uneven areas often spontaneously improve over this time window.

SPECIAL CONSIDERATIONS IN ETHNIC SKIN

Tumescent liposuction is a safe and effective procedure that is generally well tolerated in patients with ethnic skin. Given that abrasion of the epidermis or dermis is not required, the risk of widespread, confluent postinflammatory hyper- or hypopigmentation is absent. As pigmentary abnormalities are probably the most significant treatment limiting adverse event of cosmetic procedures in ethnic skin, the relatively low risk of such outcomes allows cosmetic surgeons to be optimistic and reassuring in discussing this procedure with patients. There are no known absolute contraindications to liposuction specifically applicable to patients with ethnic skin.

That being said, there are several issues that may impinge on liposuction results in non-Caucasian patients. Potential adverse events that may be more frequently seen include hypertrophic scar or keloid, as well as localized postinflammatory hyper- or hypopigmentation.

Hypertrophic scars and keloids may emerge as healing occurs at the stab incision sites created for fluid infusion and fat removal. Incisions are usually created with a no. 11 blade, and as such are 2 to 4 mm long and with negligible width. Such incisions are not typically sutured so as to permit postoperative fluid drainage, with healing by second intent proceeding spontaneously. In patients with ethnic skin, it may be prudent to place a single deep 4.0 or 5.0 Vicryl suture to approximate dermis and subcutis of the larger stab incisions and those that have been traumatically enlarged during suctioning. This may reduce the area prone to develop a hypertrophic scar in susceptible individuals by reducing overall scar without applying epidermal sutures, which can also induce scarring. When incision sites are created using punch biopsy instruments,

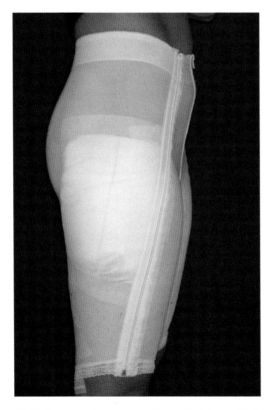

Figure 11.2 *Compression garment applied immediately after inner and outer thigh liposuction. Gauze dressings underneath are designed to wick away postprocedure fluid drainage*

the width of these apertures is near equivalent to the length and closure of the dermis and subcutis with deep sutures is highly desirable. Prior to initiating liposuction on patients with ethnic skin, it is prudent to elicit a complete history regarding prior surgeries and traumatic skin injuries. Any scars that are reported should be carefully examined by the surgeon since patients may lack the expertise to accurately designate these as hypertrophic scars or keloids. In cases where there are well-approximated surgical scars that have hypertrophied, the patient should be warned that this can recur at the liposuction incision sites, but is unlikely given the small size and low tension associated with the latter. One week following the liposuction procedure, as drainage ends and swelling diminishes, silicone-backed disposable bandages can be applied over the healing incision sites. Patients should be told that near continuous application of silicone gel sheeting for several months has been shown to flatten hypertrophic scars and may mitigate the risk of their initial eruption. In all ethnic skin patients, it is reasonable to minimize the number of incision sites. Hiding these in skin folds and in perigenital areas, if appropriate, is also encouraged. Use of longer cannulas (e.g., 9 in) can enable adequate fat removal from few entry sites.

Postinflammatory hyperpigmentation can be a telltale and unwanted mark in patients with ethnic skin. Localized to the incision points, hyperpigmentation may be more notable in lighter-skinned Indian, African American, and Asian patients. In such patients, the contrast between the background skin tone and the dark postinflammatory hyperpigmentation may highlight a series of symmetric and evenly spaced marks that are clearly man made. Patients with an array of notable pigmented macules may be self-conscious in swimwear or in intimate situations; when liposuction is on the arms or legs, marks may be difficult to conceal even in business attire. The risk of hyperpigmented macules can be assessed preoperatively by querying patients about past skin responses to scratches, burns, bruises, minor cuts, and surgeries. History of postinflammatory hyperpigmentation is not a contraindication to liposuction. Hyperpigmentation at incision sites invariably recedes, but complete resolution may be exceedingly slow, over years rather than months. As in the case of hypertrophic scars, the overall risk can be diminished by reducing the number of incision sites. Locations can also be carefully selected to maximize concealment parallel to relaxed skin tension lines, in creases and skin-folds, at the periphery of cosmetic units, and in areas usually covered by clothing or undergarments. Asymmetric positioning of incision sites can help to avoid the artifactual appearance associated with normally positioned sites that have become hyperpigmented. Number of sites may be kept constant, but slightly irregular spacing may increase the chance that any hyperpigmented macules that emerge will be perceived as moles, freckles, or some other natural skin marking. In rare instances, hypopigmentation may occur at incision sites. Hypopigmentation is much harder to remedy than hyperpigmentation, and lightening may be permanent. Excision of the hypopigmented sites can be considered, but if the initial cause of hypopigmentation is unclear, a further recurrence is possible. Depigmented patches that develop in patients with vitiligo should be treated appropriately.

It is important to reiterate to patients that liposuction is not a treatment for diabetes or a means for increasing insulin sensitivity.

While African American patients may be more prone to risk of diabetes and hypertension, neither of these are ameliorated by tumescent fat reduction. Insulin resistance has been reported to be affected by removal of very large fat volumes of 25 L or greater, but liposuction procedures of this magnitude are not within the standard of care in the United States. Safe liposuction entails infusion and removal of no more than 4 to 5 L of fluid. Very high volume liposuction can predispose patients to life-threatening fluid shifts and is strongly discouraged by most practitioners.

Liposuction on patients with ethnic skin need not lead to deleterious effects. In some cases, the outcomes may be preferable to those in Caucasian patients. For instance, Asian, Indian, and black skin may be less prone to postprocedural puckering and cellulite exacerbation, which are known risks of liposuction. While superficial suctioning of subcutis can destabilize the dermis, thereby inducing textural irregularities, ethnic skin may be less susceptible to developing the resulting fine wrinkling and crepe-like appearance postprocedure than finer and lighter skin. Similarly, some patients with ethnic skin may be less vulnerable than Caucasian patients to skin excess after liposuction. Since liposuction removes fat but not skin, a smooth postoperative contour is contingent on even and complete skin contraction. Skin elasticity sufficient to induce such contraction is more common in younger patients and often also in patients with darker skin. So ethnic skin patients receiving liposuction are often less likely to be left excess skin-fold at the site treatment, such as the abdomen or upper arms. This relative resistance to inadequate skin contraction may qualify a greater proportion of darker skinned patients as good candidates for liposuction.

DIRECTIONS FOR THE FUTURE AND CONCLUSIONS

Liposuction continues to be the most commonly performed major cosmetic procedure. Performed according to generally accepted rules, tumescent liposuction is a highly effective, extremely safe means for permanent body contour improvement. In the long run, noninvasive fat reduction techniques may displace liposuction, but these technologies remain in their infancy.

Dermatologists are uniquely qualified to refine tumescent liposuction, a procedure birthed in this specialty. Excellent references for further reading include Hanke and Sattler's *Liposuction,* the chapter on liposuction in Kaminer's *Atlas of Cosmetic Surgery,* and Narins' *Safe Liposuction and Fat Transfer.*

REFERENCES

1. Illouz YG. Body contouring by lipolysis: a 5-year experience with over 3000 cases. *Plast Reconstr Surg.* 1983;72:591-597.
2. Fournier PF. Why the syringe and not the suction machine? *J Dermatol Surg Oncol.* 1988;14:1062-1071.
3. Fournier PF. Who should do syringe liposculpturing? *J Dermatol Surg Oncol.* 1988;14:1055-1056.
4. Ostad A, Kageyama N, Moy RL. Tumescent anesthesia with a lidocaine dose of 55 mg/kg is safe for liposuction. *Dermatol Surg.* 1996;22:921-927.

5. Hanke CW, Bernstein G, Bullock S. Safety of tumescent liposuction in 15,336 patients. National survey results. *Dermatol Surg.* 1995;21:459-462.

6. Coleman IW, Hanke CW, Lillis P, Bernstein G, Narins R. Does the location of the surgery or the specialty of the physician affect malpractice claims in liposuction? *Dermatol Surg.* 1999;25:343-347.

7. Rao RB, Ely SF, Hoffman RS. Deaths related to liposuction. *N Engl J Med.* 1999;340:1471-1475.

8. Coldiron B, Fisher AH, Adelman E, et al. Adverse event reporting: lessons learned from 4 years of Florida office data. *Dermatol Surg.* 2005;31:1079-1092.

9. Hanke W, Cox SE, Kuznets N, Coleman WP III. Tumescent liposuction report performance measurement initiative: national survey results. *Dermatol Surg.* 2004;30:967-977.

10. Housman TS, Lawrence N, Mellen BG, et al. The safety of liposuction: results of a national survey. *Dermatol Surg.* 2002;28:971-978.

11. Kaplan B, Moy RL. Comparison of room temperature and warmed local anesthetic solution for tumescent liposuction. A randomized double-blind study. *Dermatol Surg.* 1996;22:707-709.

12. Yang CH, Hsu HC, Shen SC, Juan WH, Hong HS, Chen CH. Warm and neutral tumescent anesthetic solutions are essential factors for a less painful injection. *Dermatol Surg.* 2006;32:1119-1122.

13. Lawrence N, Cox SE. The efficacy of external ultrasound-assisted liposuction: a randomized controlled trial. *Dermatol Surg.* 2000;26:329-332.

14. Araco A, Gravante G, Araco F, Delogu D, Cervelli V. Comparison of power water-assisted and traditional liposuction: a prospective randomized trial of postoperative pain. *Aesthetic Plast Surg.* 2007;31:259-265.

15. Katz BE, Bruck MC, Coleman WP III. The benefits of powered liposuction versus traditional liposuction: a paired comparison analysis. *Dermatol Surg.* 2001;27:863-867.

16. Katz BE, Bruck MC, Felsenfeld L, Frew KE. Power liposuction: a report on complications. *Dermatol Surg.* 2003;29:925-927.

17. Prado A, Andrades P, Danilla S, Leniz P, Castillo P, Gaete F. A prospective, randomized, double-blind, controlled clinical trial comparing laser-assisted lipoplasty with suction-assisted lipoplasty. *Plast Reconstr Surg.* 2006;118:1032-1045.

18. Kim KH, Geronemus RG. Laser lipolysis using a novel 1064-nm Nd:YAG Laser. *Dermatol Surg.* 2006;32:241-248.

19. Rubin JP, Bierman C, Rosow CE, et al. The tumescent technique: the effect of high tissue pressure and dilute epinephrine on absorption of lidocaine. *Plast Reconstr Surg.* 1999;103:990-996.

20. Rubin JP, Xie Z, Davidson C, Rosow CE, Chang Y, May JW Jr. Rapid absorption of tumescent lidocaine above the clavicles: A prospective clinical study. *Plast Reconstr Surg.* 2005;115:1744-1751.

Vic A. Narurkar, MD, FAAD

INTRODUCTION

Nonsurgical tightening with devices has been reported with unipolar radio frequency, bipolar radio frequency, and combined unipolar and bipolar radio-frequency devices, combined radio-frequency devices and laser, broadband infrared light sources, long-pulsed infrared lasers, and fractional laser resurfacing. The common feature for all these devices is that they are "color-blind" in theory, and should not pose significant risks for darker skin, as they do not interfere with the chromophore melanin. Specific studies addressing dark skin patients with these devices is limited and it is generally assumed that because of the lack of competing chromophores, skin tightening with all the aforementioned devices should be safe in skin of color. The bigger controversy is the actual efficacy of these devices in actual three-dimensional skin tightening, regardless of the color of the skin. This chapter will review the various devices utilized for skin tightening, their mechanisms of actions, issues regarding skin of color, and potential complications.

MONOPOLAR RADIO FREQUENCY

Monopolar capacitive radio frequency is the most widely studied device for nonsurgical skin tightening and was the first modality launched specifically for this indication.[1–3] The mechanism of action involves selective heating of the dermis and subcutaneous tissue with monopolar capacitive radio frequency, while protecting the skin surface, thereby preserving epidermal integrity. The initial approach to monopolar radio frequency was to utilize high fluencies with single treatment or two treatments.[3–5] The literature shows small studies on patients up to skin type IV using this protocol,[4] without reported risks of any complications such as hypopigmentation or hyperpigmentation or scar formation with longevity of approximately 6 months. The high fluence protocols lost momentum for various reasons including significant discomfort, unpredictability and the potential for subcutaneous atrophy, as well as epidermal compromise[5] (Figure 12.1). Moreover, the duration of treatment was exceedingly slow, making it cumbersome and painful. To overcome these limitations, the high fluence protocol was replaced with a low-energy multiple-pass technique[6] with 5700 patient assessments in a 14-Physician Multispecialty Consensus Panel. This is the largest series of any tissue tightening device to this date. Parameters assessed with the newer protocol, included[1] patient feedback on heat sensation as a method for optimal energy selection[2], the use of multiple passes at moderate energy settings to yield more reproducible and consistent outcomes, and[3] treatment to a clinical endpoint of visible tissue tightening for more predictable results. In comparison to the original algorithm of high fluence, single pass treatment, which showed skin tightening in 54% of the patients and significant pain in 45% of patients, the new algorithm of multiple passes with lower fluencies, showed tightening in 92% of patients and significant pain in 5% of patients. Therefore, it appears that multiple pass lower fluence monopolar capacitive radio frequency is now the preferred modality for noninvasive skin tightening, with the largest series of treatments and most widely peer reviewed studies. Specific ethnic skin studies with this device have not been conducted, but many of these studies have included darker skin types.

COMBINATION BIPOLAR RADIO FREQUENCY AND LIGHT ENERGIES (ELECTRO-OPTICAL SYNERGY TECHNOLOGY)

Combination bipolar radio frequency and light energy devices employ combined bipolar radio frequency and optical energy with a 900-nm diode laser in a single pulse or combined bipolar radio frequency and broadband infrared light (700-2000 nm) in a single pulse. This was the second device to be introduced for nonsurgical skin tightening.[7] This technology addressed skin of color issues with the following premis—the bipolar radio frequency component of the device enables the use of lower fluencies of the optical component of the device (either laser of broadband light). This would reduce the risk from optical energy and therefore be safer for all skin types. Moreover, the optical component was believed to enable the bipolar radio frequency energy to concentrate where the optical energy has selectively heated the target. Three to six treatment sessions have been reported to achieve clinical efficacy.[8] The combined bipolar radio frequency and broadband light source has been specifically studied in Asian skin[9] with patient satisfaction rates being higher than masked observer photographic assessments and no adverse effects. As with monopolar radio-frequency device studies, long term (greater than 6 months data) is absent.

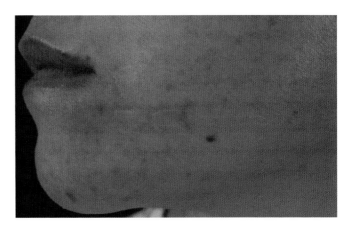

Figure 12.1 *Subcutaneous atrophy with unipolar radio-frequency device in skin type IV*

BROADBAND INFRARED LIGHT AND FRACTIONAL BROADBAND INFRARED LIGHT SOURCES

The pain and cost of original monopolar radio-frequency devices prompted the development of an alternative modality for nonsurgical skin tightening leading to the development of broadband light sources which emit in the infrared spectrum. The first device utilized a filtered 1100-1800-nm broadband light source with contact cooling and was demonstrated ultrastructurally to produce similar changes seen with capacitive monopolar radio-frequency device. Initial clinical studies showed improvement to be more dramatic in patients whose skin envelope draped separately from deeper soft tissue.[10] A multicenter study of a larger patient database of 42 patients[11] showed a mean of 50% improvement with two treatments spaced 1 month apart and included darker skin types. Two specific studies with Asian skin have been performed with this device.[12,13] The first study[12] demonstrated 51% improvement in skin laxity at 3 months follow-up in 13 Chinese patients and the second[12] demonstrated 38% significant improvement at 6-month follow-up.[13] The only reported side effect was isolated superficial blistering in a few cases.[13] However, because of bulk heating with this device, epidermal compromise leading to full-thickness scars has been seen regardless of the color of the patient (Figure 12.2). To reduce bulk heating, an alternative modality of delivering broadband light in this range has been to use a fractionated mode of dermal delivery using a fractionated broadband light source showing similar clinical effects and theoretically less risks of epidermal compromise.

LONG-PULSED 1064-nm LASERS

The rationale behind using the long pulsed 1064-nm laser for skin tightening was to determine whether a single treatment, similar to the

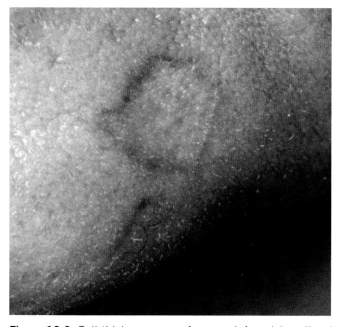

Figure 12.2 *Full-thickness scars from an infrared broadband light source*

original monopolar radio-frequency device protocol, was achievable with reduced discomfort, lack of adverse events, and less cost. Since the 1064-nm wavelength is poorly absorbed by competing chromophores of melanin, it is considered one of the safest wavelengths in treating skin of color. The proposed mechanisms of high fluence 1064 nm for skin tightening were identical to those for all nonablative skin tightening devices, with the 1064-nm laser producing selective dermal heating leading to ultrastructural collagen neogenesis and skin tightening. Two studies[14,15] compared, monopolar radio frequency with high fluence 1064-nm laser in the same patient. In both studies, the high fluence 1064-nm laser produced greater skin tightening than monopolar radio frequency (47.5% vs. 29.8% and 30% vs. 15%).

NONABLATIVE FRACTIONAL LASER RESURFACING AND ABLATIVE FRACTIONAL RESURFACING

Traditional ablative laser resurfacing produced significant treatment of skin laxity but lost momentum because of the side effects and high risks of hypopigmentation and was never considered an option in ethnic skin. The risks of ablative laser resurfacing led to the development of the aforementioned "skin tightening" devices such as radio frequency, broadband light, and long pulsed 1064-nm lasers. However, the feature which is common to all these noninvasive skin tightening modalities is the variability in response and modest results, with no studies having longer than 6-month follow-ups. This leads to the important question—can one achieve noninvasive skin tightening without resurfacing regardless of the skin type? Therefore, an alternative modality for nonsurgical skin tightening is to view it as a secondary gain to resurfacing. Two approaches have been developed to overcome limitations of traditional ablative resurfacing—the more widely studied nonablative fractional resurfacing[16–18] and the recently introduced ablative fractional resurfacing.[19] With both modalities, the primary target is not skin laxity, but dyschromia, rhytids, and scars—with improvement of skin laxity being a secondary benefit. There is much confusion about true versus "pseudo" nonablative fractional resurfacing. True nonablative laser resurfacing must meet the following three criteria: (1) a nonablative modality with preservation of the majority of the stratum corneum, (2) a true resurfacing with extrusion of epidermal contents, and (3) creation of microthermal zones of dermal injury leading to de novo collagen biosynthesis. A variety of wavelengths including 1320 nm, 1440 nm, 1540 nm, and 1550 nm have been deployed for this indication and variety of patterns including stamped versus random patterns have been utilized, with the random pattern 1550-nm laser most widely studied in the literature with supporting data on ethnic skin.[20,21] Skin tightening is a delayed man infestation (Figure 12.3), usually evident at 6 to 12 months following a series of nonablative fractional laser treatments. One large study of 289 patients examined skin types I to VI with the 1550-nm fractional nonablative laser and found impressive skin tightening at an average of 9.2 months.[22] More recently, an ablative mode of fractional resurfacing has been introduced, with the 10 600-nm wavelength most widely studied and other wavelengths such as 2790 nm and 2940 nm in development. Impressive immediate skin tightening and laxity has been observed but there is limited data on darker skin types. Initial data

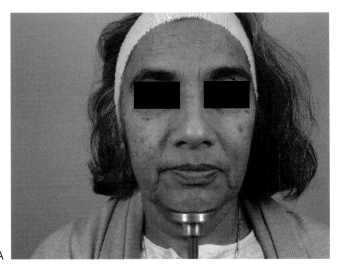 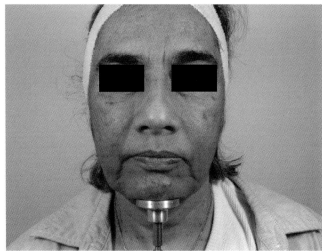

A   B

Figure 12.3 *Delayed skin tightening. Six months (A) pre- and (B) post-1550-mm fractional laser resurfacing in skin type V*

shows no evidence of hypopigmentation[19] but is limited to 3 to 6-month follow-ups.

CONCLUSIONS

There is much debate and controversy regarding the concept of nonsurgical skin tightening devices. The rationale for the development of these devices stemmed from unwanted side effects from traditional ablative resurfacing and the desire for patients to have an alternative to surgical approaches to skin tightening. In theory, all these devices are "color-blind" and offer a safe approach for all skin types. However, in practice, regardless of skin color, complications such as subcutaneous atrophy and full-thickness scars have been reported when using higher fluencies and suboptimal cooling. The most widely studied and utilized device is capacitive monopolar radio frequency, which underwent dramatic changes from a single treatment high fluence protocol to multiple passes and moderate fluence protocol, enhancing safety, patient comfort, and outcomes. There have been limited studies specifically addressing skin of color, with a few studies using filtered broadband light and devices combining bipolar radio frequency and optical energies. The common feature for all the studies for these nonsurgical skin tightening devices is limited long-term follow-ups and limited patient numbers. It is possible that a better modality for nonsurgical skin tightening may be a mode of skin resurfacing, with the advent of safer nonablative fractional resurfacing for all skin types and the recently introduced ablative fractional resurfacing. Moreover, it is becoming increasingly evident that devices are just one component on global rejuvenation, and perhaps to achieve "true" nonsurgical skin tightening in all skin colors, may require a combination of devices, fillers, and botulinum toxins.

REFERENCES

1. Lack EB, Rachel JD, D'Andrea L, Corres J. Relationship of energy settings and impedance in different anatomic areas using a radiofrequency device. *Dermatol Surg.* 2005;31(12): 1668-1670.

2. Weiss RA, Weiss MA, Munavalli G, Beasley K. Monopolar radiofrequency facial tightening: a retrospective analysis of efficacy and safety in over 600 treatments. *J Drugs Dermatol.* 2006;5(8):707-712.

3. Fritz M, Counters JT, Zelickson BD. Radiofrequency treatment for middle and lower face laxity. *Arch Facial Plast Surg.* 2004;6(6):370-373.

4. Alster TS, Tanzi E. Improvement of neck and cheek laxity with a nonablative radiofrequency device: a lifting experience. *Dermatol Surg.* 2004;30(4 Pt 1):503-507.

5. Fitzpatrick R, Geronemus R, Goldberg D, Kaminer M, Kilmer S, Ruiz-Esparza J. Multicenter study of noninvasive radiofrequency for periorbital tissue tightening. *Lasers Surg Med.* 2003;33(4):232-242.

6. Dover JS, Zelickson BD, 14-Physician Multispecialty Consensus Panel. Results of a survey of 5700 patient monopolar radiofrequency facial skin tightening treatments: assessment of a low energy multiple pass technique leading to a clinical endpoint algorithm. *Dermatol Surg.* 2007;33(8):900-907.

7. Sadick NS. Combination radiofrequency and light energies: electro-optical synergy technology in esthetic medicine. *Dermatol Surg.* 2005;31(9 Pt 2):1211-1217.

8. Doshi SN, Alster TS. Combination radiofrequency and diode laser for treatment of facial rhytides and skin laxity. *J Cosmet Laser Ther.* 2005;7(1):11-15.

9. Yu CS, Yeung CK, Shek SY, Tse RK, Kono T, Chan HH. Combined infrared light and bipolar radiofrequency for skin tightening in Asians. *Lasers Surg Med.* 2007;39(6):471-475.

10. Goldberg DJ, Hussain M, Fazeli M, Berlin AL. Treatment of skin laxity of the lower face and neck in older individuals with a broad-spectrum infrared light. *J Cosmet Laser Ther.* 2007; 9(1):35-40.

11. Taub AF, Battle EF Jr, Nikolaidis G. Multicenter clinical per-spectives on a broadband infrared light device for skin tighten-ing. *J Drugs Dermatol.* 2006;5(8):771-778.

12. Chan HH, Yu CS, Shek S, Yeung CK, Kono T, Wei WI. A prospective split face single blinded study looking at the use of an infrared device with contact cooling in the treatment. *Lasers Surg Med.* 2008;40(2):146-152.

13. Chua SH, Ang P, Khoo LS, Goh CL. Nonablative infrared skin tightening in type IV to V Asian skin: a prospective clinical study. *Dermatol Surg.* 2007;33(2):146-151.

14. Taylor MB, Prokopenko I. Split-face comparison of radiofre-quency versus long pulsed Nd-YAG treatment of facial laxity. *J Cosmet Laser Ther.* 2006;8(1):17-22.

15. Key DJ. Single treatment skin tightening by radiofrequency and long pulsed 1064 nm Nd:YAG laser compared. *Lasers Surg Med.* 2007;39(2):169-175.

16. Hantash BM, Mahmood MB. Fractional photothermolysis: a novel aesthetic laser surgery modality. *Dermatol Surg.* 2007;33(3):525-534.

17. Narurkar VA. Skin rejuvenation with microthermal fractional photothermolysis. *Dermatol Ther.* 2007;20(Suppl 1):S10-S13.

18. Geronemus RG. Fractional photothermolysis-current and future applications. *Lasers Surg Med.* 2006;38(3):169-176.

19. Hantash BM, Bedi VP, Kapadia B, et al. In vivo histological evaluation of a novel ablative fractional resurfacing device. *Lasers Surg Med.* 2007;39(2):96-107.

20. Kono T, Chan HH, Groff WF, et al. Prospective direct compari-son study of fractional resurfacing using different fluencies and densities for skin rejuvenation in Asians. *Lasers Surg Med.* 2007;39(4):311-314.

21. Chan HH, Manstein D, Yu CS, et al. The prevalence and risk factors of postinflammatory hyperpigmentation after fractional resurfacing in Asians. *Lasers Surg Med.* 2007;39(5):381-385.

22. Narurkar VA. Retrospective analysis of 877 treatments with a second generation erbium doped 1550-nm laser. *Lasers Surg Med.* 2008 (Suppl 20):27.

CHAPTER 13

Surgical Lifting and Tightening in Ethnic Skin

David J. Kouba, MD, PhD, Kee-Yang Chung, MD, PhD, and Ronald L. Moy, MD

INTRODUCTION AND DEFINITIONS

Although 75% to 80% of the planet's people are nonwhites, the majority of the cosmetic surgical literature is limited to the treatment of Caucasians. The fear of increased pigmentary and scarring complications has made cosmetic surgeons in the United States hesitant to perform elective procedures on both African and Asian patients. This fear should be replaced by knowledge of unique racial differences and modifications of surgical technique to accommodate ethnic patients who desire cosmetic surgery.

Understanding and accepting the attitudes of different cultures are extremely important for the cosmetic surgeon. Cultural traditions and resistance often have a profound psychologic influence on the nonwhite person who is contemplating cosmetic surgery. Changing ethnic appearance (e.g., "Westernization" of the Asian eyelid or reduction cheiloplasty in blacks) can cause feelings of guilt. Because elders play a dominant role in many nonwhite societies, their acceptance or rejection of cosmetic procedures has a psychologic influence on the ethnic patient. Altering shape while preserving the ethnicity of the nonwhite patient is a challenge to the cosmetic surgeon.

The surgeon who contemplates performing procedures in nonwhite patients should have an understanding of the morphologic differences between white and nonwhite skin, specifically in patients of African and Asian descent. The most apparent difference between white skin and black skin is the amount of epidermal melanin.[1] Although there is no difference in the quantity of melanocytes between the two groups,[2] the concentration of melanin within the melanosomes is increased in African skin compared with white skin (Table 13.1). In addition, the degradation rate of melanosomes within the keratinocytes of African skin is slower

than that of Caucasian skin. Although the increased melanin affords protection from the harmful effects of ultraviolet light, both the melanocytes and mesenchyma in African skin seem to be more vulnerable to trauma and inflammatory conditions than those in Caucasian skin. Post-traumatic or postinflammatory dyspigmentation can take the form of either darkening, or hyperpigmentation (Figure 13.1) or lightening of the skin, or hypopigmentation. Increased mesenchymal reactivity can result in hypertrophic scars (Figure 13.2) or even keloids (Figure 13.3), raised scars that have expanded beyond the boundaries of the original wound.[1]

The stratum corneum or outermost layer of the epidermis in African skin has a similar thickness to the same layer in Caucasian skin, but cell number and lipid content differ. Specifically, the stratum corneum in African skin has a greater number of cell layers, as well as higher lipid content. In addition, the reactivity of blood vessels is decreased in African skin, leading to less apparent erythematous reactions after chemical exposure.[3] The dermis of Asian and African skin is considerably thicker than the dermis of Caucasian skin, with thickness being proportional to the degree of pigmentation. This has ramifications for flap thickness and SMAS plication during facelifts as well as adjustments that need to be made during ablative resurfacing procedures. This increased dermal thickness may account for a lower incidence in facial rhytids in Asians and Africans. Similar to African skin, Asian skin (even the lighter variations) has a greater tendency toward hypertrophic scarring. Asians may also have a greater tendency toward prolonged redness during scar maturation than white skin.[4]

In this chapter, we will be alluding to these differences as we discuss surgical tightening and lifting techniques. The majority of tightening of the skin—defined as measurable contraction of the skin, involves methods that lead to enhanced dermal collagen production. Most of the modalities that produce skin tightening are, by

TABLE 13.1 ■ Histologic Differences Between Caucasian and Ethnic Skin Types*

Caucasian	Asian and African
	More diversely mixed apocrine/eccrine ducts
— Melanosomes	Larger, and more dispersed melanosomes
Thinner dermis	Thicker dermis
— Melanin	++ Melanin from increased melanocyte activity
++ Age-related solar elastosis	— Solar elastosis with age
— Dermal fibroblasts	Larger and ++ dermal fibroblasts

*Data compiled from Montagna W, Carlisle K. The architecture of black and white facial skin. *J Am Acad Dermatol.* 1991;24:929-937.
—, decreased in number; ++, increased in number.

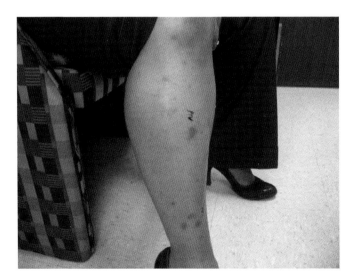

Figure 13.1 *PIH on the leg of an African American female patient*

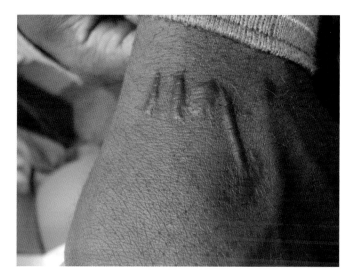

Figure 13.2 *Hypertrophic scarring on the dorsal hand of an African American patient*

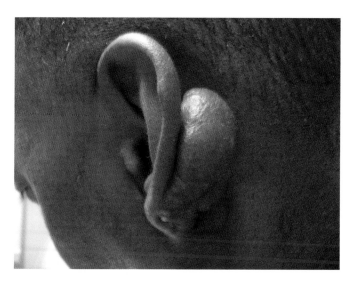

Figure 13.3 *Keloid scar resulting from ear piercing. The keloid had been previously excised without steroid injection or pressure cuff resulting in recrudescence of the keloid*

nature, destructive in different ways. In contrast, for the most part, lifting of the skin usually involves surgical manipulation. In the proceeding sections, we will focus primarily on the head and neck and discuss the anatomical and cultural differences between ethnic and Caucasian patients with regards to browlift, blepharoplasty (eyelift), and rhytidectomy (facelift) procedures.

▧ Tightening Techniques

To avoid complications when using techniques to tighten the skin, a few important inherent risks need to be appreciated when dealing with higher Fitzpatrick skin types (Table 13.2). The most common side effects to be cognizant of are postinflammatory hyperpigmentation (PIH) and keloid formation, the latter of which becomes more important in the discussion of surgical modalities (to follow). The keys to avoiding these complications involve taking a comprehensive preoperative history that includes a family history of keloids, hypertrophic scars or PIH, as well as a thorough preoperative physical examination. In this chapter, the nonsurgical tech-

niques we will be dealing with involve chemical peeling agents, dermabrasion, and laser resurfacing techniques.

One of the most common and time-tested in-office, nonsurgical procedures involves chemical peels. The various agents available for use as well as the methods used for applying them determine the depth of skin injury. Of course, there is a direct relationship between the depth of skin injury and the degree of potential tightening and consequently, the potential risk of complications. Agents such as glycolic acid peels and salicylic acid peels, when used in standard dose ranges, generally induce superficial injury that is confined to the epidermis. The risk of permanent injury from these agents is low, and consequently the risk of PIH and keloid formation in darker skin types is lower. Once the dermal–epidermal junction (DEJ) has been breached, the risk of PIH increases dramatically because of pigment incontinence, where melanin drops into the dermis and can become permanent, or semipermanent. Chemical peeling agents that commonly cause injury to the DEJ or injury extending through the DEJ into the dermis include trichloroacetic acid (TCA) peels or phenol-based peels (Figure 13.4). A common sequelae of phenol peels, even in Caucasians, is persistent hypopigmentation, making these peels an even less attractive option in ethnic skin. However, concentrated TCA can be used safely to elevate atrophic scars in Asian skin when delivered in a focal manner.[5,6]

Although dermabrasion has been largely supplanted by fractional laser resurfacing, it is still being practiced today, largely under a more limited scope. When used in this day and age, it is mainly used for acne scarring and the treatment of wrinkles and to improve the appearance of surgical scars.[7] In general, many investigators have reported disappointing results with dermabrasion used in the treatment of pigmented skin. Initial hypopigmentation over the first month, followed by hyperpigmentation, is a common complication of the procedure.[8] This hyperpigmentation may be more noticeable in lighter-skinned blacks.[8] Patients should be advised to reduce exposure to sunlight for 6 months after dermabrasion because such exposure will contribute to alterations in

---

TABLE 13.2 ▪ Fitzpatrick Skin Phototypes

Type I. Always burns easily, shows no immediate pigment darkening, never tans

Type II. Always burns easily, trace immediate pigment darkening, tans minimally and with difficulty

Type III. Burns minimally, with (+) immediate pigment darkening, tans gradually and uniformly (light brown)

Type IV. Burns minimally, with (++) immediate pigment darkening, tans well (moderate brown)

Type V. Rarely burns, with (+++) immediate pigment darkening, tans very well (dark brown)

Type VI. Never burns, with (+++) immediate pigment darkening, tans profusely (black)

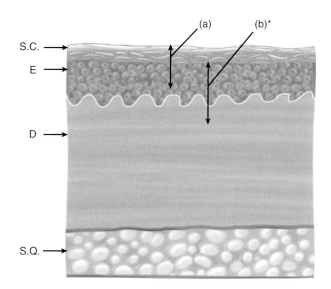

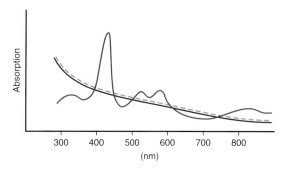

Figure 13.5 *Comparison of the absorption spectra of oxyhemoglobin (solid line) and melanin (solid line with dashed line)*

Figure 13.4 *Schematic demonstrating the potential depth of penetration of peeling agents. (A), α-Hydroxy acids and β-Hydroxy acids; (B), TCA and phenol. *The depth of penetration of these agents depends greatly on the strength of the denaturing agent applied as well as on the number of coats and the vigor with which the agent is rubbed into the skin. SC, stratum corneum; E, epidermis; D, dermis; SQ, subcutaneous*

pigmentation. Corrective cosmetics may be used to camouflage the depigmented areas.

Laser resurfacing poses other challenges that are not dissimilar from those of deeper chemical peeling agents. The interaction of light with tissue depends on chromophores to absorb incident laser light. Selective photothermolysis occurs when selective tissue absorption of laser light leads to selective destruction of the absorbing tissue.[9] In cutaneous laser surgery, the key chromophores are oxyhemoglobin, hemoglobin, water, and melanin. Advances in selective lasers have focused on designing laser delivery systems that are specific for the wavelengths for biologically active chromophores (Table 13.3). In pigmented skin, interference with melanin poses significant challenges for laser therapy. The classification of skin types based on response to ultraviolet irradiation was developed by Fitzpatrick. Laser therapy is safest in skin types I to III. Skin types IV to VI present significant challenges because of greater damage to melanin, resulting in hypopigmentation, hyperpigmentation, depigmentation, and streaky pigmentation.[10] Many cutaneous lasers have significant overlap with the absorption spectrum of melanin (Figure 13.5). Changes in pigmentation may not

be apparent for several months after laser therapy. Therefore, when treating pigmented skin, test sites and long-term follow-up are recommended before performing laser treatment.

Current laser delivery systems used for skin tightening can be divided into three general types: (1) field ablation of the target tissue, (2) deep tissue heating, and (3) those that utilize the concept of fractional photothermolysis (FP). While controlled clinical trials that demonstrate measurable tightening are lacking for FP, case records do demonstrate some evidence to support the claim that these lasers tighten the skin.[11-13]

The field of cutaneous resurfacing with lasers has witnessed unparalleled growth. The first reports of skin resurfacing were performed with carbon dioxide (CO_2) lasers in the superpulsed modes.[14] Because of unwanted thermal damage, results were not optimal and carried a significant risk of scarring (Figure 13.6). The development of pulsed CO_2 laser delivery systems and CO_2 lasers using optomechanical shutters to reduce tissue dwell time[15] has enabled laser skin resurfacing to gain widespread acceptance. The two most widely studied laser delivery systems are the Ultrapulse laser and SilkTouch systems.[16] Both modes allow for selective and controlled thermal destruction of the epidermis and dermis without significant thermal damage to the surrounding tissue.

In pigmented skin, the majority of requests for skin resurfacing are for acne scarring and rhytids. There are a handful of reports demonstrating the efficacy of using pulsed CO_2 lasers for acne scarring in Asian patients.[17] Hyperpigmentation can often be corrected by using bleaching agents before and after laser treatment. However, depigmentation and hypopigmentation are generally not reversible.

TABLE 13.3 ■ Typical Skin Chromophores and their Corresponding Peak Absorption Wavelengths

Chromophore	Approximate peak absorption wavelengths (nm)	Typical laser sources (wavelength in nm)
Melanin	*	KTP (532)/alexandrite (755)/Nd:YAG (1064)/Ruby (694)
Hemoglobin	430, 555	KTP (532)/tuneable pulsed dye (585-600)
Water	3000, 12000, 2000	CO_2 (10600)/erbium:YAG (1540)

*Melanin absorption curve lacks defined peaks.
KTP, potassium titanyl phosphate; YAG, Yttrium aluminum garnet; CO_2, carbon dioxide.

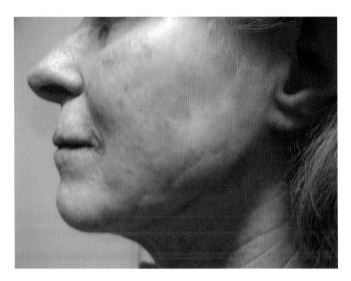

Figure 13.6 *Scarring on the face of a Caucasian patient who underwent CO$_2$ resurfacing done by a plastic surgeon*

▨ Lifting Techniques

With few exceptions, Caucasians and persons of ethnic skin types all seek relief from similar cosmetic effects of aging. While some practices might believe that certain groups do not seek cosmetic procedures, they are likely influenced by their practice's population bias. Many ethnic groups share a common misconception that only physicians from their own shared background could possibly understand their perceived unique needs. As a result, for example, many African Americans will preferentially seek dermatologists or dermasurgeons that are also African American. Consequently, Caucasian dermasurgeons may feel that African American patients

just do not seek the same procedures. Aside from that misconception based on population bias, however, there are differences in the procedures that certain groups seek or require, based on anatomic and cultural differences. While the cosmetic surgery market in the United States is dominated by Caucasian consumers, the number of ethnic patients seeking rejuvenation is dramatically increasing and it cannot be stated firmly enough that people of all ethnic groups seek surgical lifting and tightening.

Upper lid blepharoplasty in Indians, Hispanics, and African Americans are not measurably different than in Caucasians. Blepharoplasty surgery in Asians, however, requires a working knowledge of the anatomic differences between the upper eyelids of Caucasians and Asians (Figure 13.7). Absence of the superior palpebral fold produces a "single eyelid" appearance in approximately 50% of the Asian population (Figure 13.8). Asians without a superior palpebral fold lack the dermal attachments between the levator aponeurosis and/or the tarsal plate that are responsible for the crease in the upper eyelids of whites. The periorbital fat in Asians is more abundant than in the eyelids of whites, extending inferiorly anterior to the tarsal plate. The lack of the superior palpebral fold, excess skin, and abundance of periorbital fat contribute to the characteristic puffiness of the Asian upper eyelid (Figure 13.9). The epicanthal fold is a web of skin over the medial canthus and is present in approximately 90% of the upper eyelids of Asians (Figure 13.10). The size and shape of the epicanthal fold are highly variable, and therefore, several different techniques are available for modification of the fold.[18]

When discussing blepharoplasty with Asian patients, the size and shape of the new eyelid and the modification of the epicanthal fold should be ascertained. Most, if not all Asian patients are very particular about the shape of the eyelid (round vs. oval) and whether the new superior palpebral fold should be continuous with the epicanthal fold ("inside fold") or extend medial to the epicanthal

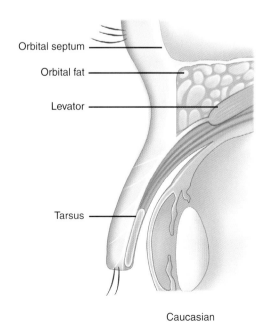

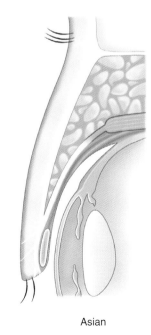

Orbital septum

Orbital fat

Levator

Tarsus

Caucasian

Asian

Figure 13.7 *Schematic demonstrating the anatomic differences between Asian and Caucasian upper eyelids (seen in cross section)*

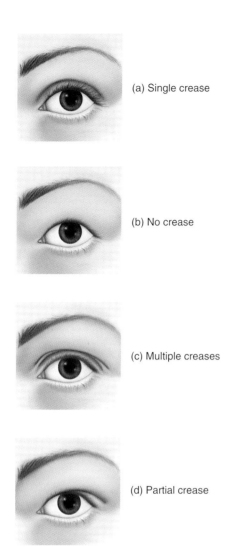

(a) Single crease

(b) No crease

(c) Multiple creases

(d) Partial crease

Figure 13.8 *Asian upper eyelid variations. (A) With single crease. (B) With no crease. (C) Multiple creases. (D) Partial crease*

fold ("outside fold"). Technical modifications of procedures commonly used on white patients include the following: (1) creation of a superior palpebral fold by skin excision and fixation sutures to the levator aponeurosis to form a "double eyelid," (2) excision of the central and medial periorbital fat pads, and (3) epicanthoplasty by simple advancement, half Z-plasty, or W-plasty.[19–21] Complications are not uncommon with blepharoplasty in Asians; up to 10% will require revision procedures. Complications that are of special concern with blepharoplasty in Asians include eyelid asymmetry, loss

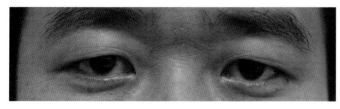

Figure 13.9 *Heavy, thick Asian upper eyelid (Used with permission from Kee-Yang Chung, MD, PhD)*

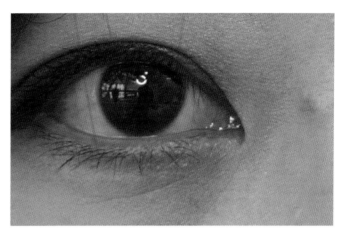

Figure 13.10 *Epicanthal fold in an Asian patient*

of the palpebral fold, laxity of pretarsal skin, retraction of the upper eyelid, hypertrophic scars, and excessive fat removal.[4]

Body contouring surgery via suction-assisted removal of fat is a well-established technique. Although similar techniques are used regardless of the ethnic origin of the patient, dysmorphic obesity has a special preference for certain people. The different tendencies to develop adipose deposits have been described as follows: Hispanics have a tendency to develop rolls on the hips with a short and inverted subgluteal crease. Caucasians develop hip rolls in continuity with an abdominal roll. Fat deposits in Asians extend from the waist to the chest and arms.[1] Undesirable complications do not differ, except for a slightly higher rate of keloids and hypertrophic scars at the site of cannula insertion (Figure 13.11) and hyperpigmentation over the treated sites in blacks.

In a general sense, liposuction or liposculpture does not quantifiably tighten the skin; however, the fibrotic changes to the subcutis that occur postoperatively can give the appearance of tightening, especially in areas such as the neck (Figure 13.12). Especially in

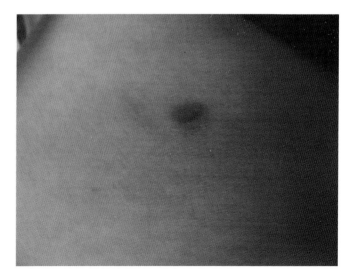

Figure 13.11 *Hyperpigmented and slightly hypertrophic cannula insertion site scar on the trunk of a 30-year-old Asian female who underwent tumescent liposuction*

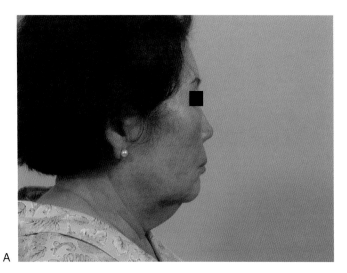
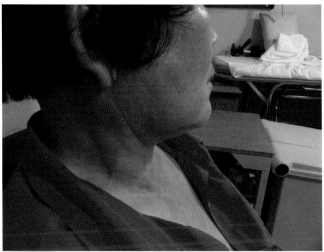

A   B

Figure 13.12 *(A)Pre- and (B) postoperative views of a middle-aged female Asian patient who had neck liposuction and platysmal plication*

this area, the purposeful fibrosis and scarring of the skin and superficial fat to the platysma and strap muscles of the anterior neck can give the appearance of tightening simply by sharpening the cervicomental angle. So while traditional liposuction does not tighten in the strictest definition (by causing dermal contraction), newer liposculpture techniques, such as laser-assisted SmartLipo™ (Cynosure Corp, MA) are attempting to fill that void.

Surgical lifting in persons of ethnic skin can be immensely different than that in Caucasians. Examination of the bony structure, fibrous attachments to the skin, the size and distribution of fatty deposits, and the histologic differences in the dermis, all play a role in the approach to lifting ethnic skin. In general, Asian skin has a thicker dermis than Caucasians, and Asian faces have, on average, smaller chin, weaker bony support structures, and larger and therefore heavier malar fat pads.[22] In addition, usually less neck work needs to be done in Asians, making a minimal incision facelift, or S-lift (as opposed to a full rhytidectomy) an attractive option for these patients. All these anatomic differences need to be recognized and adjusted for during surgical lifting procedures.

LITERATURE REVIEW

In general, evidence-based analysis of cosmetic techniques is lacking in the medical literature, let alone in the subset of cosmetic lifting and tightening techniques in ethnic skin. However, review of the safe use of these devices and surgical techniques can easily be applied to our experiences in using them to treat Asian, African and Hispanic patients. Most practitioners would agree that the sliding scale of increasing efficacy of tightening (which correlates well with increasing risk of complications) starts with radio frequency (RF) devices, followed by FP and continues with plasma resurfacing before Erbium:YAG and finally CO_2 ablative resurfacing. Use of these modalities to tighten and lift ethnic skin can be performed comfortably at the RF end and with extreme caution at the CO_2 end of the spectrum.

Nonsurgical tightening can most safely be performed using RF heating devices, such as the monopolar Thermacool™ device.

Weiss et al.[23] recently performed a retrospective review of their experience with RF heating in more than 600 patients and found greater efficacy, lower side effect profile, and higher patient satisfaction when multiple passes at lower fluences are used. A smaller case series by Alster and Tanzi[24] confirmed findings by our group[25] in a split face and by Fitzpatrick in a 6-month longitudinal full face study[26] showing measurable lifting of brow position after monopolar RF treatments. While these studies were not limited to patients of ethnic skin, the results do not highlight any increased complication rate in ethnic skin types and mirror our own findings that RF devices appear quite safe in darker skinned patients.

While FP is an emerging technology; early studies show that it is a relatively safe modality for use in ethnic skin. In a recent study of 10 patients with melasma, only one patient developed PIH after FP treatment and 60% of patients achieved between 75% and 100% clearing of their melasma. The population consisted of patients exclusively of Fitzpatrick III, IV, and V skin type.[27] Further, a recent study by Lin and Chan[28] on 16 Asian patients found that higher energy densities was not very effective in clearing hyperpigmentation and only served to increase the rate of PIH.

CLINICAL EXAMINATION AND PATIENT HISTORY

History and examination that are pertinent to the decisions of how to use nonsurgical tightening modalities center on the propensity for keloid formation as well as PIH. While the modalities mentioned above (RF heating, chemical peels, dermabrasion, laser, and plasma resurfacing), all cause tightening, they are associated with different risks of scarring and PIH in ethnic skin. Certainly, a history of healing after prior procedures is important, but in the absence of a procedure history, inquiring about healing after acne lesions or superficial abrasions is important. Equally important is a history of keloid formation, for example, after ear piercings (Figure 13.3) or a family history of keloid formation. We will frequently have patients

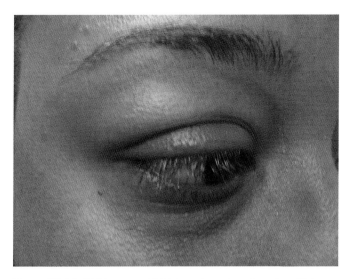

Figure 13.13 *Thirty-year-old African American female with heavy upper lid and lateral upper eyelid fullness. Lacrimal gland prolapse should be a consideration in this patient prior to performing upper lid blepharoplasty*

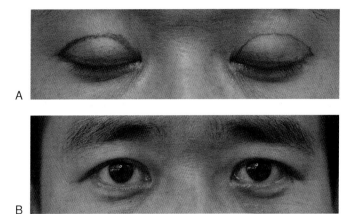

Figure 13.14 *Typical upper lid blepharoplasty in Asian male with single crease, heavy lids, and slight lateral hooding. (A) Preoperative markings; (B) three-month postoperative result (Used with permission from Kee-Yang Chung, MD, PhD)*

of color who show us scars that they have secondary to minor trauma in order to examine just how well they heal. With respect to nonsurgical tightening techniques, physical examination and history is similar across all ethnicities.

Thorough physical examination in advance of upper lid blepharoplasty is critical in Asian patients, but less so for African or Hispanic patients. While more abundant intraseptal fat and a propensity for lacrimal gland prolapse are common in patients of African descent (Figure 13.13), in general, an upper lid blepharoplasty in black or Hispanic patients does not diverge significantly from those in Caucasians. The upper lateral lid should be palpated for the presence of fullness, which if present may be because of the lacrimal gland prolapse and, as in all patients, a history of sicca symptoms should be elicited.

In the Asian upper lid, a thorough preoperative counseling should focus on goals for the eyelid after surgery. Several questions need to be raised with the patient. Namely, do they want a very subtle improvement (Figure 13.9 and 13.14) that will be hardly recognized (this is common in older Asian patients)? Do they have a single, or double eyelid crease that needs to be addressed (Figure 13.15)? Alternatively, do they want a more dramatic change that westernizes the eye (which is less common but more often requested by younger Asian patients)? More specifically, do they want the epicanthal fold reduced? Do they want the crease raised to match that of Caucasians? What are their expectations after surgery and if they decide to try to westernize the eye—are they going to be happy in the long run? Our experience tells us that most Asian patients probably will not be happy. In addition, the anatomy of the Asian eye is such that completely westernizing the eye is not a realistic goal and we frequently dissuade patients from embarking on this type of cosmetic surgery.

Certain conditions and medications are relative or absolute contraindications to blepharoplasty in all patients (Table 13.4). Smoking in any patient or ethnicity predisposes to poor healing and

patients should be encouraged to discontinue smoking for 2 weeks prior to and 2 weeks after surgery. Autoimmune disease predisposes patients to postoperative sicca syndrome and these patients should be excluded from elective blepharoplasty. The most feared complication of blepharoplasty is blindness, secondary to retro-orbital hematoma. This risk is more pronounced once the surgeon opens the orbital septum to alter the orbital fat pads. However, because of the grave nature of this specific complication, anticoagulant use that cannot be discontinued (such as Aspirin, Warfarin, Clopidogrel, or Heparin) is a contraindication to even the superficial skin-only cosmetic upper lid blepharoplasty. Patients should also be counseled to stop herbal medicines known to impair platelet function (Table 13.5). Likewise, uncontrolled hypertension is also a risk for postoperative hemorrhage and these patients should not be considered for this elective procedure.

Lower lid blepharoplasty in ethnic patients is not very different from that of Caucasians. Preoperative assessment should focus on the presence or absence of a tear trough deformity and the degree of fat pad pseudoherniation. In addition, the degree of lower lid laxity should be assessed by the snap test (Figure 13.16A and B). If prominent laxity is present, adjunctive canthopexy should be considered. While prominent crinkling of the lower lid skin is more common in Caucasians, the degree of looseness plays a major role in the decision for a transcutaneous versus transconjunctival approach to lower lid blepharoplasty. Many African patients will not have prominent loose skin to warrant the transcutaneous, or subcilliary incision and furthermore, many patients of African descent are more at risk for ectropion, which is always a concern of the subcilliary blepharoplasty.

Liposuction technique in ethnic patients is not different from that performed in Caucasian patients; however, what differs are expectations and cultural norms for weight and locations of certain fat deposits. The surgeon should not assume that the liposuction patient wants certain areas of fat reduced because if they make an incorrect assumption, the patient may lose confidence in their ability to understand their needs. A safer approach is to ask the patient, "what bothers you about your appearance," and allow them to direct the interview toward certain areas they are unhappy with.

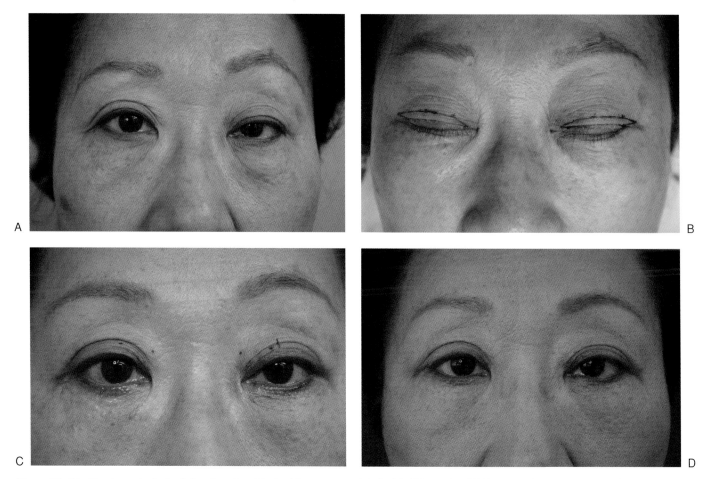

Figure 13.15 *Blepharoplasty in Asian female with double crease and left side lid ptosis. (A) Preoperative appearance. (B) Preoperative markings. (C) One-month postoperative result. (D) Three-month postoperative result (Used with permission from Kee-Yang Chung, MD, PhD)*

When performing neck liposuction, it is important to consider adjunctive augmentation mentoplasty to correct a commonly encountered slightly hypoplastic jaw in Asian patients or as well the age-related bony resorption of the mandible that occurs in all races (Figure 13.17). The patients should be photographed in profile while sitting in the neutral position. A commonly accepted degree of chin protrusion should lie in the same vertical plane as the fore-head (Figure 13.18). If jaw hypoplasia exists, it should be brought to the patient's attention as an excellent way to enhance submental liposculpture to further define the cervicomental angle. However, the patients should also be warned about the risk of PIH in the sub-mental incision scar.

A working knowledge of both the anatomy and cultural norms are all important during the preoperative facelift or browlift interviews.

TABLE 13.4 ■ Contraindications of Cosmetic Blepharoplasty

Relative contraindication	Absolute contraindication
Medically required immunosuppressant medications	Patients unable to discontinue anticoagulants because of medical indication
Sicca syndrome	History of bleeding diathesis
History of keloid formation	Unstable angina pectoris
Diabetes	Thyroid disorder and associated opthalmopathy
Glaucoma	
	Acute narrow angle glaucoma
	Unilateral blindness
	Uncontrolled hypertension
	Recent myocardial infarction
	Multiple sclerosis

TABLE 13.5 ▪ Prescription* and Nonprescription Agents that Increase the Risk of Bleeding

Prescription	Over-the-counter and Herbals
Coumarin	Aspirin (salicylic acid)
Dipyridamole	Garlic supplements
Heparin	Ginko biloba
Clopidogrel	Ginseng
Ticlopidine	Ginger
	Green tea extract
	Feverfew
	Fish oil
	Vitamin E

*U.S. Food and Drug Administration-approved prescription drugs.

Here, the discovery of history or physical examination findings, consistent with hypertrophic or keloidal scars, is imperative prior to rhytidectomy. It is also important to gauge the degree of facial lipoatrophy before performing a facelift in a patient with pronounced age-related fat loss in the midface which can make their face appear gaunt and more hollowed. Thickening the skin with agents such as poly-L-lactic acid (Sculptra™) will help to add volume and a more youthful appearance after a facelift.[29] During the examination, the heaviness and degree of ptotic cheek tissue should be assessed as this can be pronounced in patients of Asian or African descent and may affect the amount of SMAS plication needed during rhytidectomy.

Anatomic considerations of the African American face differ from those of the Caucasian and Asian face. The underlying bony differences in the orbit, maxilla as well as the mandible, combined with differences in malar fat, dermal thickness and supporting ligaments all contribute to differences in aging. For example, African Americans more commonly show changes in the periorbital area

and upper midface before showing signs of brow ptosis and jowling that are common early in the Caucasian face.[30] Commonly, patients of African and Asian descent will complain of excess skin of the upper eyelid (Figure 13.13), bagging under the eyes with hollowing and dark rings under the eyes. This can also be accompanied by rounding of the lateral canthus.[31] While the upper eyelid blepharoplasty in African Americans is not significantly different than that in Caucasians, there is a propensity towards prolapsed lacrimal gland and commonly a need for more aggressive sculpting of upper eyelid fat pads in both Africans and Asians.[32]

DEVICE/TREATMENT SELECTION

The decision between nonsurgical tightening techniques and a surgical approach is relatively straightforward and involves a combination of physical examination findings along with patient preference. With respect to the latter, the decisions are fairly straightforward. If a patient presents, for example, with only moderate nondynamic facial rhytids and laxity and could easily benefit from tightening by either rhytidectomy or resurfacing, the decision should be the patient's to make—after the surgeon has presented an accurate assessment of discomfort and recovery time after either procedure. This consideration of the patient's inherent comfort level is important, as some patients are gravely fearful of any surgery while others want the best result in the fastest time period regardless of perioperative discomfort.

For those patients who desire facial skin tightening, there are many options. When compared to other groups of patients, the balance between effectiveness and potential risks is more exaggerated. For those procedures where significant tissue destruction is purposefully used, a much higher risk of PIH, keloid or hypertrophic scar formation is possible. So while TCA peeling, CO_2 resurfacing and plasma resurfacing can be used in Asians, Hispanics and light-skinned African patients, they should all be used far more judiciously for fear of complications. Fortunately, darker skinned

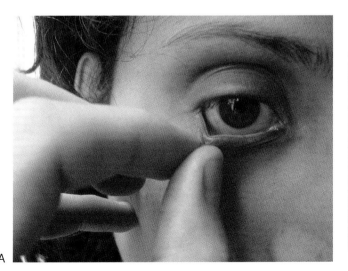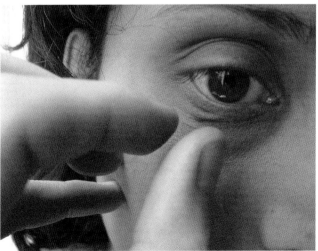

A   B

Figure 13.16 *Snap test to determine the extent of lid laxity. (A) The lower lid is gently retracted and then (B) released. The time to snap back to the globe and the tightness of the lid determines the degree of laxity. In this young Indian female, there is a good snap, connoting no lid laxity*

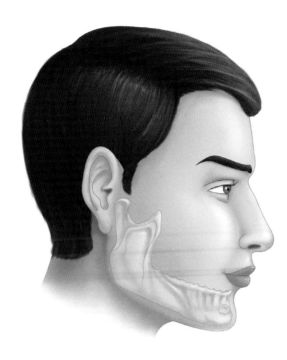

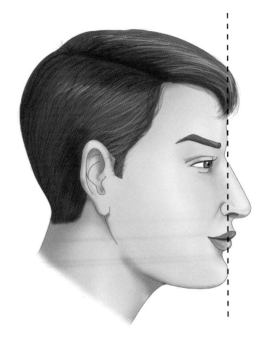

Figure 13.18 *Chin protrusion in the ideal profile. A vertical line should extend from the forehead to the chin when the patient is in the neutral position*

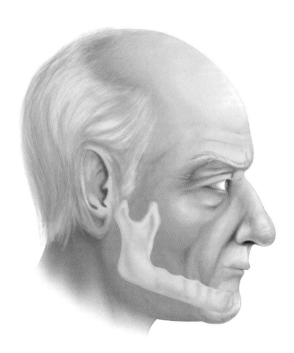

Figure 13.17 *Schematic of age-related mandibular bony resorption from youth (top) compared with old age (bottom)*

devices appear to be safe for use in Fitzpatrick skin types I to V with minimal risk.[27] Increased treatment density, however, may be associated with a greater risk of PIH.[28] This gradual resurfacing is useful for treating dyspigmentation, scars and fine rhytids and is an excellent nonsurgical alternative.[28] With respect to all FP devices, the Cynosure Affirm (1440 nm) may be safer to use on ethnic skin than the Fraxel 1550 nm (Reliant Corp) or Starlux (Palomar Corp.) because it does not penetrate as deeply. Newer devices under development include a fractionated CO_2 laser which

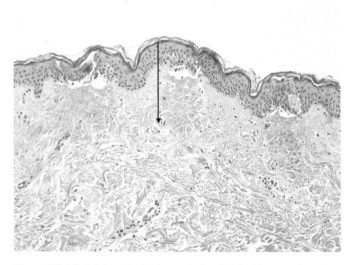

Figure 13.19 *Histopathologic analysis of skin biopsy taken after FP treatment demonstrating a single microscopic thermal zone of damage extending 300 μm. A fractionated 1440-nm Nd:YAG device was used (Affirm^{TM}, Cynosure Corp., MA)*

patients usually have less actinic damage than their Caucasian counterparts, and requiring less tightening on average.

A relatively new modality has recently emerged in the past 3 to 4 years based on the concept of FP. These devices are ablative lasers, but they create only microscopic zones of thermal damage, ranging from a few 100-μm deep, to 1 mm in depth (Figure 13.19). Depending on the device and the treatment parameters, usually between 250 and 1000 of these microscopic treatment zones are placed per square centimeter, resulting in transient, sunburn-like erythema that can last between 1 to 3 days.[11] These

reportedly has slightly increased posttreatment downtime of 3 to 5 days but may deliver as an option that increases tightening more than current FP lasers. No data yet exists on safety in darker skin types. Cynosure Corp. has developed a newer dual fractionated laser at 1320 nm and 1440 nm that fires the two sources with a 3-ms delay between bursts. While preliminary studies regarding tightening are ongoing, the combination of a deeper penetrating 1320-nm device, coupled with their more superficial 1440-nm laser may provide safety in ethnic skin while delivering modest tightening needed in this population.

Upper eyelid skin redundancy or blepharochalasia, if mild, can be treated either surgically or nonsurgically. Nonsurgical modalities include the time-tested TCA peel or CO_2 laser resurfacing. Both have similar recovery periods and can be performed comfortably (although one must be wary of being overly aggressive) in Asian, Hispanic and fair-skinned African patients. Similar results can be obtained with plasma resurfacing (Portrait PSR3®) although settings should be far less aggressive in ethnic patients than in Caucasians. A safer tightening modality that can be used comfortably in darker Fitzpatrick skin types IV to VI is RF heating. Monopolar RF devices such as Thermacool (Thermage Corp.) have adapted their tip sizes to treat the thin skin of the upper eyelid. Nothing more than modest results should be expected from this modality, but if proper protective eyeshields are worn by the patient, risks are minimal in any skin type.

METHOD OR TREATMENT APPLICATION

Darker skin, up through Fitzpatrick type IV can safely tolerate lower levels of most resurfacing devices. While older modalities such as medium depth peeling and dermabrasion are relatively contraindicated in skin types III and IV because of their lack of predictability, leading to increased risk of scar and PIH complications, newer tightening devices, such as FP, plasma resurfacing and RF heating can be used with confidence at lower energies. Treatments that need to be adjusted the least for ethnic skin are the monopolar and bipolar RF deep dermal heating devices. In general, settings only slightly lower than those used on Caucasian skin can be used safely in Asian and African patients. Our experience with several FP devices has been one of significant tolerance in ethnic skin. We find that some Asian patients appear to tolerate even higher energies than Caucasian patients, perhaps because of their thicker dermis (unpublished observations). Plasma resurfacing, however, should be approached with caution in darker skin types. Plasma resurfacing boasts a shorter downtime than traditional CO_2 resurfacing, and many of these patients get impressive results. However, this modality exists on a risk/benefit spectrum just below CO_2 or erbium resurfacing and significantly more effective and less risky than FP. So, just as we would approach CO_2 or erbium resurfacing in ethnic skin types with caution using lower energies and less passes, we would approach plasma resurfacing in ethnic patients in the same regard.

Surgical lifting techniques should be modified for specific techniques and specific ethnic groups. While brow-lifting techniques in themselves do not differ significantly in ethnic patients compared to Caucasian patients, blepharoplasty and rhytidectomy techniques do need to be altered. These differences are mainly based upon anatomical and cultural considerations.

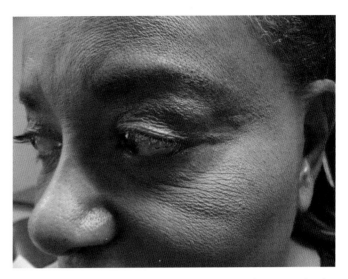

Figure 13.20 *Upper blepharoplasty preoperative consultation photo in a middle-aged African American patient. Bulge in the upper lateral lid should raise suspicions for lacrimal gland prolapse (Used with permission from Kee-Yang Chung, MD, PhD)*

Profound blepharoptosis cannot be treated well without surgery. Upper eyelid blepharoplasty in an African American patient (Figure 13.20) should start with preoperative markings at the existing eyelid crease, noting that on average, the crease in African Americans is usually 6 to 8 mm above the lid margin, which is slightly lower than that of Caucasians (usually 8 to 10 mm in Caucasian females). The amount of skin taken depends on the degree of blepharochalasia and it is important, however, to leave roughly 8 to 10 mm of upper lid skin as measured from the superior incision line to the inferior margin of the eyebrow.[30] As mentioned previously, once a small orbicularis muscle strip is harvested and the septum is entered, more fat sculpting may be necessary as compared to Caucasians and care should be taken to examine bulges at the lateral aspect of the upper to investigate lacrimal gland prolapse. If present, the lacrimal gland can be gently repositioned using an orbital rim pexing suture that then passes only through the lacrimal gland capsule.

Upper lid blepharoplasty in Asians is usually not complicated. Most Asian patients want to maintain the Asian eye characteristics and usually desire improvement that even people close to them will not notice. In these cases, the key is identifying the eyelid crease. The crease is usually 3 to 6 mm above the lash margin. The lower incision should be made at that spot and the remainder of the procedure is not different from blepharoplasty in other patients (Figure 13.21). However, if no crease is present, the incision should be made immediately above the lid margin (Figure 13.22). Asian upper lid blepharoplasty becomes more complicated when the patients want to alter the inherent characteristics of their eyelids (usually to westernize the eye). These are usually the minority of patients, and in our experience, tends to be younger patients.

Lower lid blepharoplasty in African Americans should, whenever possible, be performed using the transconjunctival approach so as to avoid the complications of PIH or even scar hypertrophy that can be associated the subcilliary approach in darker skinned patients. Care should be taken in performing lower lid blepharoplasty in

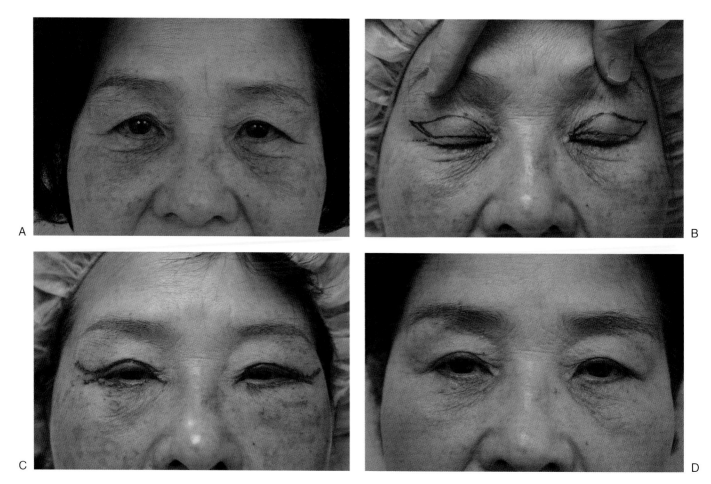

Figure 13.21 *Upper lid blepharoplasty in Asian female with single crease and prominent lateral hooding and lower lid laxity (A) Preoperative appearance. (B) With the brow elevated manually, the incision lines are drawn with a sterile gentian violet marking pen. Note the lateral flare to compensate for the lateral hooding. (C) Immediate postoperative result. (D) Note the subcilliary approach to tighten the skin of the lower lids (Used with permission from Kee-Yang Chung, MD, PhD)*

African American patients as the proptosis that is common when African American patients age, as well as the infraorbital hypoplasia that occurs, puts these patients at risk for lid retraction.[33] Canthopexy, or lid tightening procedures, may be necessary to augment the lower lid blepharoplasty in order to prevent postoperative ectropion.[31] Asian patients can have more hypertrophic orbital fat pads, so that some removal of fat may be necessary in addition to any transposition of fat pads into the nasojugal groove.

Midface descent with accentuation of the melolabial fold and a deepening of the tear trough deformity, is commonly encountered

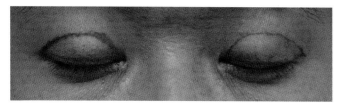

Figure 13.22 *Asian patient who lacks an eyelid crease. Here the incision line proposed is directly above the lash margin (Used with permission from Kee-Yang Chung, MD, PhD)*

in the aged African American face. Correction of the tear trough deformity can be accomplished through either subperiosteal or subcutaneous filling agents such as hyaluronic acid based fillers or fat injections, or with transposition of the medial fat pad during transconjunctival blepharoplasty. Special considerations should be made when attempting to correct the combination of inframalar lipoatrophy and ptosis of the soft tissues of the midcheek which serve to accentuate the melolabial fold. Surgical correction involving either the open approach (rhytidectomy) should not be taken lightly as unacceptable scarring and/or keloid formation may occur if facelift incisions are secured under tension (Figure 13.23). Alternative approaches would include the variety of minimally invasive suture suspension techniques, which can be performed in exactly the same manner as in Caucasian patients.

Neck rejuvenation in ethnic patients is not significantly different than in Caucasians, except that neck sagging is not as prominent in ethnic skin and the risk of postauricular keloid formation may be higher in black patients. One aspect to consider is mandibular hypoplasia and the added benefit that augmentation mentoplasty would bring to neck liposculpture. Newer techniques such as SmartLipo (Cynosure Corp, MA) may add the benefit of tightening

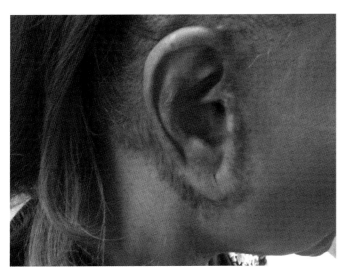

Figure 13.23 *African female who had a facelift performed by a plastic surgeon 4 years prior. Note the significant spreading and dyspigmentation of the rhytidectomy scars. She has had numerous intralesional steroid injections to help flatten the hypertrophic scarring on the postauricular portion*

to fat removal. This device uses a 1064-nm laser-tipped cannula, which has a 6-μs pulse width laser to rupture adipocytes in the deeper fat compartments (Figure 13.24). The surgeon is also directed to scrape the laser-tipped cannula against the dermis of the overlying skin. The theory behind this device is that in addition to liquefying the fat in the area of localized adiposity, the dermis contracts in response to the photothermal effect that causes tissue coagulation. No studies have yet shown if ethnic skin patients are at any greater risk with this aspect of the device, although in our hands we have not yet had any PIH when treating even African American patients.

In summary, both lifting and tightening of ethnic skin poses certain challenges for the dermasurgeon that need to be addressed from both an anatomical and cultural perspective. In general, the complication rate from tightening techniques in ethnic skin will be higher if exactly the same parameters are used as in Caucasian patients. However, once those techniques are adjusted for by the differences in ethnic skin, then efficacy and side effect profiles can be comparable to those in Caucasians. Lifting techniques in ethnic skin also pose certain challenges that are more dependent on anatomical differences, but those differences should not stop the practitioner from helping these patients. With the help of this chapter, dermasurgeons should be better equipped to master the anatomy needed to successfully perform blepharoplasty, rhytidectomy and liposuction on ethnic patients.

REFERENCES

1. Grimes PE, Hunt SG. Considerations for cosmetic surgery in the black population. *Clin Plast Surg.* 1993;20:27-34.
2. Montagna W, Carlisle K. The architecture of black and white facial skin. *J Am Acad Dermatol.* 1991;24:929-937.
3. Berardesca E, Maibach HI. Sensitive and ethnic skin. A need for special skin-care agents? *Dermatol Clin.* 1991;9:89-92.
4. McCurdy JA Jr. *Cosmetic Surgery of the Asian Face.* New York, NY: Thieme Medical Publishers; 1990.
5. Cho SB, Park CO, Chung WG, et al. Histometric and histochemical analysis of the effect of trichloroacetic acid concentration in the chemical reconstruction of skin scars method. *Dermatol Surg.* 2006;32:1231-1236.
6. Lee JB, Chung WG, Kwahck H, et al. Focal treatment of acne scars with trichloroacetic acid: chemical reconstruction of skin scars method. *Dermatol Surg.* 2002;28:1017-1021.
7. Swinehart JM. Case reports: surgical therapy of acne scars in pigmented skin. *J Drugs Dermatol.* 2007;6:74-77.
8. Pierce H, Brown L. Laminar dermal reticulopathy and chemical peeling in the black patient. *J Dermatol Surg Oncol.* 1980;12:69-73.
9. Anderson RR, Parish JA. Selective photothermolysis: precise microsurgery by selective absorption of pulsed radiation. *Science.* 1983;220:524-527.
10. Fitzpatrick TB. The validity and practicality of sun-reactive skin types I through VI. *Arch Dermatol.* 1988;124:869-871.
11. Hantash BM, Mahmood MB. Fractional photothermolysis: a novel aesthetic laser surgery modality. *Dermatol Surg.* 2007;33:525-534.
12. Narurkar VA. Skin rejuvenation with microthermal fractional photothermolysis. *Dermatol Ther.* 2007;20(Suppl 1):S10-S13.
13. Laubach HJ, Tannous Z, Anderson RR, et al. Skin responses to fractional photothermolysis. *Lasers Surg Med.* 2006;38:142-149.
14. David LM, Lask GP, Glassberg E, et al. Laser abrasion for cosmetic and medical treatment of facial actinic damage. *Cutis.* 1989;43:583-587.
15. Lowe NJ, Lask G, Griffin ME, et al. Skin resurfacing with the UltraPulse carbon dioxide laser. Observations on 100 patients. *Dermatol Surg.* 1995;21:1025-1029.

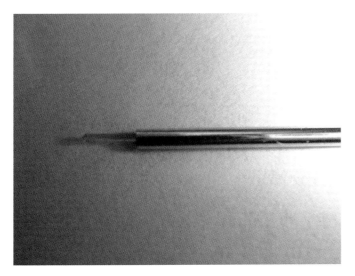

Figure 13.24 *Smartlipo 1064-nm fiber optic laser-tipped cannula*

16. Lask G, Keller G, Lowe N, et al. Laser skin resurfacing with the SilkTouch flashscanner for facial rhytides. *Dermatol Surg.* 1995;21:1021-1024.

17. Ho C, Nguyen Q, Lowe NJ, et al. Laser resurfacing in pigmented skin. *Dermatol Surg.* 1995;21:1035-1037.

18. McCurdy JA. Blepharoplasty in the oriental eye. *Am J Cosmet Surg.* 1985;2:29.

19. Zhang H, Zhuang H, Yu H, et al. A new Z-epicanthoplasty and a concomitant double eyelidplasty in Chinese eyelids. *Plast Reconstr Surg.* 2006;118:900-907.

20. Park JI. Modified Z-epicanthoplasty in the Asian eyelid. *Arch Facial Plast Surg.* 2000;2:43-47.

21. Park JI. Root Z-epicanthoplasty in Asian eyelids. *Plast Reconstr Surg* 2003;111:2476-2477.

22. Shirakabe Y, Suzuki Y, Lam SM. A new paradigm for the aging Asian face. *Aesthetic Plast Surg.* 2003;27:397-402.

23. Weiss RA, Weiss MA, Munavalli G, et al. Monopolar radiofrequency facial tightening: a retrospective analysis of efficacy and safety in over 600 treatments. *J Drugs Dermatol.* 2006;5:707-712.

24. Alster TS, Tanzi E. Improvement of neck and cheek laxity with a nonablative radiofrequency device: a lifting experience. *Dermatol Surg.* 2004;30:503-507.

25. Nahm WK, Su TT, Rotunda AM, et al. Objective changes in brow position, superior palpebral crease, peak angle of the eyebrow, and jowl surface area after volumetric radiofrequency treatments to half of the face. *Dermatol Surg.* 2004;30:922-928.

26. Fitzpatrick R, Geronemus R, Goldberg D, et al. Multicenter study of noninvasive radiofrequency for periorbital tissue tightening. *Lasers Surg Med.* 2003;33:232-242.

27. Rokhsar CK, Fitzpatrick RE. The treatment of melasma with fractional photothermolysis: a pilot study. *Dermatol Surg.* 2005;31:1645-1650.

28. Lin JY, Chan HH. Pigmentary disorders in Asian skin: treatment with laser and intense pulsed light sources. *Skin Therapy Lett.* 2006;11:8-11.

29. Kouba DJ, Fincher EF, Moy RL. An algorithmic approach to esthetic facial volume restoration. *Dermatol Ther.* 2007;20 (Suppl 1):S14-S15.

30. Matory WE Jr. *Ethnic Considerations in Facial Aesthetic Surgery.* Philadelphia, PA: Lippincott-Raven Publishers;1998.

31. Harris MO. The aging face in patients of color: minimally invasive surgical facial rejuvenation-a targeted approach. *Dermatol Ther.* 2004;17:206-211.

32. Bosniak SL, Cantisano Zilkha M. *Cosmetic Blepharoplasty and Facial Rejuventation.* Philadelphia, PA: Lippincott-Raven Publishers; 1999.

33. McCord CD, Groessl SA. Lower-lid dynamics: influence on blepharoplasty and management of lower-lid retraction. *Op Tech Plast Reconstr Surg.* 1998;5:99-108.

CHAPTER 14 Cosmeceuticals in Ethnic Skin

Zoe Diana Draelos, MD

INTRODUCTION

Skin cosmeceuticals represent an interesting realm between dermatologic drugs and cosmetics. Traditional drugs are products designed to treat skin disease available only by prescription. On the other hand, cosmetics are used to scent, adorn, and color the skin without the intent of altering its structure or function. New understandings of skin physiology, novel raw materials, clever formulations, and increased consumer awareness of skin aging have resulted in a poorly defined category of dermatologics known as cosmeceuticals. Cosmeceuticals are of particular interest in the ethnic population, since skin ashiness, facial skin shine, antiaging photoprotection, and irregular pigmentation are of key importance. Improvement in all of these appearance related areas could only be achieved through an understanding of the ingredients combined to deliver an identified skin benefit. This chapter focuses on the use of cosmeceuticals in ethnic skin.

COSMECEUTICAL TREATMENT ALTERNATIVES

Cosmeceutical treatment alternatives for ethnic skin can be divided into the basic hygiene activities of cleansing and moisturizing and skin health activities consisting of photoprotection and skin lightening. The unique melanin distribution of ethnic skin creates formulation challenges for optimal skin functioning, since inflammation of any sort results in undesirable darkening of the skin color, known as postinflammatory hyperpigmentation. While mild skin irritation may be tolerable in minimally pigmented skin, since the resulting erythema is short lived and not accompanied by hyperpigmentation, any product-induced inflammation in ethnic skin may cause prolonged pigmentary change. Thus, cleansers designed to produce mild exfoliation and improve skin surface texture in Caucasian skin, may produce postinflammatory hyperpigmentation in African America skin. Similarly, antiaging moisturizers with hydroxy acids designed to induce edema and minimize facial fine lines in Caucasian skin may also produce pigmentary changes in African American skin. It is for this reason that the reader must understand unique ethnic skin needs in terms of cleansing and moisturizing while addressing important skin issues in terms of photoprotection and skin lightening.

▨ Cleansing

Cleansing of the skin is important, both for optimal appearance and good hygiene. The cleansing of ethnic skin presents some unique challenges because of the adverse effects of over or under cleansing the skin. To understand how cleansing affects skin appearance, it is important to understand how the human eye assesses skin

beauty. Visible light reaches the skin surface and is either reflected back to the eye from the stratum corneum or enters the skin and is then reflected back to the eye from collagen fibers, blood vessels, and melanosomes. In ethnic skin, the desquamating corneocytes contain pigment. This brown skin scale appears gray when viewed, as a result of the air interface behind the scale and gives rise to the term "ashy," which is used to describe the appearance of dry skin in darker complected population. The term likens the skin scale to the gray appearance of ashes after combustible material has been consumed by fire. Ashy skin is equated with dry skin and is considered unattractive because of the suboptimal skin color viewed as light bounces off of the stratum corneum.

Visible light may also enter ethnic skin, which contains abundant pigment, for subsequent reflection to the eye. If the pigment is evenly distributed, the skin appears an even brown color. If the melanin is present in clumps, the skin will appear unevenly lighter and darker depending on the pigment distribution (Figure 14.1). In Fitzpatrick skin types I, II, and III, unevenness in skin color is caused by the irregular distribution of vascular structures and collagen, giving the skin undesirable red and yellow colors. The effects of collagen breakdown and the formation of telangiectatic vascular structures are not of primary concern in ethnic skin, making pigmentary change the single most important measure of skin attractiveness.

Thus, a good cleanser must remove enough sebum for the skin to appear clean, but not too much sebum to create ashy skin scale. There are a variety of cleansers that have been developed for facial and body cleansing to meet various skin needs. These include bar soaps, liquid cleansers, lipid-free cleansers, cleansing creams, exfoliating cleansers, and cleansing clothes. The value of each of these cleanser types is discussed in the context of ethnic skin needs.

Soaps and cleansers

The most common type of cleanser used for face and body cleaning in the marketplace is the bar soap (Table 14.1). However, not all

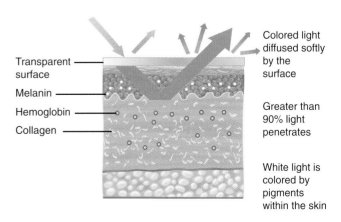

Figure 14.1 *Skin color perceptions. Light is reflected from the skin surface and within the skin from hemoglobin, collagen, and melanin.*

TABLE 14.1 ■ Cleanser Types

Cleanser type	Advantages	Disadvantages	Example
Soap	Excellent sebum removal	High pH, most irritating	Ivory (Procter & Gamble)
Syndet	Less sebum removal, neutral pH	Less skin cleansing	Dove (Unilever)
Combar	Antibacterial properties	Moderately irritating	Irish Spring (Colgate-Palmolive)

bar products contain soap. Soap technically refers to a chemical composition created by a reaction between a fat and an alkali resulting in a fatty acid salt with a pH of 9 to 10.[1] The original mass market soap conforming to this chemical composition was Ivory (Procter & Gamble), which is still sold today. This bar soap has excellent sebum and environmental dirt removal capabilities, but cleansing habits have changed from the once weekly family bath to daily bathing for purposes beyond personal hygiene. Many people shower for relaxation, the enjoyment of warm water running over the body, or aromatherapy. Facial cleansing has also increased for purposes of removing facial cosmetics or creating a clean skin surface for the application of medications. These are skin needs that were not present when Ivory soap was originally created. It is this frequent facial and body washing that led to the need for a cleanser with less detergent qualities for individuals with lower sebum production, but the desire to frequently wash.

This newer type of cleanser was labeled a synthetic detergent, also known as a syndet, because it did not have the traditional chemistry of a soap. Instead, synthetic detergents contained less than 10% soap with a pH adjusted to 5.5 to 7. It was theorized that this more neutral cleanser pH would produce less skin irritation and dryness than the true soaps formulated with a higher alkaline pH. This may or may not be true and is still rather controversial, since the ability of a cleanser to complex with the stratum corneum and the completeness with which the cleanser can be rinsed from the skin appear to be important secondary cleanser mildness considerations. Popular synthetic detergent bar cleansers include Dove bar (Unilever), Oil of Olay bar (Procter &Gamble), and Cetaphil® bar (Galderma). These bar cleansers remove less sebum and are less likely to damage the intercellular lipids, thus preventing the formation of ashy skin in an ethnic population with dry skin.

A third type of bar cleanser, extremely popular in ethnic skin, is known as a combar. It contains both true alkaline soap and synthetic detergents to create a bar with better sebum removal abilities, but decreased likelihood of inducing intercellular lipid damage.[2] Popular examples of combars include Dial (Dial Corp.), Irish Spring® (Colgate-Palmolive), and Coast (Colgate-Palmolive). Many of the combar cleansers also contain an antibacterial, such as triclosan, to decrease body odor by reducing the bacterial count present on the skin surface. Combars are extremely popular among ethnic individuals with oily skin and abundant apocrine secretions. Pigmented skin appears much shinier than Caucasian skin with a minimal amount of sebum. This is caused by wetting effects of the sebum on the stratum corneum and the elimination of the air/corneocyte interfaces. A minimal amount of sebum increases light reflection back to the eye creating the appearance of shiny skin, which is considered to be oily unattractive skin by many ethnic individuals. Combar cleansers offer the benefit of sebum removal to

reduce facial shine while preventing ashiness from over-removal of intercellular lipids.

Tremendous market diversity has created cleansers that do not fit into the strict categories outlined above. For example, syndet bar cleansers are available with triclosan for odor control purposes in formulations such as Lever 2000 (Unilever). The triclosan is slightly drying and irritating on the skin surface, but this irritation is balanced by the less-thorough sebum removal of the syndet cleanser. In addition, soaps, syndets, and combars are now available in liquid formulations with the same name as the soap for consumers, who prefer to wash with a liquid rather than a bar. The attributes of the liquid cleanser are the same as the bar cleanser, except that it is easier to overuse a liquid cleanser by applying too much to the skin surface and removing more sebum and intercellular lipids from the skin surface than desired.

There is one new area of liquid cleanser development worth discussing that offers a unique benefit to ethnic individuals with extremely dry ashy skin. This type of liquid cleanser is known as a high petrolatum depositing body wash and must be applied to the body with a woven mesh, known as puff (Olay Ribbons, Procter & Gamble). These cleansers are designed to take advantage of new emulsion technology allowing water-soluble and oil-soluble ingredients to be combined in one continuous liquid phase. In this type of cleanser, a synthetic detergent is placed in the water-soluble phase and petrolatum, dimethicone, and soybean oil are placed in the oil-soluble phase. When the cleanser is placed on the puff, the water-soluble phase mixes with the shower water and removes sebum and environmental dirt from the skin surface for rinsing down the drain. As the concentration of water on the skin increases with rinsing, the oil-soluble phase coats the skin surface leaving behind a thin layer of petrolatum, dimethicone, and soybean oil. These ingredients smooth down the skin scale created by cleansing and reduce the appearance of ashiness. This new technology offers an important skin benefit for ethnic individuals who wish to bathe frequently without concerns of ashy skin. It is anticipated that new cleansers for the ethnic skin care market will focus on combining skin hygiene with the varying personal needs for bathing.

There are other cleansing technologies that fulfil specific bathing and hygiene needs. These variants are listed in Table 14.2 and discussed next.

Lipid-free cleansers

There are ethnic individuals who possess extremely dry skin, possibly created by the presence of dermatologic disease, who cannot bathe with water and soap, syndet, or combar cleansers previously discussed. For this unique skin care need, lipid-free cleansers were developed, which are liquid products that clean without fats distinguishing them from the cleansers previously discussed. Lipid-free

TABLE 14.2 ■ **Cleanser Formulations**

Type	Advantage	Disadvantage	Example
Bar	Inexpensive, excellent cleansing	No moisturizing qualities	See Table 14.1
Liquid	Less messy, no soap dish	More expensive, can use too much product	Soft soap (Colgate-Palmolive)
Lipid-free	Less drying, used without water	Leaves behind thin film, no antibacterial properties	Cetaphil (Galderma) CeraVe cleanser (Coria)
Cleansing Cream	Removes cosmetics, nondrying	Leaves behind thick film, no antibacterial properties	Cold cream (Ponds)
Abrasive Scrub	Exfoliant, improves skin texture	Irritating, may cause hyperpigmentation	Seventh day scrub (Clinique)
Cleansing Cloth	Gentle exfoliation, disposable cleansing	Mildly irritating, expensive	Daily facial cloths (Olay)

cleansers are applied to dry or moistened skin, rubbed to produce lather, and rinsed or wiped away (Cetaphil® Cleanser, Galderma; CeraVe™ Cleanser, Coria). These products may contain water, glycerin, cetyl alcohol, stearyl alcohol, sodium laurel sulfate, and sometimes propylene glycol. They leave behind a thin moisturizing film, but do not have strong antibacterial properties and may not remove odor from the armpit or groin. For facial cleansing and cosmetic removal, lipid-free cleansers are ideal for ethnic dry skin.

Cleansing cream

Cleansing creams are an older cleanser formulation, popular for cleaning extremely dry ethnic skin. Cleansing creams are composed of water, mineral oil, petrolatum, and waxes.[3] Cold cream, a variant of cleansing cream, is created by adding borax to the formulation.[4] These products are excellent at removing cosmetics in persons with extremely dry skin. They are wiped on the face and then wiped off without water. It is the wiping that removes the oil-soluble and water-soluble materials from the face. Cleansing cream would not be recommended in ethnic population with acne or oily skin, but are an alternative for cleansing extremely dry ashy facial skin.

Abrasive scrub

A very popular facial cleanser is known as the abrasive scrub. These products contain syndet cleansers and a particulate designed to physically remove the stratum corneum from the face to improve skin texture. The particulate material may be polyethylene beads, aluminum oxide, ground fruit pits, or sodium tetraborate decahydrate granules to induce various degrees of exfoliation.[5] The most abrasive scrub is produced by aluminum oxide particles and ground fruit pits and the least aggressive abrasion of the skin is found in products that contain sodium tetraborate decahydrate granules, which soften and dissolve during use. These products can cause irritation when used on sensitive ethnic skin resulting in postinflammatory hyperpigmentation. In general, it is better to use a mild cleanser followed by a moisturizer to improve the appearance of ashy skin rather than an abrasive scrub to remove the skin scale.

Disposable cleansing cloth

A more appropriate method of removing skin scale from ethnic skin is the disposable cleansing cloth. The cloths are less abrasive than an abrasive scrub and composed of a combination of polyester, rayon, cotton, and cellulose fibers held together via heat through a technique known as thermobonding. Additional strength is imparted to the cloth by hydroentangling the fibers. This is achieved by entwining the individual rayon, polyester, and wood pulp fibers with high pressure jets of water, which eliminates the need for adhesive binders, thereby creating a soft, strong cloth. These cloths are packaged dry and impregnated with a cleanser that foams modestly when the cloth is moistened. The type of cleanser in the cloth depends whether strong sebum removal is required by oily skin or modest sebum removal is required by dry skin. Humectants and emollients can also be added to the cloth to decrease barrier damage with cleansing or to smooth the skin scale present in xerosis.

In addition to the composition of the ingredients preapplied to the dry cloth, the weave of the cloth will also determine its cutaneous effect. There are two types of fiber weaves used in facial products: open weave and closed weave. Open weave cloths are so named because of the 2- to 3-mm windows in the cloth between the adjacent fiber bundles. These cloths are used in persons with dry and/or sensitive skin to increase the softness of the cloth and decrease the surface area contact between the cloth and the skin yielding a milder exfoliant effect. Closed weave cloths, on the hand, are designed with a much tighter weave and provide a more aggressive exfoliation. Ultimately, the degree of exfoliation achieved is dependent on the cloth weave, the pressure with which the cloth is stroked over the skin surface, and the length of time the cloth is applied. Cleansing cloths should be used gently in ethnic population to avoid irritation resulting in postinflammatory hyperpigmentation.

The goal of all cleansers is to remove sebum from the skin surface and leave the intercellular lipids intact. This is a lofty goal for any cleanser, which accounts for the tremendous growth in the moisturizer market, designed to minimize cleanser-induced dry skin.

■ Moisturizing

Moisturizers are deigned to improve the texture, feel, and appearance of the skin. From a medical standpoint, moisturizers must increase the water content of the skin (moisturization), make the skin feel smooth and soft (emolliency), and protect injured or

TABLE 14.3 ■ Moisturizer Classification

Type	Advantages	Disadvantages	Example
Occlusive	Most effective reduction of water loss	Thick, greasy	Petrolatum, lanolin, mineral oil
Humectant	Attract water to the dehydrated stratum corneum	Can enhance water loss if barrier defective	Glycerin, sorbitol, propylene glycol, hyaluronic acid
Hydrophilic Matrix	Physical barrier to water loss	Film must remain intact for efficacy	Colloidal oatmeal, proteins

exposed skin from harmful or annoying stimuli (skin protectant). For the water content of the skin to increase, barrier repair must be initiated, dermal–epidermal water diffusion must occur, and the synthesis of intercellular lipids must proceed.[6] It is generally thought in the cosmetics industry that a stratum corneum containing between 20% and 35% water will exhibit the softness and pliability of normal stratum corneum.[7]

Occlusive moisturizers

There are three primary mechanisms by which the stratum corneum can be rehydrated: occlusives, humectants, and hydrophilic matrices (Table 14.3).[8] Occlusive agents are oily substances that place a water impermeable coating over the stratum corneum to create an artificial barrier until true barrier repair can occur (Table 14.4). The most occlusive moisturizer is petrolatum.[9] It reduces water loss through the damaged stratum corneum by 99%, allowing 1% water loss to continue, thus providing the signal for barrier repair to be transmitted.[10] Petrolatum is the most effective moisturizer known as it permeates throughout the interstices of the stratum corneum mimicking the intercellular lipids.[11] It is highly effective at reducing the appearance of ashy ethnic, but its poor aesthetics have created a need for other occlusive moisturizing ingredients.

Another major category of occlusive moisturizers is oils. These can be mineral, vegetable, or other synthetic oils. Mineral oil is the second most commonly used moisturizing ingredient behind petro-

TABLE 14.4 ■ Occlusive Moisturizing Ingredients by Category

1. Hydrocarbon oils and waxes: petrolatum, mineral oil, paraffin, squalene
2. Silicone oils: dimethicone, cyclomethicone
3. Vegetable and animal fats: soybean oil, grape seed oil, almond oil
4. Fatty acids: lanolin acid, stearic acid
5. Fatty alcohol: lanolin alcohol, cetyl alcohol
6. Polyhydric alcohols: propylene glycol
7. Wax esters: lanolin, beeswax, stearyl stearate
8. Vegetable waxes: carnauba, candelilla
9. Phospholipids: lecithin
10. Sterols: cholesterol

latum. It is less sticky and has better aesthetics, but still leaves behind a greasy skin film. This has led to the search for other thinner oils that still retard stratum corneum water loss, also known as transepidermal water loss. Lighter vegetable oils, such as soybean oil, grape seed oil, and sesame seed oil, are alternatives used in less occlusive moisturizer formulations. The newest and most aesthetically pleasing oils used in moisturizers are the silicone oils, such as dimethicone and cyclomethicone. These silicone products are the basis for many of the oil-free formulations that do not contain traditional mineral and vegetable oils. They do not impart a greasy feel to the skin; yet provide excellent reduction in transepidermal water loss.

A typical moisturizer will combine petrolatum, water, and oils to yield the thickness and aesthetics desired for the intended user and the body area of application. Thus, a moisturizer for ethnic skin would be aimed at smoothing down skin scale to eliminate ashiness. Since ashiness reduction is accomplished primarily by occlusive moisturizing ingredients, many ethnic moisturizers contain highly occlusive agents such as cocoa butter, lanolin, shea butter, and mineral oil.

Humectant moisturizers

Another mechanism of moisturization is the use of humectants. Humectants are substances that absorb water.[12] In moisturizer formulation, humectants attract water from the dermis to the dehydrated epidermis.[13] This water is then held in the skin by the occlusive ingredients that prevent loss until the skin barrier can be repaired. Most quality moisturizers contain both humectant and occlusive ingredients. Popular humectants used in moisturizers include glycerin, honey, sodium lactate, urea, propylene glycol, sorbitol, pyrrolidone carboxylic acid, gelatin, hyaluronic acid, and vitamins.[14,15] Humectants are not as commonly used in ethnic moisturizers, as in moisturizers designed for Fitzpatrick skin types I, II, and III. This is because humectants can increase the appearance of ashy skin if the concentration of occlusives is not sufficient.

Hydrophilic moisturizers

The final and least important method of moisturization is the use of hydrophilic matrices. Hydrophilic matrices are large molecular weight substances that physically prevent evaporation of water from the damaged stratum corneum. The original hydrophilic matrix used in dermatology was the oatmeal bath. The colloidal oatmeal was placed in the bath to form a protective coating over the skin and prevent evaporation. Oatmeal baths are sometimes recommended by dermatologists for persons with atopic dermatitis to prevent enhanced dryness from bathing. Other hydrophilic matrices used in moisturizers include the newer engineered proteins that can form a thin film over the skin surface altering both its ability to hold water and optical characteristics. These proteins form the basis for many of the antiaging moisturizers designed for all skin colors since the protein film is invisible on the skin surface.

Emolliency

As mentioned previously, one of the most important attributes of moisturizers designed for ethnic skin is the ability to reduce the appearance of ashy skin by smoothing down skin scale. This is a quality known as emolliency. Emolliency is the ability to create a smooth skin surface by temporarily filling the spaces between the desquamating skin scales with oil droplets.[16] These same oils that smooth down skin scale may also function as occlusive moisturizers. Commonly used emollients in ethnic moisturizers include di-isopropyl dilinoleate, isopropyl isostearate, propylene glycol, jojoba oil, isostearyl isostearate, octyl stearate, dimethicone, and cyclomethicone.[17]

Moisturizer formulation

There are two basic moisturizer formulations: oil-in-water and water-in-oil emulsions. Oil-in-water emulsions are the most popular moisturizers and contain primarily water, in which the oil is dissolved. Water-in-oil emulsions, on the other hand, contain primarily oil in which the water is dissolved. Oil-in-water emulsions can be identified by their cool feel and nonglossy appearance while water-in-oil emulsions can be identified by their warm feel and glossy appearance.[18] Oil-in-water emulsions dominate the marketplace because they are less greasy and leave a thinner film on the skin surface because of evaporation of the dominant water phase, but they also provide less moisturizing.

The tremendous number of moisturizers in the ethnic marketplace can be created by varying the amount of water and oil in the formulation and the specialty ingredients designed to impart some unique skin benefit. Daytime moisturizers for ethnic skin are generally composed of mineral oil, propylene glycol, and water in sufficient quantity to form a lotion to which sunscreen may be added. If the lotion is labeled as an oil-free formulation, the mineral oil will be replaced with dimethicone. Night creams are typically thicker and more moisturizing and may be composed of mineral oil, lanolin alcohol, petrolatum, and water to form a cream. Body lotions generally contain 10% to 15% in the oil phase and 75% to 85% in the water phase. Humectants, such as glycerin, are added in a 5% to 10% concentration to make the remainder of the formulation. Hand creams have 15% to 40% in the oil phase, 45% to 80% in the water phase, and 15% humectants, making them the thickest of all the moisturizer formulations.[19]

To understand how a moisturizer is constructed, it is worthwhile to consider the formulation of a common inexpensive body lotion designed for ashy skin is typically composed of water, mineral oil, propylene glycol, stearic acid, and petrolatum or lanolin. Humectants, such as glycerin or sorbitol, may be included in addition to specialty ingredients, such as vitamins A, D, and E or aloe and allantoin. Specialty ingredients can be used for marketing purposes or to impart unique skin benefits to the formulation. For example, vitamin E is an excellent emollient imparting smoothness to rough scaly skin. Vitamin E is used to add shine to deeply pigmented ethnic skin. Allantoin, on the other hand, is a naturally occurring anti-inflammatory obtained from the comfrey root that can be used to prevent postinflammatory hyperpigmentation in easily irritated skin.

Photoprotection

One of the major cosmeceutical categories includes products designed to prevent aging of the skin. While skin aging is not as prominent in ethnic skin as in Caucasian skin, it represents the second appearance concern behind irregular pigmentation, the next topic of discussion. Most of the antiaging claims in cosmeceuticals are supported by the inclusion of sunscreen ingredients in the formulation. Sunscreen formulation in ethnic skin is challenging because of the postinflammatory hyperpigmentation that accompanies irritation and the appearance of white sunscreen ingredients on pigmented skin. These issues will be further examined as the various categories of sunscreens are reviewed.

Sunscreens can provide photoprotection by reflecting or absorbing UV radiation. Physical sunscreens, also known as inorganic sunscreens, reflect UV radiation across the complete spectrum. Inorganic sunscreens are white particulates, such as zinc oxide or titanium dioxide, which are suspended in a lotion applied to the skin surface. Chemical sunscreens, also known as organic sunscreens, function by absorbing UV energy and transforming it to heat, which is radiated from the skin surface. Organic sunscreens are colorless, but share a common phenolic ring structure, such that they are chemically altered as part of the photoprotection process. These sunscreens are consumed during wearing, but new advancements have prolonged the longevity of organic sunscreens. A discussion of these two sunscreen categories in the ethnic population follows.

Inorganic sunscreens

As mentioned previously, zinc oxide and titanium dioxide, comprise the main inorganic sunscreen ingredients in the marketplace. They are available in variety of particle forms: micronized, microfine, colorless, and nanoparticle. Titanium dioxide is typically used in the micronized particle form. Here the particles are a variety of different shapes and sizes, some large and some small. This provides optimal photoprotection, since there are many different surfaces to reflect the UV radiation; however, the larger particle size is visible to the human eye creating a white film appearance. For this reason, micronized titanium dioxide may be a problematic sunscreen ingredient in ethnic skin.

Smaller particles are found in microfine formulations, typically composed of zinc oxide, which are formulated for daywear in the form of sunscreen-containing moisturizers. However, even microfine particles can create a subtle white film in darker complected ethnic skin. This has led to the development of "colorless" zinc oxide, which is indeed invisible on the skin, but the photoprotective qualities of the ingredient are also reduced. The newest form of zinc oxide to enter the marketplace, for ethnic skin photoprotection, is nanoparticle zinc oxide, but there are some unresolved health issues regarding nanoparticle skin safety.

Nanoparticles possess a diameter between 1 and 100 nm and are found in the environment as a byproduct of fire, internal combustion engines, and air pollution exhaust. These particles are invisible to the human eye, but can penetrate the skin and lung tissues, gaining access to the lymphatics and blood circulation. From there, these particles can be widely distributed throughout the body. Once these particles enter the body, they cannot be removed. Concern has been voiced in the medical community that metal nanoparticles might be responsible for neurologic disease, yet others have wondered if the chronic inflammation induced by nanoparticles, as manifested by unusually high levels of interleukins 8 and 12 in nanoparticle containing skin, might not cause other degenerative diseases. At present, the main concern regarding nanoparticle zinc oxide is its ability to enter the skin either through the pilosebaceous orifices, between the corneocytes, or through the corneocytes via passive diffusion. While nanoparticle zinc oxide would be a perfect ingredient for ethnic skin photoprotection because of its ability to prevent dyspigmentation, its invisible skin characteristics, and the lack of heat production, its safety requires further investigation.

Organic sunscreens

The other group of sunscreen ingredients to provide photoprotection is known as organic sunscreens because they undergo a chemical reaction, known as resonance delocalization. During resonance delocalization, the phenol ring, which contains an electron-releasing group in the ortho and/or para position, absorbs UV radiation and transforms it to heat. The reaction and is irreversible rendering the sunscreen inactive once it has absorbed the UV radiation. There are many more organic than inorganic sunscreens. Organic sunscreens are in general more appropriate for ethnic skin, since they are colorless when applied yet providing excellent prevention of hyperpigmentation.

Organic sunscreen ingredients can be divided into UVA absorbers (320–360 nm), including avobenzone, ecamsule, and oxybenzone and UVB absorbers (290–320 nm), such as the salicylates and cinnamates. UVA photoprotection is extremely important in ethnic skin to prevent unwanted tanning and decrease the incidence of photo-induced postinflammatory hyperpigmentation. One of the main UVA photoprotectants for ethnic skin is avobenzone, also known as Parsol 1789. Unfortunately, avobenzone is highly photounstable with 36% of the avobenzone destroyed shortly after sun exposure. It is estimated that all the avobenzone is gone from a sunscreen after 5 hours or 50 J of exposure necessitating frequent reapplication. Avobenzone is also chemically incompatible with other commonly used inorganic filters, such as zinc oxide and titanium dioxide. However, avobenzone has assumed new importance as a proprietary sunscreen complex, known as Helioplex™ (Neutrogena®), has been introduced that combines avobenzone with oxybenzone and 2,6-diethylhexylnaphthalate to create a photostable avobenzone with long-lasting UVA photoprotectant qualities. Ecamsule, better known as Mexoryl™ (L'Oréal), also stabilizes avobenzone.

UVB photoprotection is important in ethnic skin to prevent sunburn. Both the salicylates and the cinnamates can be used because of their colorless transparent nature. The salicylate class includes octyl salicylate (Octisalate) and homomenthyl salicylate (Homosalate), which absorb UVB radiation because of internal hydrogen bonding at 300–310 nm. Approximately 56% of the sunscreens in the current marketplace use the salicylates as a secondary sunscreen active, since they have an excellent safety record with minimal allergenicity. The cinnamates, on the other hand, are the most popular sunscreen category currently used in antiaging cosmeceuticals for ethnic skin. 86% of products with an SPF rating contain octyl methoxycinnamate, also known as Octinoxate, which has maximal absorption at 305 nm. Octyl methoxycinnamate has excellent photostability with only 4.5% degradation after UVB exposure.

Pigment Lightening

Facial hyperpigmentation is the most common sign of photoaging found in ethnic skin. It may present in the form of small lentigenes across the lateral cheeks, usually begins approximately at 25 to 30 years of age, depending on cumulative sun exposure, with continued accumulation of lesions throughout life. Pigmentation can also present in the form of melasma with reticulated pigmentation over the sides of the forehead, lateral jawline, and upper lip. Unique ethnic pigmentation can also occur in the periorbital area, especially in persons of Indian descent. Lastly, hyperpigmentation can present following any injury to the skin, such as acne lesions, thermal burns, or repeated mechanical trauma. Cosmeceutical treatments for hyperpigmentation are problematic. A successful treatment must remove existing pigment from the skin, shut down the manufacture of melanin, and prevent the transfer of existing melanin to the melanosomes. This section examines the ingredients currently used in cosmeceutical preparations to lighten pigment, such as hydroquinone, retinoids, mequinol, azelaic acid, arbutin, kojic acid, aleosin, licorice extract, ascorbic acid, soy proteins, and N-acetyl glucosamine. This section examines the efficacy and safety of each of these ingredients.

Hydroquinone

The gold standard ingredient for hyperpigmentation therapy in the United States is hydroquinone (Figure 14.2). It is found in many over-the-counter (OTC), physician dispensed, and prescription skin lightening preparations. Hydroquinone predated formation of the U.S. Food and Drug Administration (FDA), thus many formulations currently on the market have never been studied for safety and efficacy. These formulations include those that contain 2% hydroquinone, the maximum concentration allowed in OTC drugs and physician-dispensed products, and some of the generic 4% hydroquinone formulations, only available by prescription. Other proprietary hydroquinone-containing drugs, which have undergone FDA scrutiny through the investigational new drug pathway, have well-established safety and efficacy validated through carefully designed large-scale vehicle controlled clinical trials. Many new hydroquinone formulations have appeared in the last 2 years in physician-dispensed lines, but these products have not undergone clinical study. It is this plethora of hydroquinone-containing creams for sale in many different markets that has caused health concerns

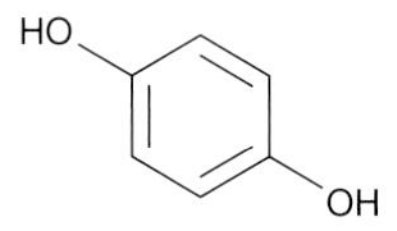

Figure 14.2 *Chemical structure of hydroquinone. Hydroquinone is the most effective pigment-lightening agent*

and the present FDA controversy regarding the removal of hydroquinone from the marketplace.

There are several important health issues that need to be considered before determining the safety of hydroquinone in ethnic population. For many years, it has been known that hydroquinone can cause ochronosis.[20] Ochronosis is a characteristic blue/black discoloration of the skin seen in deeply pigmented ethnic population where high concentration hydroquinone has been used for a prolonged period on the face. Whether this is caused by the effect of hydroquinone alone or other substances present in the formulation or higher concentrations of hydroquinone or interaction with other oral medications is unknown. Additional concern arose when oral hydroquinone was reported to cause cancer in rodents fed large amounts of the substance, yet human carcinogenicity has not been established.[21] While oral consumption probably is not related to topical application, hydroquinone remains controversial because it may be toxic to melanocytes.

Hydroquinone, a phenolic compound chemically known as 1,4 dihydroxybenzene, functions by inhibiting the enzymatic oxidation of tyrosine and phenol oxidases. It covalently binds to histidine or interacts with copper at the active site of tyrosinase. It also inhibits RNA and DNA synthesis and may alter melanosome formation, thus selectively damaging melanocytes. These activities suppress the melanocyte metabolic processes inducing gradual decrease of melanin pigment production.[22] Issues regarding the topical toxicity of hydroquinone arise because it is a strong oxidant rapidly converted to the melanocyte toxic products p-benzoquinone and hydroxybenzoquinone. These byproducts may cause depigmentation.

Hydroquinone is very difficult to formulate in a stable preparation. It is a highly reactive oxidant that rapidly combines with oxygen. Typically, hydroquinone skin-lightening creams are a creamy color, which changes to a darker yellow or brown as oxidation occurs. As the discoloration progresses, the activity of the hydroquinone decreases. Products with any off-color change should be immediately discarded as they may be irritating to the skin and do not contain active hydroquinone to inhibit pigment formation.

Prescription of hydroquinone products have tried to increase the skin lightening potency of formulations by adding penetration enhancers such as glycolic acid or tretinoin as a supplemental pigment-lightening agent. Other prescription formulations have added microsponges to create time delivery of hydroquinone to the skin, while others have placed the hydroquinone in a special one-way airtight dispenser. Some formulations have added sunscreen ingredients to the hydroquinone to prevent UV-induced pigment darkening. It is very important to select a formulation for ethnic skin that minimizes irritation, which will prove to be counterproductive to pigment lightening. Thus, testing the product for several weeks on a limited hyperpigmented site may be valuable in preventing an untoward result.

The future of hydroquinone in the United States is still uncertain as of this writing. Apparently, some of the controversy arose when the FDA asked industry to perform some collaborative self-funded studies on the safety of hydroquinone and submit a written report detailing the findings. The report was not submitted as requested and the FDA acted by stating that it would withdraw all OTC 2% hydroquinone preparations and prescription formulations that were not studied as investigational new drugs once currently manufactured supplies are depleted. Whether this ruling will be enforced and how it will be enforced is unknown. More details regarding the future of hydroquinone in the United States should be forthcoming shortly.

The potential withdrawal of hydroquinone from some of the U.S. markets and its removal from European and Japanese markets has spurred interest in developing pigment lightening alternatives. This has spurred the cosmetics and pharmaceutical industry to focus on other pigment-lightening ingredients and their efficacy. There can be no doubt that skin-lightening products will become a larger and larger worldwide ethnic cosmeceutical market.

Mequinol

The primary prescription lightening alternative to hydroquinone is mequinol, approved for use in the United States and Europe. Mequinol is chemically known as 4-hydroxyanisole. Other names include methoxyphenol, hydroquinone monomethyl ether, and p-hydroxyanisole. Mequinol is available in the United States in a 2% concentration and is commercially marketed as a prescription skin lightener in combination with 0.01% tretinoin, functioning as a penetration enhancer, and vitamin C, in the form of ascorbic acid and ascorbyl palmitate, to enhance skin lightening. These active agents are dissolved in an ethyl alcohol vehicle.

The exact mechanism of action accounting for the skin lightening properties of mequinol is unknown; however, it is a substrate for tyrosinase thereby acting as a competitive inhibitor in the formation of melanin precursors. It does not damage the melanocyte like hydroquinone, but is not generally felt to be as effective. Mequinol has been observed to cause longstanding depigmentation in some Caucasian patients, but repigmentation generally occurs with time. The tretinoin in combination with the mequinol may cause postinflammatory hyperpigmentation in some African American patients, but again the skin darkening lightens with time when the product is discontinued.

At present, the product is marketed in a tube with a small sponge tipped applicator for limited area use. The sponge is designed for dabbing on lentigenes and focal areas of hyperpigmentation. It is not packaged for overall facial application, an important distinction in the treatment of ethnic skin pigmentation from the previously discussed hydroquinone creams.

Retinoids

Retinoids have been used both directly and indirectly as pigment-lightening agents (Table 14.5). The prescription retinoids used for direct improvement in skin pigmentation are tretinoin and tazarotene.[23,24] These retinoids have an effect on skin pigmentation as demonstrated by a decrease in cutaneous freckling and lentigenes.[25] It is the irregular grouping and activation of melanocytes that accounts for the dyspigmentation associated with photoaging,[26] which is normalized by retinoids.[27] While this effect is more dramatic with prescription topical tretinoin and tazarotene, topical OTC retinol has been thought to provide similar effects as a cosmeceutical.

Retinol, the dietary form of vitamin A, induces changes in the skin similar to those produced by tretinoin, but with out the irritation of retinoic acid.[28] Retinol has been shown to convert to retinoic acid in a two-step oxidation process in the skin. Although retinol has a lower potency than retinoic acid and requires tenfold higher

TABLE 14.5 ■ **Retinoid categories***

Vitamin A Metabolites	Vitamin A	Vitamin A Esters
Retinoic acid $R{=}COOH$	Retinol $R{=}CH_2OH$	Retinyl acetate $R{=}CH_2OOCCH_3$
Retinoldehyde $R{=}CHO$		Retinyl propionate $R{=}CH_2OOCC_2H_5$
Tazarotene		Retinyl palmitate $R{=}CH_2OOCC_{15}H_{31}$

*Retinol and retinyl esters are found in the OTC market as cosmeceuticals.

concentrations to produce similar epidermal effects, it can be effective in improving the appearance of photodamage.[29] The main challenge to retinol formulations has been the successful development of high-concentration stabilized formulas. Retinol is not nearly as effective as tretinoin or tazarotene in pigment lightening.

Retinoids are sometimes used to indirectly lighten dyspigmentation. In this case, the retinoids are used as penetration enhancers. A side effect of retinoids is an irritant dermatitis characterized by erythema, dryness, and scaling.[30,31] These cutaneous changes damage the skin barrier allowing increased access of other pigment-lightening agents, such as hydroquinone and mequinol, to the melanocytes. Some preparations that combine tretinoin and hydroquinone must also incorporate a potent topical corticosteroid to prevent excess irritation resulting in decrease patient compliance and/or postinflammatory hyperpigmentation. These corticosteroid-containing formulations are important in the ethnic population where retinoid irritation may cause pigment darkening instead of enhanced pigment lightening. Ashiness, or the presence of loose scale on the skin surface, may also be induced by retinoid irritation requiring the use of a moisturizer to obtain an acceptable cosmetic appearance. It is these challenges that have spurred the development of alternative botanical skin lightening ingredients for the ethnic population.

Azelaic acid

The irritation profiles of hydroquinone and retinoids have led to the search for other pigment lightening ingredients in the prescription realm. One such ingredient is azelaic acid. Azelaic acid is available currently as a 15% gel approved in the United States for the treatment of rosacea. It is a 9-carbon dicarboxylic acid obtained from cultures of Pityrosporum ovale. Although its lightening effects are mild, several large studies done with a diverse ethnic background population have compared its efficacy to that of hydroquinone.[32,33] It interferes with tyrosinase activity too, but may also interfere with DNA synthesis. It appears to have a specificity for abnormal melanocytes, and for this reason it has been used to suppress the progression of lentigo maligna to lentigo maligna melanoma.

Azelaic acid has an excellent safety profile, but may cause short-lived stinging when topically applied in some individuals. It can be safely combined with retinoids to yield an additive benefit, but it is not as effective as hydroquinone in treating dyschromias. Thus, hydroquinone, mequinol, and azelaic acid are the only three prescription-active ingredients used for pigment lightening, which is

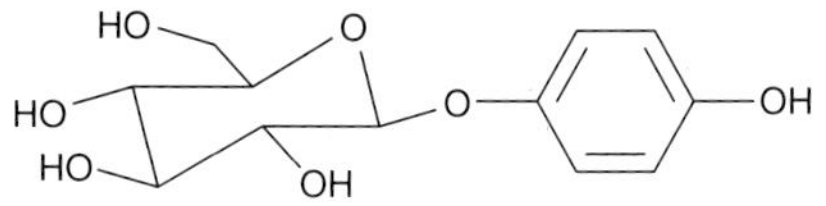

Figure 14.3 *Chemical structure of arbutin. Arbutin is chemically similar to hydroquinone*

remarkable given the size of the dyschromia market. All the other ingredients used for pigment lightening are found in the OTC realm, the next topic of discussion.

Arbutin

The most effective OTC pigment-lightening ingredients are botanicals that contain a structure similar to hydroquinone. Arbutin is one of these ingredients obtained from the leaves of the bearberry plant, but also found in lesser quantities in cranberry and blueberry leaves (Figure 14.3). It is a naturally occurring gluconopyranoside that causes decreased tyrosinase activity without affecting messenger RNA expression.[34] It also inhibits melanosome maturation. Arbutin is not toxic to melanocytes and is used in a variety of pigment-lightening preparations in Japan at concentrations of 3%. Higher concentrations are more efficacious than lower concentrations, but a paradoxical pigment darkening may occur because of postinflammatory hyperpigmentation in ethnic skin. At present, a synthetic form, known as deoxyarbutin, is available with greater inhibition of tyrosinase than the botanically derived chemical.[35] Deoxyarbutin is probably the most effective pigment-lightening agent in the OTC realm.

Kojic acid

The second most effective OTC skin-lightening agent is kojic acid, chemically known as 5-hydroxymethyl-4 H-pyrane-4-one (Figure 14.4). It is a hydrophilic fungal derivative obtained from *Aspergillus* and *Penicillium* species. It is the most popular agent employed in the Orient for the treatment of melasma,[36]; however, it is somewhat controversial as it has been disallowed and then reinstated as an acceptable pigment-lightening agent. It is a known sensitizer and has been shown to be mutagenic in cell culture studies. The activity of kojic acid is attributed to its ability to prevent tyrosinase activity by binding to copper.[37]

Aleosin

After deoxyarbutin and kojic acid, the available skin-lightening ingredients decrease in efficacy. For this reason, many manufacturers combine multiple ingredients in one formulation hoping to inhibit pigment production by interrupting melanogenesis at multiple steps along the pathway. Aleosin is a low-molecular-weight

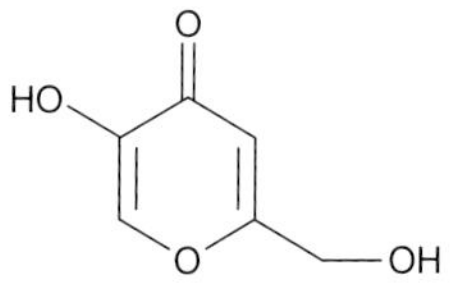

Figure 14.4 *Chemical structure of kojic acid. Kojic acid is the most common pigment-lightening agent used in cosmetics*

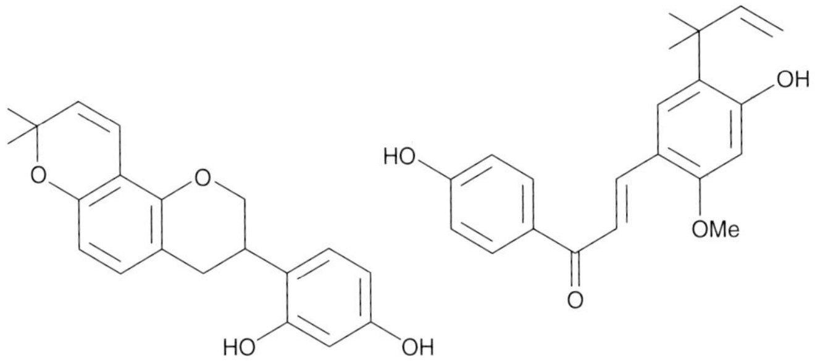

Figure 14.5 *Chemical structure of licorice extract. A variety of licorice extracts have been developed for pigment lightening. This is an example of one extract*

glycoprotein obtained from the aloe vera plant. It is a natural hydroxymethylchromone functioning to inhibit tyrosinase by competitive inhibition at the DOPA oxidation site.[38,39] In contrast to hydroquinone, it shows no cell cytotoxicity, however, it has a limited ability to penetrate the skin because of its hydrophilic nature. It is commonly used in combination with arbutin or deoxyarbutin to decrease tyrosinase activity through several different mechanisms.

Licorice extract

The safest pigment-lightening agents with the fewest side effects are the licorice extracts (Figure 14.5). It is for this reason that licorice extract is the most commonly used agent in cosmetics for brightening skin. Licorice extract can be incorporated into facial foundations or moisturizers. In addition, the licorice extract has topical anti-inflammatory properties theoretically helpful in decreasing skin redness and postinflammatory hyperpigmentation. The active agents are known as liquiritin and isoliquirtin, which are glycosides containing flavenoids.[40] Liquiritin induces skin lightening by dispersing melanin. It is typically applied to the skin in a dose of 1 g per day for 4 weeks to see a clinical result, however, the extract is quite expensive and the concentration used in most cosmetics is modest.

Ascorbic acid

Many times the licorice extract is combined with ascorbic acid, also known as vitamin C (Figure 14.6). Ascorbic acid interrupts the production of melanogenesis by interacting with copper ions to reduce dopaquinone and by blocking dihydrochinindol-2-carboxyl acid oxidation.[41] However, ascorbic acid is rapidly oxidized and is of limited stability making biologically active formulations challenging. It is a poor skin-lightening agent when used alone and is usually combined with licorice extracts and soy, the next topic of discussion, to create a minimally effective skin-lightening product sold as a cosmeceutical, since these ingredients have excellent safety profiles.

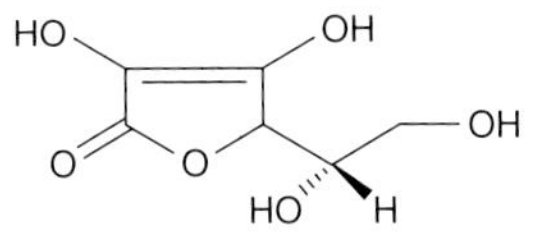

Figure 14.6 *Chemical structure of ascorbic acid. Ascorbic acid, also known as vitamin C, is a minimally-effective pigment-lightening agent*

Soy proteins

The most commonly used skin-lightening agent in cosmeceutical moisturizers is a soy extract known as soybean trypsin inhibitor. Soybean trypsin inhibitor inhibits the activation of a pathway necessary for keratinocyte phagocytosis of melanosomes and melanosome transfer.[42] This pathway, known as the protease-activated receptor 2 (PAR-2) pathway, can be inhibited after 3 weeks of raw soy milk application. The inhibition of melanosme transfer is reversible, thus side effects are minimal and the safety profile excellent.[43] However, the pigment lightening effect is not as pronounced as with hydroquinone, since only melanosome transfer is inhibited and not melanin production.

N-Acetyl glucosamine

The newest cosmeceutical pigment-lightening agent to be introduced this past year was *N*-acetyl glucosamine, an amino-monosaccharide produced by the body through the addition of an amino group to glucose.[44] It has many roles within the body including functioning as a substrate for the production of hyaluronic acid, heparan sulfate, and proteoglycans. These substances are important in maintaining the water content of the dermis by serving as humectants. *N*-Acetyl glucosamine also inhibits the glycosylation of tyrosinase, an important enzyme in melanin production, accounting for its pigment lightening abilities.[45] A randomized double blind clinical study utilizing topical 2% *N*-acetyl glucosamine applied twice daily for 8 weeks in a cosmeceutical moisturizer showed modest pigment lightening.[46]

Pigment lightening is an important part of ethnic dermatologic therapy and a recognized segment of the cosmeceutical and cosmetics market. This discussion has served to highlight the paucity of effective ingredients able to lighten skin. The major themes that have emerged are the melanocyte toxicity, carcinogenic potential, irritation profile, and sensitizing abilities of the existing ingredients. Most agents with excellent pigment-lightening effects also have increased side effects. No single agent has achieved the delicate balance between interrupting melanogenesis effectively without causing other cellular damage or inflammation.

Hydroquinone remains the most effective pigment-lightening agent discovered to date, but it does not have a clean safety profile making it the subject of controversy. It is unclear exactly how the FDA will rule regarding the future of hydroquinone. Nevertheless, formulations should be carefully tested for stability, since it is the oxidative by products of hydroquinone that are most toxic to melanocytes. This is achieved through proper manufacturing, low oxygen exposure packaging design, expiration dating of products, and a formulation with robust antioxidants. Hydroquinone can be safely used in ethnic skin under the direction of a dermatologist.

FUTURE DIRECTIONS AND CONCLUSIONS

The unique needs of ethnic skin are related to the desire to prevent inflammation, minimize photodamage, decrease dyspigmentation, and avoid ashiness. These problems can be improved or magnified by proper or improper product selection. Products designed for Fitzpatrick skin types I, II, and III may not meet these needs. The prevention of inflammation is necessary to avoid inducing unnecessary pigment darkening that may take months to resolve.

Pigmentary changes are only magnified by photodamage in the form of temporary UVA-induced tanning or the more permanent formation of lentigenes. Since dyspigmentation is unavoidable, most persons with ethnic skin will use a pigment-lightening formulation either from the OTC or prescription market at some point in their lives. Selecting an effective, nonirritating product assumes great importance. Finally, the presence of ashiness, caused by the pigmented desquamating corneocytes on the skin surface, must be reduced or eliminated through the use of moisturizers with emollients and oils designed to smooth the scale back onto the skin surface until desquamation occurs. An understanding of these concepts will allow the dermatologist to better care for the skin of the growing worldwide ethnic population.

REFERENCES

1. Wortzman MS. Evaluation of mild skin cleansers. *Dermetol Clin.* 1991;9:35-44.

2. Wortzman MS, Scott RA, Wong PS, Lowe MJ, Breeding J. Soap and detergent bar rinsability. *J Soc Cosmet Chem.* 1986;37: 89-97.

3. deNavarre MG. Cleansing creams. In: deNaarre MG, ed. *The Chemistry and Manufacture of Cosmetics.* Vol 3. 2nd ed. Wheaton, Illinois: Allured Publishing Corporation;1975:251-264.

4. Jass HE. Cold creams. In: deNaarre MG, ed. *The Chemistry and Manufacture of Cosmetics.* Vol. 3. 2nd ed. Wheaton, Illinois: Allured Publishing Corporation;1975:237-249.

5. Mills OH, Kligman AM. Evaluation of abrasives in acne therapy. *Cutis.* 1979;23:704-705.

6. Jackson EM. Moisturizers: What's in them? How do they work? *Am J Contact Dermatitis.* 1992;3(4):162-168.

7. Reiger MM. Skin, water and moisturization. *Cosmet Toilet.* 1989;104:41-51.

8. Baker CG. Moisturization: new methods to support time proven ingredients. *Cosmet Toilet.* 1987;102:99-102.

9. Friberg SE, Ma Z. Stratum corneum lipids, petrolatum and white oils. *Cosmet Toilet.* 1993;107:55-59.

10. Grubauer G, Feingold KR, Elias PM. Relationship of epidermal lipogenesis to cutaneous barrier function. *J Lip Res.* 1987;28:746-752.

11. Ghadially R, Halkier-Sorensen L, Elias PM. Effects of petrolatum on stratum corneum structure and function. *J Am Acad Dermatol.* 1992;26:387-396.

12. Rieger MM, Deem DE. Skin moisturizers II The effects of cosmetic ingredients on human stratum corneum. *J Soc Cosmet Chem.* 1974;25:253-262.

13. Idson B. Dry skin: moisturizing and emolliency. *Cosmet Toilet.*1992;107:69-78.

14. de Groot AC, Weyland JW, Nater JP. *Unwanted Effects of Cosmetics and Drugs Used in Dermatology.* 3rd ed. Amsterdam, The Netherlands: Elsevier, 1994:498-500.

15. Spencer TS. Dry skin and skin moisturizers. *Clin Dermatol.* 1988;6:24-28.

16. Wehr RF, Krochmal L. Considerations in selecting a moisturizer. *Cutis.* 1987;39:512-515.

17. Brand HM, Brand-Garnys EE. Practical application of quantitative emolliency. *Cosmet Toilet.* 1992;107:93-99.

18. Idson B. Moisturizers, emollients, and bath oils. In: Frost P, Horwitz SN, eds. *Principles of Cosmetics for the Dermatologist.* St. Louis, MO: CV Mosby; 1982:37-44.

19. Schmitt WH. Skin-care products. In: Williams DF, Schmitt WH, eds. *Chemistry and Technology of the Cosmetics and Toiletries Industry.* London, UK: Blackie Academic & Professional;1992: 121.

20. Lawrence N, Bligard CA, Reed R. et al. Exogenous ochronosis in the United States. *J Am Acad Dermatol.* 1988;18:1207-1211.

21. Nordlund JJ, Grimes PE, Ortonne JP. The safety of hydroquinone. *J Eur Acad Dermatol Venerol.* 2006;20(7):781-787.

22. Halder RM, Richards GM. Management of dischromias in ethnic skin. *Dermatol Ther.* 2004;17:151-157.

23. Kligman AM, Grove GL, Hirose R, Leyden JJ. Topical tretinoin for photoaged skin. *J Am Acad Dermatol.* 1986;15(4):836-859.

24. Kligman AM. The treatment of photoaged human skin by topical tretinoin. *Drugs.* 1989;38(1):1-8.

25. Weinstein GD, Nigra TP, Pochi PE, et al. Topical tretinoin for treatment of photodamaged skin. *Arch Dermatol.* 1991;127: 659-665.

26. Gilchrest BA, Blog FB, Szabo G. Effects of aging and chronic sun exposure on melanocytes in human skin. *J Invest Dermatol.* 1979;73:141-143.

27. Bhawan J, Serva AG, Nehal K, et al. Effects of tretinoin on photodamaged skin a histologic study. *Arch Dermatol.* 1991;127: 666-672.

28. Kang S, Duell EA, Voorhees JJ, et al. Application of retinol to human skin in vivo induces epidermal hyperplasia and cellular retinoid binding proteins characteristic of retinoic acid but without measurable retinoic acid levels of irritation. *J Invest Dermatol.* 1995;105(4):549-556.

29. Duell EA, Kang S, Voorhees JJ. Unoccluded retinol penetrates human skin in vivo more effectively than unoccluded retinyl palmitate or retinoic acid. *J Invest Dermatol.* 1997;109(3): 301-305.

30. Weinstein GD, Nigra TP, Pochi PE, et al. Topical tretinoin for treatment of photodamaged skin. *Arch Dermatol.* 1991;127: 659-665.

31. Green CK, Griffiths CEM, Finkel LJ, et al. Topical retinoic acid (tretinoin) for melasma in Black patients. *Arch Dermatol.* 1994;130:727-733.

32. Fitton A, Goa KL. Azelaic acid: a review of its pharmacological properties and therapeutic efficacy in acne and hyperpigmentary skin disorders. *Drugs.* 1991;5:780-798.

33. Balina LM, Graupe K. The treatment of melasma. 20% azelaic acid versus 4% hydroquinone cream. *Int J Dermatol.* 1991;30 (12):893-895.

34. Hori I, Nihei K, Kubo I. Structural criteria for depigmenting mechanism of arbutin. *Phytother Res.* 2004;18:475-469.

35. Boissy RE, Visscher M, DeLong MA. Deoxyarbutin: a novel reversible tyrosinase inhibitor with effective in vivo skin lightening potency. *Exp Dermatol.* 2005;14(8):601.

36. Lim JT. Treatment of melasma using kojic acid in a gel containing hydroquinone and glycolic acid. *Dermatol Surg.* 1999;25:282-284.

37. Garcia A, Fulton JE Jr. The combination of glycolic acid and hydroquinone or kojic acid for the treatment of melasma and related conditions. *Dermatol Surg.* 1996;22(5):443-447.

38. Choi S, Lee SK, Kim JE, et al. Aloesin inhibits hyperpigmentation induced by UV radiation. *Clin Exp Dermatol.* 2002;27: 513-515.

39. Jones K, Hughes J, Hong M, et al. Modulation of melanogenesis by aloesin: a competitive inhibitor of tyrosinase. *Pigment Cell Res.* 2002;15:335-340.

40. Amer M, Metwalli M. Topical Liquiritin improves melasma. *Int J Dermatol.* 2000;39(4):299-301.

41. Espinal-Perez LE, Moncada B, Castanedo-Cazares JP. A double blind randomized trial of 5% ascorbic acid vs 4% hydroquinone in melasma. *Int J Dermatol.* 2004;43(8):604-607.

42. Seiberg M, Paine C, Sharlow E, et al. Inhibition of melanosome transfer results in skin lightening. *J Invest Dermatol.* 2000;115(2):162-167.

43. Paine C, Sharlow E, Liebel F, et al. An alternative approach to depigmentation by soybean extracts via inhibition of the PAR-2 pathway. *J Invest Dermatol.* 2001;116:587-595.

44. Bissett DL. Glucosamine: an ingredient with skin and other benefits. *J Cosmet Dermatol.* 2006;5(4):309-315.

45. Bissett DL, McPhail SJ, Farmer TL, et al. Topical N-acetyl glucosamine affects pigmentation-relevant genes in in vitro genomics testing. *Pig Cell Res.* 2006;19:373.

46. Bissett DL, Robinson L, Li J, Miyamoto K. Topical N-acetyl glucosamine reduces the appearance of hyperpigmented spots on human facial skin. *J Am Acad Dermatol.* 2006;54: AB54.

Jennifer Y. Lin, MD, Joyce Teng Ee Lim, MD, FRCPI, FAMS, and Henry Hin-Lee Chan, MD, FRCP

INTRODUCTION

Acquired hyperpigmentation disorders of the skin are among the most common complaints in a general dermatology clinic, especially in patients with skin of color. Among those, melasma is known both for causing significant psychosocial stress and for its difficulty to treat. Melasma is classically characterized by symmetric facial hyperpigmented macules and patches commonly affecting the forehead, malar eminences, periorbital areas, and the upper lip. Despite the advent of powerful pigment-targeting lasers, the treatment for melasma remains challenging. This chapter reviews what is currently understood about the pathogenesis, discusses evidence-based treatments, and offers clinical pearls on difficult-to-treat cases.

INCIDENCE

In the United States alone, approximately 5 to 6 million individuals are afflicted with melasma, with a higher incidence worldwide. In Asia, it is a common diagnosis in any dermatology clinic and can reach an incidence of 0.25% to 4% of cases seen in any dermatology institution.[1] Melasma is much more commonly seen in women, although men can also be affected (reported 10%),[2] suggesting a hormone-related etiology. This strong linkage between melasma and hormones is demonstrated by an increased incidence in the setting of pregnancy, in which case melasma can also be termed chloasma, or "the mask of pregnancy." In addition, the use of birth control pills or estrogen replacement therapy, ovarian or thyroid dysfunction, and ovarian tumors have also been associated with the onset of melasma.

Although all skin types can be affected, melasma is seen at a much higher incidence in darker skin phototypes (Fitzpatrick Skin Phototypes IV to VI) with extensive ultraviolet radiation (UV) exposure. This in combination with the appearance of melasma in sun-exposed areas and the presence of solar elastosis on histology all point to a UV-mediated process.

Medications and other systemic illnesses have also been reported to be associated with the onset of melasma, including phototoxic and photoallergic medications, antiepileptic medications, cosmetics, altered nutrition, and hepatic disease.[1]

CLINICAL PRESENTATION

Onset of melasma typically occurs in a woman's childbearing years (20s through 30s). The appearance of pigment is heightened in the summer when UV exposure is more common.

At least three clinical patterns have been described: centrofacial (64%), malar (27%), and mandibular (9%). The course is typically chronic, fading when UV exposure is diminished.

From a treatment standpoint, determining the distribution of pigment in the skin layers is critical. Increased pigment can be seen in either the epidermis (presenting as a brown-to-black pigment) or dermis (presenting as a blue-gray pigment), or both. A Wood's lamp (365 nm) can be useful in separating the types of pigmentation: increased reflectance will be seen in epidermal hyperpigmentation versus none in dermal hyperpigmentation. In one study of 210 patients, using a Wood's lamp, melasma was classified into epidermal (70%), dermal (10% to 15%), and mixed (20%).[3] The presence of dermal pigment can make these lesions difficult to separate from acquired bilateral nevus of Ota-like macules (ABNOM) and there is likely overlap between these entities.

PATHOPHYSIOLOGY

The pathophysiology of melasma is unknown and most theories stem from known risk factors: UV, hormones, and genetics.

Histologically, increased melanin can be seen in the basal and suprabasal keratinocytes (epidermal pigmentation) and in the dermis (dermal pigmentation). Most studies have not demonstrated an increase in the number of melanocytes; however, melanocytes are "activated" in appearance by their larger size and increase in dendricity.[4] This suggests that melasma is primarily a problem of increased melanin production and distribution rather than of melanocyte proliferation. The increase in dermal melanin has been more difficult to characterize and is contained in either macrophages (termed melanophages)[5] or dermal dendrocytes.

Solar elastosis is also often increased in lesional skin, which suggests a common process in the dermis or may represent a marker for the degree of accumulated UV damage required for melasma formation.[6]

◼ Ultraviolet Radiation

The role of UV exposure has been strongly associated with melasma, illustrated by the location of melasma commonly on sun-exposed areas of the face. Therefore, strict sun avoidance is an important part of the therapeutic regimen. Both UVA and UVB have been implicated in the pathogenesis. Signaling factors in response to UVB-mediated tanning have begun to be elucidated and have also been found to be expressed in higher levels in lesional melasma skin as compared to perilesional skin. This includes melanocyte-stimulating hormone (MSH), c-kit, and endothelin-1.[7,8] These growth factors are secreted by the keratinocyte in response to UV and may be deranged in the setting of melasma. Understanding these pathways further may lead to improved targeted therapies.

◼ Hormone Involvement

Melasma has been associated with female sex hormones given its association with oral contraceptives and pregnancy. In one study examining 400 pregnant women in Iran, the incidence of melasma was 15.8% but it was not associated with pregnancy trimester.[9] There have also been reported cases of hyperpigmentation on arms (atypical sites) after initiation of hormone replacement therapy.[10]

Genetic Predisposition

As many as 54% of patients have a family history of melasma, strongly suggesting a genetic predisposition.[9] One pair of identical twins reported developing melasma, while other siblings under similar conditions did not.[6]

TREATMENT OF MELASMA

Therapeutic Goals and Options

The goals of melasma therapy are basically twofold: the removal of existing pigments and the prevention of the formation of new pigments. Any form of therapy should be targeted at the etiology of melasma as previously discussed (Figure 15.1). These involve a combination of sun protection with topical therapies (aim to reduce melanin formation and/or to inhibit the transfer of melanosomes from the melanocytes to the keratinocytes) and procedural therapies (to accelerate cell turnover and, in the presence of ABNOM, to remove the dermal melanocytes).

As melasma can persist for several decades, maintenance therapy is essential. Optimal treatment therefore involves an intensive phase and a maintenance phase using a combination of topical and procedural therapies and the avoidance of aggravating factors.

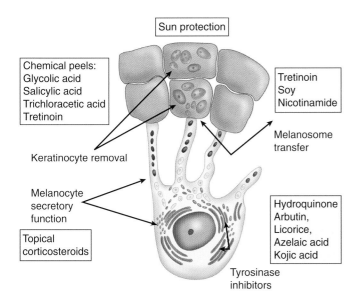

Figure 15.1 *Medical treatment of melasma. Therapeutic agents for hyperpigmentation act at various parts of the pigmentary system, including: keratinocyte removal (chemical peel—glycolic acid, salicylic acid, trichloracetic acid, retinoic acid [tretinoin]); melanosome transfer (tretinoin); tyrosinase inhibitors (hydroquinone [primary agent], mequinol, azelaic acid, kojic acid); melanocyte secretory function (topical corticosteroids—mechanism not fully elucidated)*

Sun Protection

An important factor in the pathogenesis of melasma is UV light exposure. All patients seeking treatment for melasma should practice daily sun protection, usually using a combination of sunscreens, physical protection, and, in some countries, oral sunblock. A broad-spectrum sunscreen should be worn during the day, and physical protection in the form of hats, sunglasses, umbrellas, or protective clothing is advisable when outdoors. An oral sunblock containing *Polypodium leucotomos* (a fern extract marketed as Helioblock) can be taken 30 minutes prior to sun exposure. This acts as an antioxidant and an immune modulator, prevents actinic erythema, and increases the skin's tolerance to the effects of UV radiation.[11]

Topical Therapy

A variety of topical agents are used to treat melasma. These agents act as tyrosinase inhibitors (hydroquinone, azelaic acid, kojic acid, arbutin, licorice extracts, mulberry, bearberry) or prevent the transfer of melanosomes to keratinocytes (nicotinic acid, niacinamide, soy, tretinion) or accelerate cell turnover in the epidermis, thereby reducing the amount of time cells have to acquire pigment (alphahydroxyacids, betahydroxyacids, tretinion).

During the intensive phase, combination topical therapy is used and there are many different combinations used in different parts of the world. The most frequently used combination formulation is that proposed by Kligman and Willis[12] in 1975, which combined hydroquinone 5%, tretinoin 0.1%, and dexamethasone 0.1% or variations of the original formulation with dermatologists substituting different corticosteroids and modifying the concentrations of the tretinoin and hydroquinone.[13,14] Using this formula, Kligman and Willis[12] were able to depigment the skin of African American volunteers almost completely within 5 to 7 weeks. None of the agents used singly resulted in more than slight skin lightening and omitting one component greatly reduced the level of therapeutic efficacy.[12] Hydroquinone blocks melanogenesis by competitive tyrosinase inhibition, inhibits DNA and RNA synthesis in melanotic cells, degrades melanosomes, and destroys melanocytes.[15,16] Tretinoin causes dispersion of pigment granules in keratinocytes, interferes with pigment transfer, accelerates epidermal transfer, and accelerates cell turnover in the epidermis. It also decreases the rate of transfer of melanosomes to the keratinocytes. The steroid suppresses the biosynthetic and secretory function of melanocytes, thus suppressing melanin production without destroying the melanosomes.[17,18] In the triple combination, tretinoin overrides the atrophy-promoting and antimitotic effect of the corticosteroid and the tretinoin-induced irritation may facilitate epidermal penetration of hydroquinone and also prevent its oxidation. The corticosteroid antagonizes the thinning effect of tretinion and reduces tretinoin-induced irritation. The combination is used daily. A variation of the triple combination cream containing 5% hydroquinone, 0.1% tretinoin, and 1% hydrocortisone was used twice weekly instead of daily to treat 25 Korean women with melasma.[14] Clinical and histological improvements were seen in 40% of patients after 4 months of therapy. In this study, 72% of patients had irritant dermatitis even though the cream was used twice weekly.

A more stable hydrophilic triple-combination commercially available cream containing hydroquinone 4%, tretinion 0.05%, and fluocinolone acetonide 0.01% (Triluma Cream, Galderma, France) has also been shown to be effective in treating melasma. In two multicenter trials that enrolled 641 patients with moderate-to-severe facial melasma, 29% achieved complete clearing in 8 weeks while 77% achieved complete or near-complete clearing in 8 weeks.[19] Clinical improvement was evident as early as 4 weeks after starting therapy. Treatment-related adverse events seen at 8 weeks were erythema, desquamation, burning, dryness, and pruritus. No patient had skin atrophy. A similar 8-week study was undertaken in Asia; 260 Asian patients with moderate-to-severe melasma from nine centers (from Korea, Singapore, Hong Kong, the Philippines, and Taiwan) were treated with this triple combination. Results were not as impressive compared to the multicenter trials—50% achieved complete or near-complete clearing in 8 weeks (Figure 15.2). The cream was better tolerated among Asian patients with a lower incidence of erythema, desquamation, burning, and dryness (data presented at Pigmentary Research meeting, July 2007, Singapore). A large community-based trial of 1290 patients using this triple-combination cream (Triluma cream) showed rapid improvement of melasma among all skin types, including whites, Hispanics, blacks, Asians, American Indians, Alaskan natives, and Pacific Islanders.[20]

There are concerns regarding the mutagenicity or carcinogenicity of hydroquinone. In Europe and in some countries in Asia, hydroquinone is available as a prescription drug. Irritant reactions are common. The incidence of irritant reactions in monotherapy with hydroquinone varies from 0% to 70% of patients, and the incidence rises to 10% to 100% in combination therapy.[21] Allergic contact dermatitis is rare. Chronic use of hydroquinone has been associated with ochronosis and nail discoloration.[22–24] The incidence of cutaneous ochronosis outside Africa is rare. There are many postulations why this is so. One postulation is that the hydroquinone used outside Africa does not contain resorcinol or hydroethanolic

compounds. As for carcinogenicity, concerns arose when rodents that were administered large oral doses of hydroquinone developed cancer; however, there are no known associations of cancer development in humans related to the use of topical hydroquinone.

Another combination therapy for the treatment of melasma is the use of 20% azelaic acid and 0.05% tretinion.[25] In a study to compare the efficacy of this double combination to azelaic acid monotherapy, 50 Asian patients were treated with either a double-combination cream (20% azelaic acid and 0.05% hydroquinone) or a 20% azelaic acid cream over a 6-month period. Both treatments yielded approximately 73% good to excellent results. However, the double-combination cream showed a faster response and a more pronounced improvement during the first 3 months and had a higher rate of excellent results at the end of 6 months (34.8% for the combination cream compared to 5.3% for the monotherapy). Azelaic acid (1,7-heptanedicarboxylic acid) is a competitive inhibitor of tyrosinase and produces ultrastructural damage to normal melanocytes.[26,27] The efficacy of 20% azelaic acid monotherapy had been compared with 4% hydroquinone monotherapy. Three hundred twenty-nine women with melasma were treated with either cream more than a 24-week period.[28] Both creams were applied twice daily—65% of patients using azelaic acid had good to excellent results compared with 73% of patients using 4% hydroquinone. No significant treatment differences were observed between the two groups with regard to overall rating, reduction in lesion size, and pigmentary intensity. Eighteen patients on azelaic acid had itching or burning compared to one patient on hydroquinone who had burning. However, in another study involving 155 melasma patients, 20% azelaic acid was superior to 2% hydroquinone in clearing melasma.[29] Azelaic acid monotherapy had been compared with sequential therapy of 0.05% clobetasol propionate cream for 8 weeks followed by 20% azelaic acid for 16 weeks. Seventy percent of patients on the combination cream had more than 66% clearance of their melasma compared to 3% in the group using 20% azelaic acid alone.[30]

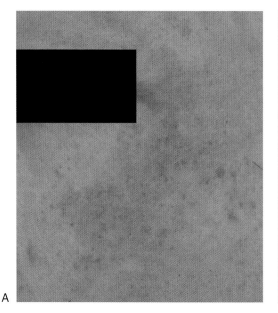
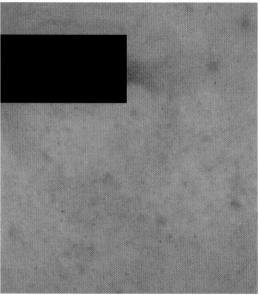

A   B

Figure 15.2 *(A) Before and (B) after one month treatment with triple combination therapy*

Tretinoin, alone or in combination with other agents, has been used for treating melasma. A combination therapy of 0.1% tretinion with 5% hydroquinone (without steroid) improved melasma by 66% in 20 Hispanic patients when the cream was applied twice daily.[31] Another combination therapy involved the use of 0.1% tretinion gel applied twice a day, along with 4% hydroquinone and 7% lactic acid, in Japanese patients. Melasma improved as early as 4 weeks.[32] A more aggressive treatment involving a two-phase treatment protocol—a bleaching phase and a healing phase—was reported in 18 Japanese patients.[33] Here a 10% all-*trans* retinol gel was applied to the pigmented areas followed by a 5% hydroquinone–7% lactic acid ointment over the whole face for 2 to 6 weeks until the pigmentation was sufficiently reduced. This was followed by the healing phase where a 5% hydroquinone–7% ascorbic acid ointment was used for 4 to 6 weeks. Improvement was seen in 16 of the 18 patients after an average treatment period of 11.3 weeks, and in six patients, the pigmentation was almost clear. Side effects included erythema and scaling during both the bleaching and the healing phase.

Kojic acid, a fungal metabolic product, inactivates tyrosinase by the chelation of copper and suppresses the tautomerization from dopachrome to 5,6-dihydroindole-2-carboxy acid. It is commonly found in cosmetic lightening products sold in Asia. Kojic acid is not used as a monotherapy for melasma as it is less effective than 2% hydroqunone.[34] It is often used in combination with other skin lighteners like arbutin or licorice in cosmetic products. A triple combination of 2% kojic acid, 10% glycolic acid, and 2% hydroquinone has been shown to be superior to a double combination of 10% glycolic acid and 2% hydroquinone.[35] A comparative study of kojic acid/glycolic acid gel on one side of the face and hydroquinone-glycolic acid gel on the other side applied daily for 3 months showed equivalent results in pigment reduction.[36]

Another popular skin lightener found in cosmetic product is niacinamide. Niacinamide had no effect on tyrosinase or melanogenesis. In a study by Minwalla,[37] niacinamide gave a 35% to 68% inhibition of melanosome transfer in a keratinocyte/melanocyte coculture model and reduced cutaneous pigmentation in a pigmented reconstructed epidermal model. In clinical studies, it significantly decreased hyperpigmentation and increased skin lightness compared with vehicle alone after 4 weeks of use.[37]

A less effective agent, calcium D-pantetheine-S-sulfonate, has depigmenting effects on human melanocytes. It modifies glycoyslation of tyrosinase and tyrosinase-related protein 1.[38] In a vehicle-controlled clinical study,[39] 20 patients with melasma were treated with a 10% calcium D-pantetheine-S-sulfonatecream while 13 patients were treated with a 5% calcium D-pantetheine-S-sulfonatecream. In the group using the 10% cream, 12 of 20 patients showed lightening of the melasma compared to the placebo site, while in the group using the 5% cream, 10 of 13 patients showed improvement. The 10% cream was more effective than the 5% cream. Side effects were minimal with two patients having stinging and itchiness on both the active and placebo sites.

■ Procedural Therapy

Melasma is a therapeutic challenge for the dermatologist. Since most Asian patients with melasma have both epidermal and dermal pigmentation (as well as clinically undetected ABNOM), topical therapy alone is often insufficient to clear their melasma. Chemical peels, microdermabrasion, lasers, and intense pulse light are often used in combination with topical therapy.

Chemical peels

Different types of peeling agents have been used to improve or clear melasma. Among these are glycolic acid, trichloroacetic acid, Jessner's solution, lactic acid, salicylic acid, phenol, and tretinoin. When using chemical peels on patients with skin of color, it is safer to use lower concentrations of peeling agents and to use only superficial peeling agents to avoid the risk of causing postinflammatory hyperpigmentation. The two most common peeling agents used in treating melasma are glycolic acid and salicylic acid.

Glycolic acid peels are often performed during the intensive phase. In a study of Chinese women in Singapore, glycolic acid peels (20% to 70%) were performed every 3 weeks on one-half of the face while the other half did not receive any skin peeling. A total of eight peels were performed, and at the end of the study, the side that received the peels improved compared to the side that did not received any peeling.[40] Glycolic acid peels are shown to be safe and effective in treating people with Fitzpatrick skin type IV. Twenty-five women with melasma from India were pretreated with 10% glycolic acid lotion at night 2 weeks prior to skin peeling.[41] Each woman received 50% glycolic acid peels monthly for 3 months. After the third peel, 15 patients had moderate-to-good response. Two patients did not have any improvement. Side effects were minimal, with one patient having hyperpigmentation over the eyebrows. Salicylic acid 20% to 30% at two weekly intervals had been performed on 25 patients, 6 of whom had melasma. The patients were treated with 4% hydroquinone for 2 weeks prior to receiving the peels. A total of five peels were done for each patient. Results indicated moderate-to-significant improvement in 88% of patients. Minimal to mild side effects were noted in 16%.[42] Another peeling agent that is useful for treating melasma is trichloroacetic acid. However, this has a higher risk of postpeel hyperpigmentation in patients with skin of color. Tretinoin peels are also used to treat melasma. In a study of 10 Indian women with melasma, one-half of the face was treated with a 1% tretinoin peel (1% tretinoin in 95% isopropyl alcohol base and 5% chloroform with antioxidant 1-butylated hydroxytuolene), while the other half was treated with a 70% gylcolic acid peel.[43] Each patient received the peels at weekly intervals for 12 weeks. At the end of the study, the 1% tretinoin peel was as effective as the 70% glycolic acid peels in lightening moderate-to-severe melasma. Side effects were minimal and the peels were well tolerated.

Microdermabrasion

Microdermabrasion is safe and effective in lightening melasma in all skin types. It is done at 1- to 2-week intervals for a total of six treatments. Patients should continue with their topical lightening agents. Microdermabrasion improves melasma indirectly by enhancing the penetration of topical agents as well as by allowing light to reflect better from the smooth surface. In treating patients with skin of color, one should not be too aggressive in treatment, to prevent epidermal injury, which may lead to worsening of the skin pigmentation.

Vitamin C iontophoresis

Ascorbic acid is known to both inhibit melanin formation and reduce oxidized melanin. However, it does not easily penetrate the skin and is quickly oxidized. Magnesium-L-ascorbyl-2-phosphate is stable in an aqueous solution but easily dissociates to anions, making it difficult to enter the skin. Suzuki first introduced vitamin C iontophoresis in 1998 to treat melasma.[44] A randomized double-blind placebo-controlled trial of vitamin C iontophoresis was carried out by Huh et al.[45] to show its effectiveness in treating melasma. Twenty-nine Korean patients with melasma had vitamin C solution (Magnesium-L-ascorbyl-2-phosphate) applied to one-half of the face while distilled water was applied on the other half prior to iontophoresis. Patients were treated twice weekly for 12 weeks. At the end of the study period, the melasma improved on the side receiving the vitamin C solution as evidenced from photographs and a reduced L value measured by a colorimeter, which was statistically significant. However, patients' self-assessment showed that both the vitamin C solution side and the placebo were effective. Further studies are needed before recommending vitamin C iontophoresis as a standard treatment for melasma.

▦ The Use of Laser and Intense Pulsed Light in the Treatment of Epidermal and Mixed-Type Melasma

The results of previous studies have discouraged the use of laser in the treatment of epidermal and mixed-type melasma. Early work by Grekin et al.[46] concluded that pulsed dye 510-nm laser could not remove melasma and could increase pigmentation. Another study also indicated that melasma was resistant to treatment with a Q-switched (QS) ruby laser, regardless of fluence (7.5 to 15 J/cm^2).[47] There was no permanent improvement and, in some cases, hyperpigmentation occurred.

The cause for such unwanted effects is likely related to the pathogenesis of melasma. As mentioned earlier, melanocytes in lesional skin are hyperactive; sublethal laser damage by pigment-targeting lasers can increase the production of melanin from these melanocytes and result in hyperpigmentation. Therefore, to use laser or IPL for the treatment of melasma should be considered as a second-line treatment among patients who already have received at least 3 months of topical treatments.

If laser or intense pulsed light source is to be used for the treatment of melasma, the operator should ensure a minimal degree of inflammation postoperatively to avoid an increase in pigmentation. Previous studies examined the use of IPL (570-nm and 590- to 615-nm filters at 4-week intervals for a total of four treatments) for the treatment of melasma and indicated that melasma improved by 39.8% compared to only 11.6% improvement in the control group.[48] Two patients in the intense pulsed light group experienced transient postinflammatory hyperpigmentation, and partial repigmentation was noted 24 weeks after the last treatment session. Patient expectation should include microcrust formation 2 to 3 days after irradiation with resolution within 1 to 2 weeks. Negishi et al.[49] treated four patients with melasma with the intense pulse light and showed improvement in pigmentation and texture. No mention was made about the type of melasma. Patients were on bleaching agents after the third treatment session and there was no control in this study.[49] In a more recent study, 89 patients with melasma were treated with an intense pulse light source device

with a uniform pulse profile. They were able to achieve excellent results (77.5% of treated subjects had more than 50% improvement 3 months after treatment) with low risk of increase in pigmentation (3%). This was despite the lack of topical bleaching agents during the study period. Their findings differ significantly from previous data, although the uniform profile of this IPL device may be one of the reasons for such observation as suggested by the investigators. Other factors that may contribute to the differences in clinical outcome include geographical location of the test site and recruitment criteria.

Long-pulsed pigment lasers can also be used to treat epidermal/mixed-type melasma. The clinical end point is an ashen gray appearance of the treated skin, and a test area should be performed to identify those who develop increase in pigmentation, which in the author's (H.C.) experience is approximately 10%. QS 1064-nm Nd:YAG laser (8-mm spot size, 2.3 J/cm^2) can also be used for the treatment of melasma. Mild erythema can be used as the clinical endpoint and patients will require once- to twice-monthly treatments. Depigmentation has been seen among patients who received too frequent treatments (Figure 15.3).

Resurfacing lasers have also been used with some success in the treatment of melasma. The aim of the ablative laser is to remove only the abnormal melanocytes that are thought to be along the basal layer of the epidermis. The melanocytes along the appendageal structures are normal. Manaloto and Alster treated 10 patients with refractory melasma with Er:YAG laser.[50] Significant improvement was seen 3 to 6 weeks later but biweekly glycolic acid peels were required. Angsuwarangsee and Polnikorn compared combined CO$_2$ laser and QS alexandrite laser (QSAL) versus QSAL alone in the treatment of refractory melasma.[51] The combined approach yielded better results but was associated with more adverse effects including PIH that occurred in 2 of 6 patients. These findings suggest that the functionally abnormal melanocytes are unlikely to be confined to the epidermal basal layer.

Fractional skin resurfacing involves the use of a 1540-nm laser to create microscopic spots of thermal injury that are surrounded by healthy skin tissue.[52] As the area of thermal injury is very small, the lateral migration of keratinocytes occurs rapidly, which leads to the complete reepithelialization of the epidermis within 24 hours. Studies have indicated that it can be used effectively for the treatment of epidermal melasma with significant improvement in 60% and mild improvement in 30% of treated patients[53,54] (Figure 15.4). However, approximately 10% of patients developed generalized increase in pigmentation, which can be most undesirable (Figure 15.5).

Regardless of the type of laser/IPL devices, the main issues are recurrence and in approximately 10% of cases, increase in pigmentation. As a result, laser/IPL should be considered as a second-line treatment and test areas should be performed prior to full-face treatment.

▦ The Use of Laser for the Treatment of ABNOM (Figure 15.6)

The use of QS lasers can be most effective in the treatment of ABNOM. Previous work with the QS Ruby (fluence 7-10 J/cm^2 at

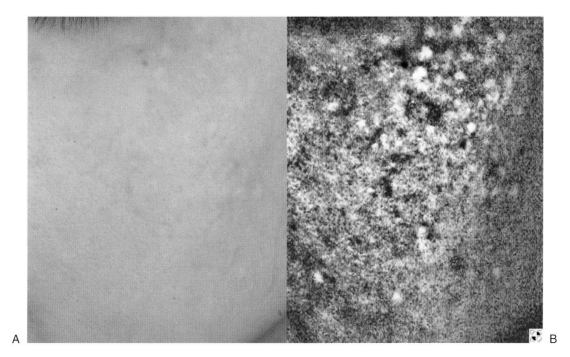

Figure 15.3 *Depigmentation after the use of QS 1064 nm Nd:YAG laser for the treatment of melasma as shown in cross polarized and ultraviolet lightening mode*

a repetition rate of 1 Hz and spot size of 2-4 mm) indicated that complete clearance could be obtained in more than 90% of patients treated.[55] There was no recurrence after 6 months to 4.3 years (with a mean of 2.5 years) of follow up. Postinflammatory hyperpigmentation was common and affected 7% of patients. The QS 1064 nm Nd:YAG laser is also effective but postinflammatory hyperpigmentation affects 50% to 73% of patients.[56,57] Another retrospective analysis of 32 female Chinese patients treated with QSAL (755 nm, 3-mm spot size, 8 J/cm^2) concluded that 80% of patients had more than 50% clearance and more than 28% had complete clearance.[58] Hyperpigmentation occurred in 12.5% of the patients, but resolved in all cases following treatment with hypopigmenting topical medication.

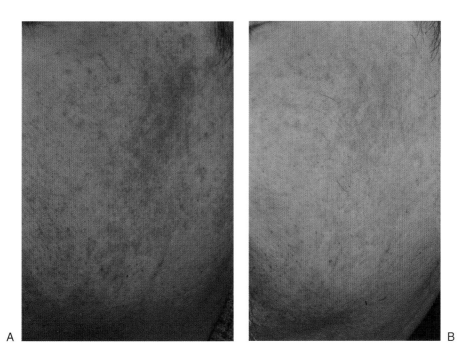

Figure 15.4 *Improvement of melasma (A) before and (b) after treatment with fractional resurfacing*

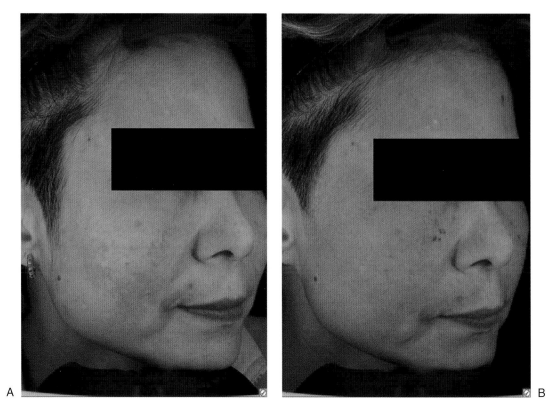

Figure 15.5 *Uniform hyperpigmentation (A) before and (B) after treatment of melasma with fractional resurfacing*

SUMMARY

Medical treatment of melasma consists of sun protection, the avoidance of aggravating factors like oral contraceptives and a combination of topical therapies and procedural therapies. During the intensive phase, a triple-combination cream, either Kligman's or modified Kligman's formulation (including Triluma), is used at night with 4% hydroquinone monotherapy and a sunblock in the day. If the melasma improvement is slow, chemical peels, intense pulse light, and microdermabrasion are added until the melasma clears. Once better, the improvement is maintained with monotherapy of either hydroquinone, kojic acid, niacinamide, or arbutin.

If ABNOM is suspected or unmasked during treatment it can be effectively eradicated using the QS ruby, alexandrite, or Nd:YAG lasers, with the latter being the safest for Asian persons. In refractory melasma, ablative lasers are often used but patients are warned about the risk of transient postlaser hyperpigmentation. Often patients may have "very subtle epidermal melasma," which is invisible to the naked eye under normal light but can be diagnosed by UV photography. Such melasma may become prominent during treatment with intense pulse light.

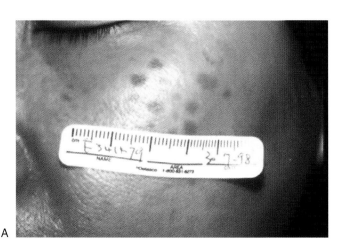

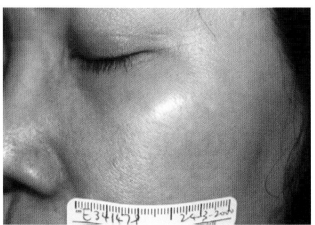

Figure 15.6 *Treatment of ABNOM with QSAL*

REFERENCES

1. Goh CL, Diova CN. A retrospective study on the clinical presentation and treatment outcome of melasma in a tertiary Dermatological Referral Centre in Singapore. *Sing Med J.* 1999;40:455-458.

2. Nicolaidou E, Antoniou C, Katsambas AD. Origin, clinical presentation, and diagnosis of facial hypermelanoses. *Dermatol Clin.* 2007;25:321-326.

3. Sanchez NP, et al. Circumscribed dermal melaninoses: classification, light, histochemical, and electron microscopic studies on three patients with the erythema dyschromicum perstans type. *Int J Dermatol.* 1982;21:25-31.

4. Katsambas A, Antoniou Ch, Katsarou A, Stratigos J. Melasma: a clinical study of 210 patients. 17th World Congress of Dermatology, 1987:177-17.

5. Grimes PE, Yamada N, Bhawan J. Light microscopic, immunohistochemical, and ultrastructural alterations in patients with melasma. *Am J Dermatopathol.* 2005;27:96-101.

6. Kang WH, et al. Melasma: histopathological characteristics in 56 Korean patients. *Br J Dermatol.* 2002;146:228-237.

7. Kang HY, et al. The dermal stem cell factor and c-kit are overexpressed in melasma. *Br J Dermatol.* 2006;154:1094-1099.

8. Im S, Kim J, On WY, Kang WH. Increased expression of alpha-melanocyte-stimulating hormone in the lesional skin of melasma. *Br J Dermatol.* 2002;146:165-167.

9. Moin A, Jabery Z, Fallah N. Prevalence and awareness of melasma during pregnancy. *Int J Dermatol.* 2006;45: 285-288.

10. Varma S, Roberts DL. Melasma of the arms associated with hormone replacement therapy. *Br J Dermatol.* 1999;141: 592.

11. Elmets CA, Singh D, Tubesing K et al. Cutaneous photoprotection from ultraviolet injury by green tea polyphenols. *J Am Acad Dermatol.* 2001: 44:425-432.

12. Kligman AM, Willis I. A new formula for depigmenting human skin. *Arch Dermatol.* 1975;111:40-48.

13. Gano SE, Gracia RL. Topical tretinoin, hydroquinone and betamethasone valerate in the therapy of melasma. *Cutis.* 1979;23:239-241.

14. Kang WH, Chun SC, Lee S. Intermittent therapy for melasma in Asian patients with combined topical agents (retinoic acid, hydroquinone and hydrocortisone): clinical and histological studies. *J Dermatol.* 1998;25:587-596.

15. Palumbo A, D'Ischia M, Misuraca G, et al. Mechanism of inhibition of melanogenesis by hydroquinone. *Biochim Biophys Acta.* 1991;1073:85-90.

16. Jimbow K, Obata H, Pathak MA, et al. Mechanism of depigmentation by hysroquinone. *J Invest Dermatol.* 1974;62:436-449.

17. Menter A. Rationale for the use of topical corticosteroids in melasma. *J Drugs Dermatol.* 2004;3(2):169-174.

18. Kanwar AJ, Dhar S, Kaur S. Treatment of melasma with potent topical corticosteroids. *Dermatology.* 1994;188:170-172.

19. Taylor SC, Torok H, Jones T, et al. Efficacy and safety of a new triple-combination agent for the treatment of facial melasma. *Cutis.* 2003;72:67-72.

20. Grimes P, Kelly P, Toork H, et al. Community-based trial of a triple-combination agent for the treatment of facial melasma. *Cutis.* 2006,77:177-184.

21. Nordlund JJ, Grimes PE, Ortonne The safety of hydroquinone. *J Eur Acad Dermatol Venereol.* 2006;20:781-787.

22. Findlay GH, Morrison JGL, Simson IW. Exogenous ochronosis and pigmented milium from hydroquinone bleaching creams. *Br J Dermatol.* 1975;93:613-622.

23. Levin Cy, Maibach H. Exogenous ochronosis. An update on clinical features, causative agents and treatment options. *Am J Clin Dermatol.* 2001;2:213-217.

24. Mann RJ, Harman RRM. Nail staining due to hydroquinone skin-lightening creams. *Br J Dermatol.* 1983;108:363-365.

25. Graupe K, Verallo-Rowell VM, Verallo V, et al. Combined use of 20% azelaic acid cream and 0.05% tretinion cream in the topical treatment of melasma. *J Dermatol Treatment.* 1996;7:235-237.

26. Nazzaro-Porro M. Azelaic acid. *J Am Acad Dermatol.* 1987;17:1033-1041.

27. Fitton A, Goa KL. Azelaic acid. A review of its pharmacological properties and therapeutic efficacy in acne and hyperpigmentary skin disorders. *Drug.* 1991;41:780-798.

28. Balina LM, Graupe K. The treatment of melasma 20% azelaic acid versus 4% hydroquinone cream. *Int J Dermatol.* 1991;30:893-895.

29. Verallo-Rowell VM, Verallo V, Graupe K, et al. Double-blind comparison of azelaic acid and hydroquinone in the treatment of melasma. *Acta Derm Venereol (Stockh).* 1989;143(suppl): 58-61.

30. Sarkar R, Bhalla M, Kanwar AJ. A comparative study of 20% azelaic acid cream monotherapy versus a sequential therapy in the treatment of melasma in dark-skinned patients. *Dermatology.* 2002;205:249-254.

31. Pathak MA, Fitzpatrick TB, Kraus EW. Usefulness of retinoic acid in the treatment of melasma. *J Am Acad Dermatol.* 1986;15:894-899.

32. Yoshimura K, Harii K, Shibuya F, et al. A new bleaching protocol for hyperpigmented skin lesions with a high concentration of all-trans-retinoic acid aqueous gel. *Aesthetic Plast Surg.* 1999;23:285-291.

33. Yoshimura K, Momosawa A, Alba E, et al. Clinical trial of bleaching treatment with 10% all trans retinol gel. *Dermatologic Surg.* 2003;29:155-160.

34. Piamphongsant T. Treatment of melasma: a review with personal experience. *Int J Dermatol.* 1998;37:897-903.

35. Lim JTE. Treatment of melasma using kojic acid in a gel containing hydroquinone and glycolic acid. *Dermatol Surg.* 1999;25:282-284.

36. Gracia A, Fulton JE. The combination of glycolic acid and hydroquinone or kojic acid for the treatment of melasma and related conditions. *Dermatolo Surg*. 1999;22:443-447.

37. Hakozaki T, Minwalla L, Ang JZ, et al. The effect of niacinamide on reducing cutaneous pigmentation and suppression of melanosome transfer. *Br J Dermatol*. 2002;147:20-31.

38. Franchi J, Coutadeur MC, Marteau C, et al. Depigmenting effects of calcium D-Pantetheine-S-Sulfonate on human melanocytes. *Pigment Cell Res*. 2000;13:165-171.

39. Hayakawa R, Matsunaga K, Ukei C, et al. Biochemical and clinical study of calcium Pantetheine-S-Sulfonate. *Acta Vitaminol Enzymol*. 1985;7(1-2):109-114.

40. Lim JTE, Tham SN. Glycolic acid peels in the treatment of melasma. *Dermatol Surg*. 1997;23:177-179.

41. Javaheri SM, Handa S, Inderjit K. Safety and efficacy of glycolic acid facial peel in Indian women with melasma. *Int J Dermatol*. 2001;40:354-357.

42. Grimes PE. The safety and efficacy of salicylic acid chemical peels in darker racial-ethnic groups. *Dermatol Surg*. 1999; 25:18-22.

43. Khunger N, Sarkar R, Jain RK. Tretinoin Peels versus glycolic acid peels in the treatment of melasma in dark skinned patients. *Dermatol Surg*. 2004;30:756-760.

44. Suzuki II. Skin lightening with iontophoresis of L-ascorbic acid-2-phosphate (in Japanese). *J Jpn Soc Aesthet Plastic Surg*. 1998;20:46-67.

45. Huh CH, Seo KI, Park JY, et al. A randomized double-blind placebo controlled trial of vitamin C iontophoresis in melasma. *Dermatol*. 2003;206:316-320.

46. Grekin RC, Shelton RM, Geisse JK, Frieden I. 510-nm pigmented lesion dye laser. Its characteristics and clinical uses. *J Dermatol Surg Oncol*. 1993;19:380-387.

47. Taylor CR, Anderson RR. Ineffective treatment of refractory melasma and postinflammatory hyperpigmentation by Q-switched ruby laser. *J Dermatol Surg Oncol*. 1994;20:592-597.

48. Wang CC, Hui CY, Sue YM, et al. Intense pulsed light for the treatment of refractory melasma in Asian Persons. *Dermatol Surg*. 2004;30:1196-1200.

49. Negishi K, Tezuka Y, Kushikata N, et al. Photorejuvenation for Asian skin by intense pulsed light. *Dermatol Surg*. 2001;27: 627-632.

50. Manaloto RM, Alster T. Erbium:YAG laser resurfacing for refractory melasma. *Dermatol Surg*. 1999;25:121-123.

51. Angsuwarangsee S, Polnikorn N. Combined ultrapulse CO_2 laser and Q-switched alexandrite laser compared with Q-switched alexandrite laser alone for refractory melasma: split-face design. *Dermatol Surg*. 2003;29:59-64.

52. Manstein D, Herron GS, Sink RK, Tanner H, Anderson RR. Fractional photothermolysis: a new concept for cutaneous remodeling using microscopic patterns of thermal injury. *Lasers Surg Med*. 2004;34:426-438.

53. Tannous ZS, Astner S. Utilizing fractional resurfacing in the treatment of therapy-resistant melasma. *J Cosmet Laser Ther*. 2005;7:39-43.

54. Rokhsar C, Fitzpatrick RE. The treatment of melasma with fractional photothermolysis: a pilot study. *Dermatol Surg*. 2005;31:1645-1650.

55. Kunachak S, Leelaudomlipi P, Sirikulchayanonta V. Q-Switched ruby laser therapy of acquired bilateral nevus of Ota-like macules. *Dermatol Surg*. 1999;25:938-941.

56. Kunachak S, Leelaudomlipi P. Q-switched Nd:YAG laser treatment for acquired bilateral nevus of Ota-like maculae: a long-term follow-up. *Lasers Surg Med*. 2000;26:376-379.

57. Polnikorn N, Tanrattanakorn S, Goldberg DJ. Treatment of Hori's nevus with the Q-switched Nd:YAG laser. *Dermatol Surg*. 2000;26:477-480.

58. Lam AY, Wong DS, Lam LK, Ho WS, Chan HH. A retrospective study on the efficacy and complications of Q-switched. Alexandrite laser in the treatment of acquired bilateral nevus of Ota-like macules. *Dermatol Surg*. 2001;27:937-941.

CHAPTER 16

Treatment of Dermatosis Papulosa Nigra

James C. Collyer, MD, and Susan Leu, MD

INTRODUCTION

Dermatosis papulosa nigra (DPN) is a benign condition first described by Castellani in 1925. It is a very common skin dermatosis that consists of multiple dark brown to black, smooth, dome-shaped papules mostly on the face, upper back, chest and neck of darkly pigmented individuals (Figure 16.1). While those affected are most commonly African American, reports of DPN have been described in Asians, Europeans, and Hispanics.

Pathogenesis is largely unknown, but many authors consider DPN to be a variant of seborrheic keratosis based on their similar histopathologic findings. DPN may be caused by a nevoid developmental defect of the pilosebaceous follicle and thus may be classified under the group of epithelial nevi.[1]

The incidence in study populations varies from 10% to 77%, with approximately 50% of patients reporting a family history of similar lesions.[1,2] Darker individuals are affected most frequently with a 2:1 predominance in females. DPN appear after puberty and slowly increase in size and number with age with a peak incidence in the sixth decade,[2] although there have been reports of patients as young as age three with the lesion.[3]

Despite the benign nature of these lesions, many patients seek out medical advice on management and treatment. The conventional treatment options include simple excision, cryosurgery, electrodessication, curettage, dermabrasion, and laser removal. While all these treatment modalities can be effective in treating DPN, there are potential side effects, such as scarring and dyspigmentation.

CLINICAL EXAMINATION AND PATIENT HISTORY

While DPN are considered completely benign, many patients are bothered by their cosmetic appearance or occasionally find them pruritic, and therefore come to the dermatologist's office seeking treatment. They are commonly referred to as "moles" and patients often want to be assured they are not malignant. Patient history usually consists of these lesions appearing after puberty and slowly increasing in size and number, which some patients feel gives them an older appearance. These papules may also become irritated by clothing, jewelry, or eyewear.

Physical examination reveals multiple, well-demarcated, firm, smooth, dome-shaped papules that vary from dark brown to black in color (Figures 16.2 and 16.3). They can also be pedunculated, resembling acrochordons.[1] They usually measure between 1–5 mm in diameter and are mostly located on the malar area of the face but can also be on the neck, trunk, and other areas of the face[1] (Figure 16.4). In a study of 93 patients, all affected patients had facial lesions with 40% having face and neck involvement and 29% with face, neck, and trunk lesions.[2] Unless recently irritated,

there is usually no evidence of scaling, crusting, or ulceration. Differential diagnosis includes seborrheic keratosis, acrochordons, melanocytic nevi, syringomas, solar lentigines, verrucae, trichoepitheliomas, and adenoma sebaceum (Table 16.1).

DPN are fairly characteristic in appearance; however if diagnosis is difficult to establish clinically, skin biopsy can be performed which will reveal mild to moderate hyperkeratosis, acanthosis, papillomatosis in the epidermis which is very similar histologically to small acanthotic seborrheic keratosis (Figures 16.5 and 16.6). Horn cysts (keratin-filled invaginations of the epidermis) can be present as well as dilatation of the hair follicles. The epidermis, especially the basal layer, shows marked hyperpigmentation when compared to adjacent epidermis. In DPN that are pedunculated, histology reveals a well-developed fibrous stalk with minimal amounts of inflammatory cells in a perivascular distribution (Figure 16.7).

TREATMENT

Treatment options are varied for DPN, but all of them are considered elective because of the benign nature of these lesions. Treatment consists of simple excision with scissors, cryosurgery, electrodessication, curettage, dermabrasion, and laser removal.

Preprocedure consultation is extremely important. This is the time to discuss the patient's medical history and medications, different treatment options, side effects, and also to determine patient expectations and goals (Table 16.2). It is therefore important for the practitioner to encourage an active conversation and determine if

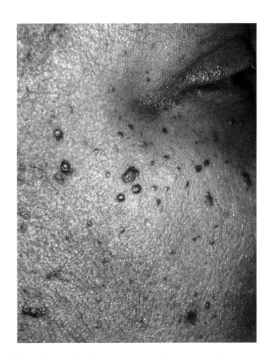

Figure 16.1 *Multiple dark brown to black, smooth, dome-shaped papules on the right cheek*

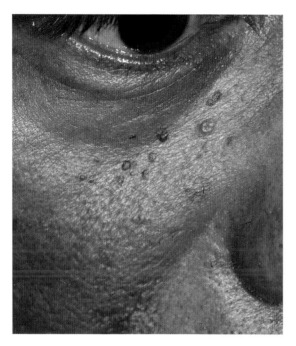

Figure 16.2 *Many well-demarcated, dark brown, smooth, dome-shaped papules*

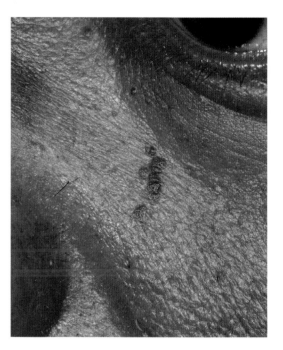

Figure 16.4 *DPN in a malar distribution*

the patient has reasonable expectations of treatment and outcome. The entire sequence of proceedings before, during, and after the procedure must be discussed, including in-depth postoperative care. As this is often a cosmetic procedure, it is important that the practitioner feels confident that there will be a desirable cosmetic outcome if treatment is to be initiated. Accordingly, a detailed physical examination must be performed. As darker pigmented skin is more susceptible to postinflammatory hypo- and hyperpigmentation and scarring, patients must be counseled on these risks. Patients must also understand that the goal of treatment is to flatten, smooth, or improve the appearance of these lesions. It is not always possible to completely remove them.

Before treatment is started, informed consent is obtained. It is also important to find out if the patient has a history of keloids or recent isotretinoin use, which has been reported to be associated with delayed re-epithelialization and hypertrophic scarring.[4] Additionally, as hereditary hemolytic diseases such as sickle cell anemia, thalassemia, and glucose-6-phosphate dehydrogenase deficiency are more prevalent in darker pigmented individuals, a detailed family and personal medical history may be beneficial. A history of HIV, viral hepatitis, or diabetes mellitus may affect postoperative healing from any type of procedure.[5] Unwanted outcomes can be limited if there is proper patient education, patient expectations are understood, and conservative measures are used in treatment. If there are extensive numbers of lesions on the face to be treated, it may be helpful to chose a "test area" and then have patients follow-up in 3 to 4 weeks. Pre- and postoperative photographs are often helpful for both patient and practitioner.

Since the surface area treated may be broad, different options for pain control, if any, can be discussed and utilized if needed during the procedure. If anesthesia is required, topical anesthetic agents are preferred. As DPN only involve the epidermis, full dermal analgesia is

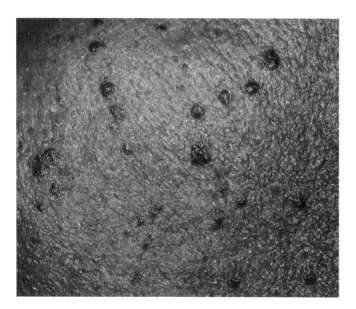

Figure 16.3 *A closer view of DPN*

TABLE 16.1 ■ Differential Diagnosis of Dermatosis Papulosa Nigrae

Acrochordons
Adenoma sebaceum
Melanocytic nevi
Seborrheic keratoses
Solar lentigines
Syringomas
Trichoepitheliomas
Verrucae

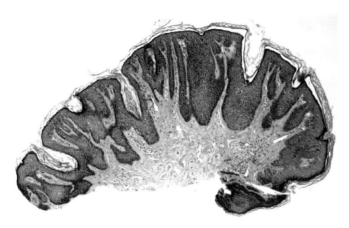

Figure 16.5 *Low-power histologic examination reveals moderate hyperkeratosis, acanthosis, papillomatosis in the epidermis*

usually not necessary. A recent study by Carter revealed that applying either EMLA (2.5% lidocaine and 2.5% procaine, AstraZeneca LP) or L.M.X.4 (liposomal lidocaine 4%, Ferndale Laboratories Inc.) under occlusion (Tegaderm) for 30 minutes provided satisfactory anesthesia for patients undergoing electrodessication for DPN.[6] Some practitioners may feel that applying topical anesthetic under occlusion is an inconvenience, so L.M.X.4 may be more beneficial. Unlike EMLA, where occlusion significantly enhances its efficacy, L.M.X.4 may not need occlusion because of its liposomal formulation. Regardless, both agents are marketed in packages with and without Tegaderm.[6] Tumescent anesthesia with a 0.05% to 0.1% lidocaine solution may be used if a large area is to be treated with dermabrasion, the CO_2 laser, or the erbium:YAG laser.

Simple excision with scissors is an effective and economical way to treat DPN, although there is risk of scar formation, especially in patients with a history of keloid formation. This procedure may or may not require topical anesthesia depending on the size of the lesion and the physician's judgment after evaluation of the patient. The gradle scissor is a short-handled scissor with curved blades

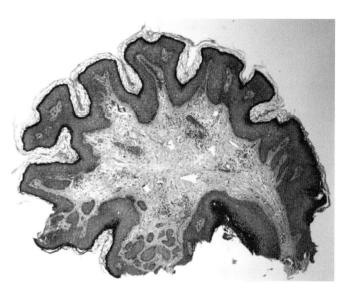

Figure 16.7 *DPN with a mild perivascular lymphocytic infiltrate and a fibrous stalk resembling an acrochordon*

and a tapered fine-pointed tip that is ideal for delicate simple excision of DPN. Hemostasis may be achieved using compression, light electrodessication, or topical hemostatics, such as caustics. Examples of topical caustics include aluminum chloride, silver nitrate, and ferric sulfate (Monsel's solution), of which the latter two may potentially stain the skin.

Electrodessication uses a high-voltage, low-amperage, high frequency current in a monoterminal fashion to cause heat generation and tissue separation with minimal tissue damage, as compared to electrocautery.[7] In electrodessication, the electrode contacts the skin, causing superficial tissue dehydration. Most damage is epidermal and there is minimal risk of scarring as long as lower power settings are used (Figure 16.8). Higher power settings may cause superficial scarring, hypopigmentation, and electric burns. Additionally, this modality may theoretically cause cardiac pacemaker and implantable cardioverter-defibrillator (ICD) malfunction. Electrodessication costs approximately $250–$500 depending on the area to be treated, but may be a painful procedure for patients. These patients should be counseled on the use of topical anesthetics before the procedure.

Another treatment option to be considered is curettage. Light abrasive curettage without local anesthesia resulted in a 50% excellent response with only 5% poor outcome as a result persistent hypopigmentation.[8] In addition, light cryosurgery may also be

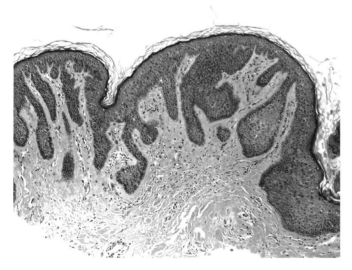

Figure 16.6 *Polypoid lesion with regular basaloid acanthosis, elongation of the rete ridges, and prominent basal layer hyperpigmentation. The underlying dermis appears normal*

TABLE 16.2A ▪ Treatment Options for DPN

Chemical peel (spot treatment)
Cryosurgery
Curettage
Dermabrasion
Electrodessication
Laser
Observation
Simple excision

TABLE 16.2B ■ **Components of the Pretreatment Consultation**

Medical history
Social history
Surgical history
Medications (including over-the-counter)
Thorough physical examination
Detailed explanation of treatments, risks/benefits of these treatments, treatment options, and informed consent

added to curettage. First, apply the cryospray on the DPN until the freeze halo covers the entire lesion. After letting it thaw for a few seconds, curettage the frozen lesion with one or two strokes.[4] However, cryosurgery (costing $250–500 depending on the area to be treated) is used cautiously as melanocytes are more susceptible to destruction than keratinocytes with this mode of treatment, and patients may be left with unsightly hypopigmented (or less likely hyperpigmented) lesions.

Dermabrasion is a resurfacing procedure that can effectively treat DPN.[4] It utilizes a rotating diamond fraise or wire brush, costing approximately $1500. Lower settings should also be incorporated when treating darker skin types. This modality is not commonly used in people of color because of the increased risk of residual dyschromia and scarring.

Laser removal is becoming a popular and effective treatment for DPN. However, an understanding of basic laser principles, particularly in ethnic skin, is critical when treating DPN, as the increased melanin content in the epidermis of darker pigmented individuals can lead to hyper- or hypopigmentation.[5] The CO_2, Er:YAG, KTP, Fraxel, Q-switched ruby, Q-switched alexandrite, and 532-nm diode lasers have been used to treat DPN.[9,10] One must be careful that the spot size does not exceed the diameter of the skin lesion to minimize any risk of damage to the surrounding skin. Another limitation to laser treatment is its expense. For example, treatment with the Fraxel laser averages approximately $1200 per treatment and KTP costs $450–850 depending on the treatment area.

When using lasers for removal of DPN in ethnic skin, lower energy settings should be used as to avoid dyspigmentation. Proposed laser settings for the Iridex 532 nm diode laser have recently been set forth.[11] DPN can be treated using a 700-nm hand-piece set at 12 J/cm², 3 W, and a 6 Hz repetition rate without anesthesia resulting in a pulse duration of 15 ms. The lesions appear ashen in color with a dry and rough texture after laser treatment. Treatments are repeated at 3-week intervals. This modality has been used successfully without residual postinflammatory hypo- or hyperpigmentation.[11]

With any treatment modality, strict posttreatment skin care is essential. Patients should be advised to cleanse the treated area with a gentle cleanser (Cetaphil or CeraVe) and avoid all abrasive cleansers. Patients must also avoid picking or scratching the treated area and to use a physically blocking, high SPF sunscreen (minimum SPF 30). Patients should return to clinic in 4 to 8 weeks for follow-up or immediately if there are any complications. In the case of postinflammatory hyperpigmentation, use of hydroquinone or topical retinoids can be used. Hypopigmentation usually resolves spontaneously after several months but may be persistent.[9]

DIRECTIONS FOR THE FUTURE AND CONCLUSIONS

In conclusion, DPN are benign lesions that do not need to be treated. However, if a patient desires treatment for these lesions there are many different treatment modalities available. Risks and benefits of each treatment must be discussed with the patient as

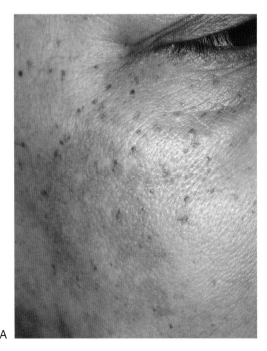 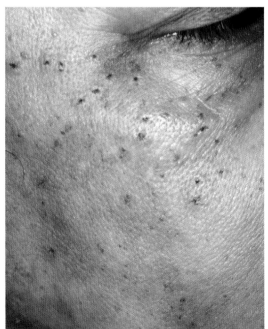

Figure 16.8 *(A) Pretreated DPN. (B) DPN immediately posttreatment with electrodessication. There is minor crusting and erythema of the treated areas*

well as discussion of the patient's expectations. The most promising frontier in treatment of DPN appears to lie in laser surgery. However, more controlled studies must be done to determine optimal settings, document treatment success, as well as complication rates.

REFERENCES

1. Hairston MA Jr, Reed RJ, Derbes VJ. Dermatosis Papulosa Nigra. *Arch Dermatol.* 1964;89:655-658.

2. Grimes PE, Arora S, Minus HR, et al. Dermatosis papulosa nigra. *Cutis.* 1983;32:385-386.

3. Bolognia J, Jorizzo JL, Rapini RP. *Dermatology.* London, UK; New York, NY: Mosby; 2003:1701-1702.

4. Robinson JK. *Surgery of the Skin: Procedural Dermatology.* Philadelphia, PA: Elsevier Mosby; 2005:195,466,592,602.

5. Jackson BA. Lasers in ethnic skin: a review. *J Am Acad Dermatol.* 2003;48:S134-S138.

6. Carter EL, Coppola CA, Barsanti FA. A randomized, double-blind comparison of two topical anesthetic formulations prior to electrodesiccation of dermatosis papulosa nigra. *Dermatol Surg.* 2006;32:1-6.

7. Fitzpatrick TB, Freedberg IM. *Fitzpatrick's dermatology in general medicine.* 6th ed. New York, NY: McGraw-Hill Medical Pubication Division; 2003.

8. Kauh YC, McDonald JW, Rapaport JA, et al. A surgical approach for dermatosis papulosa nigra. *Int J Dermatol.* 1983; 22:590-592.

9. Khatri KA. Ablation of cutaneous lesions using and erbium:YAG laser. *J Cosmet Laser Ther.* 2003;5(3-4):150-153.

10. Goldberg DJ. *Laser Dermatology.* New York, NY: Springer; 2005.

11. Lupo MP. Dermatosis papulosis nigra: treatment options. *J Drugs Dermatol.* 2007;6:29-30.

CHAPTER 17

Postinflammatory Hyperpigmentation

Yan I. Zhu, MD, PhD

INTRODUCTION, ETIOLOGY, AND DEFINITION

Postinflammatory hyperpigmentation (PIH) primarily affects dark-skinned individuals (Fitzpatrick Skin Phototype III through VI) or lighter-skinned individuals with dark irides and has no gender predilection (Figure 17.1). With the increasing ethnic diversity of the United States, dermatologists will encounter more inquiry about PIH. Postinflammatory hyperpigmentation often leads to anxiety in individuals, which is sometimes out of proportion to the severity of the condition. This anxiety is aggravated by the fact that there is no quickly effective treatment other than cosmetic cover-ups. Frequently patients are more concerned about the dyschromia and not aware of the inflammatory condition that is causing PIH (Table 17.1, Figure 17.2). The definition of postinflammatory hyperpigmentation, as its name implies, is very straightforward. Other names used for PIH include postinflammatory melanoderma. There are only a few conditions such as melasma, solar lentigo, and drug-induced hyperpigmentation that may mimic PIH. *Melasma* tends to be macular and has uniform intensity and well-defined borders, while PIH tends to follow the shape and distribution of the preceding inflammation and has irregular pigmentation intensity and indistinct or feathered borders. *Solar lentigo* appears on the sun-exposed area of a person, typically the face, dorsal arms, and hands. *Drug-induced hyperpigmentation* should be suspected in individual who have taken such medications as minocycline, chloroquine, bleomycin, mercury, or amiodarone. The pigmentation tends to be symmetrically distributed and may not correlate with preceding inflammation. In the author's opinion, hyperpigmentation at the site of fixed drug eruption should be categorized as PIH.

Why do inflammatory processes cause hyperpigmentation? The answer was first proposed to lay in the complex interaction between inflammatory cells and melanocytes in 1988.[1] Later, more specific inflammatory mediators were implicated to be involved in PIH, particularly leukotriene (LT)C_4, LTD_4, and thromboxane B_2.[2] Therefore, it is conceivable that the degree of hyperpigmentation correlates with the severity of inflammation as demonstrated in UVB-induced PIH.[3] Topical anti-inflammatory agents have been found to reduce in a parallel manner both UVB-induced erythema and subsequent PIH.[3] This is the basis of applying topical anti-inflammatory agents in preventing laser-induced PIH.

Histologically, PIH can demonstrate both epidermal and dermal pigmentation. A lighter-brown appearance suggests melanin within the epidermis, while a darker-gray or black tone indicates dermal pigmentation. One study showed that PIH associated with acne, folliculitis, eczema, or shaving showed increased melanin exclusively at basal layer of epidermis but not in the dermis.[4] However, when there is disruption of the basement membrane, pigmentary incontinence may occur, resulting in dermal deposit of melanin, as seen in hyperpigmentation in atopic dermatitis or lichenoid dermatoses.[5] The depth of the deposition of melanin helps determine which treatment modalities to choose and potentially how effective treatments can be. If the pigment deposition is dermal, topical applications are rarely effective (refer to section "General Treatment Approach and Prevention of PIH" below).

LITERATURE REVIEW/EVIDENCE-BASED SUMMARY

There are very few randomized, double-blinded, and well-controlled clinical trials conducted on PIH in the past two decades. In 1993, Bulengo-Ransby et al.[4] showed that 40 weeks of topical tretinoin in black patients significantly lightens PIH. The lightening was noticed as early as 4 weeks of application in tretinoin group, and persisted throughout the study. Through skin biopsies, the epidermal melanin content was found to decrease by 23% in tretinoin-treated lesions, while the lightening by colorimetry was much higher at 40%. The study also showed that daily application of topical tretinoin is relatively well tolerated. It did not cause pigmentary darkening in normal skin; alternatively, it was shown to lighten normal skin in black subjects. Based on these data, it is postulated that the mechanisms of efficacy of tretinoin on PIH may include inhibiting the rate of melanogenesis,[6,7] more evenly redistributing epidermal melanin, and increasing epidermal turnover.

In 1997, Burns et al.[8] conducted a randomized and controlled clinical trial on the safety and efficacy of glycolic acid peels on PIH in dark-complexioned individuals. All subjects were put on a topical regimen of hydroquinone and tretinoin. The control group applied 2% hydroquinone/10% glycolic acid gel twice daily and 0.05% tretinoin cream at night. The peel patients used the same topical regimen and, in addition, received six serial glycolic acid peels (68% maximum concentration). The subjects receiving serial glycolic acid peels showed a trend toward more rapid and greater

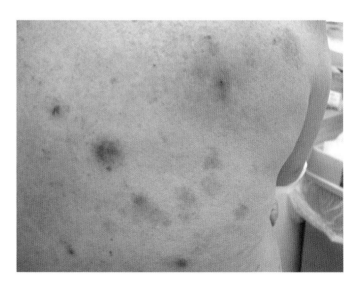

Figure 17.1 *Postinflammatory hyperpigmentation from nummular eczema on the back of an Asian man. Notice the coin-shaped lesions*

TABLE 17.1 ■ List of Inflammatory Processes or Insults to the Skin that Can Cause PIH

Acne (Figure 17.2)
Allergic or irritant contact dermatitis
Atopic dermatitis
Folliculitis
Lichen planus
Lupus erythematosus
Phytophotodermatitis
Trauma

improvement of PIH and also experienced increased lightening of the normal skin with minimal adverse effects.

In 1998, Kakita and Lowe[9] conducted a multicenter, randomized, double-blinded, parallel-controlled clinical trial comparing the efficacy of the combination of azelaic acid 20% cream (Azelex) and glycolic acid (15% first, then 20%) lotion versus hydroquinone 4% in vehicle lotion in the treatment of facial hyperpigmentation in darker-skinned patients. At week 24, overall improvement, reduction in lesion area, pigmentary intensity, and disease severity were comparable in the two treatment groups. The combination of azelaic acid 20% cream and glycolic acid 15% or 20% lotion had only a slightly higher rate of mild local irritation.

In 2006, Grimes et al.[10] conducted a double-blinded, randomized, vehicle-controlled clinical trial in 74 patients from darker racial ethnic groups who had acne, evaluating the safety and efficacy of tazarotene 0.1% cream on PIH associated with acne. They found that once-daily application of tazarotene cream for 18 weeks was effective against PIH and well tolerated. Erythema, burning, peeling, or dryness was not more than mild in either treatment group.

CLINICAL EXAMINATION AND PATIENT HISTORY

Taking a thorough history is the most important first step in diagnosis and planning a treatment regimen. When the cause is clearly

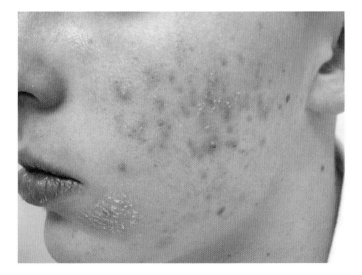

Figure 17.2 *Postinflammatory hyperpigmentation in an acne patient*

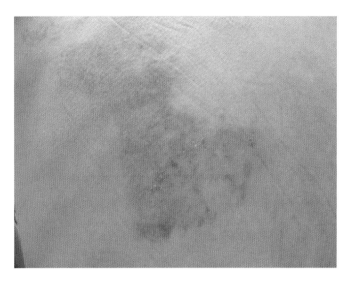

Figure 17.3 *Postinflammatory hyperpigmentation from application of ice with resulting cold injury. Notice the geometric shape of the lesion*

identified and explained to patients, their compliance with therapy will increase. When a hyperpigmented patch or macule is in the vicinity of an inflammatory eruption, the diagnosis of PIH is very clear. Sometimes a little investigation may be needed (Figure 17.3). The inciting factor of PIH associated with phytophotodermatitis from fruit or fragrance, fixed drug eruption, or cold or heat treatment may be more difficult to identify. Interestingly, PIH may provide a clue to the diagnosis of morphea when the erythema is absent but hyperpigmentation is associated with skin atrophy.

Clinical examination begins with assessing the borders, uniformity, and depth of pigmentation, facilitated by the use of a dermatoscope or a Wood's lamp. Under a Wood's lamp, epidermal lesions have an accentuated border, whereas dermal lesions lack this quality. Mixed lesions, holding both epidermal and dermal pigmentation, may only show partial accentuation.

If the pigmentation is mainly dermal, it is wise to advice patients that treatment will be challenging, and perseverance is paramount. Within the area of PIH, different regions may have different depth of pigmentation, and it is advisable to incorporate this into patient education and treatment strategy.

GENERAL TREATMENT APPROACH AND PREVENTION OF PIH

Despite many years of research, we still do not have a quick and easy treatment for PIH. It is important to discuss the difficulty of

TABLE 17.2 ■ Basic Principles of Treating PIH

1. Manage or control the underlying skin condition that causes inflammation
2. Stop all potential irritants such as fragrance, cosmeceuticals, herbal preparations, toners, astringents, witch hazel, and alcohol
3. Sunscreen and sun protection for all patients; prefer zinc- or titanium-based sun blocks to avoid irritation
4. Patience, patience, and patience

TABLE 17.3 ■ Treatment Modalities for PIH

Topical therapies	Mechanisms
Retinoid or its derivatives	Inhibits melanogenesis,[7] redistribution of epidermal melanin,[4] increase epidermal turnover
Hydroquinone	Inhibits tyrosinase, destruction of melanocytes, degradation of melanosomes, and the inhibition of the synthesis of DNA and RNA
Kojic acid	Inhibits tyrosinase through chelation of copper
Azelaic acid	Oxidizes unsaturated fatty acids to dicarboxylic acids, which competitively inhibits tyrosinase, directly cytotoxic against melanocytes, reduces free radical production
Methimazole[13]	Noncytotoxic inhibitor of melanin production of melanocytes
Chemical peels	
Salicylic acid peel	Exfoliation, anti-inflammation
Glycolic and lactic acid	Exfoliation, inhibit melanin synthesis in melanoma cells[14]
Laser/light treatment	Direct thermolysis of melanin[12]

treatment with patients before initiating therapies so that they have realistic expectations.

The basic principles of treating PIH are listed in Table 17.2 and serve as the foundation of all further treatment options that are discussed in detail in the next section. For principle 1, the choices of therapies depend on the underlying skin conditions. For example, if the cause is because of atopic dermatitis or nummular eczema, then topical steroid or nonsteroidal anti-inflammatory agents will be the treatment of choice. If the cause is inflammatory acne, then managing the papules, pustules, nodules, or cysts with topical or oral agents is the first step. Principle 2 is based on stopping any topical that causes burning or stinging, which may lead to further inflammation and PIH. Principle 3 hallmarks that strict sun protection must be followed while under treatment for PIH or further dyschromia will likely occur. Finally, principle 4 emphasizes the need to educate the patient that the treatment of PIH requires time and patience.

Special Situations: When dermal pigmentation is present, it is wise to advise patients that there is not yet an ideal therapy to reach the melanin deep in the skin, and a tincture of time is recommended. When both epidermal and dermal pigmentation are present, reducing epidermal pigmentation with topicals or laser may allow for deeper penetration of pigment-targeting lasers.

To prevent PIH when using laser or light therapy in patients with darker skin, especially if erythema develops during treatment, applying a medium- to high-potency topical steroid immediately after treatment with repeat applications within 24 hours has been very effective in preventing PIH in the author's experience. Epidermal cooling devices allow higher fluences to be used and lowers the risk for dyspigmentation.[11] For postlaser hyperpigmentation, topical bleaching agents such as hydroquinone and tretinoin have been effective.[12]

DETAILED ASSESSMENT OF BENEFITS AND LIMITATIONS OF TREATMENT APPROACHES

It is prudent to offer patient multiple treatment options and discuss the risks and benefits of each option. Involving patients in the decision-making is the most effective way of ensuring compliance and

patience. The combination of strict sun protection and topical hydroquinone continues to be one of the most popular treatment modalities for PIH.

Table 17.3 lists many treatment modalities that have been reported in the literature for PIH and their mechanisms of action.

Kojic acid is a chemical produced by several species of fungus, especially *Aspergillus oryzae*, which has the Japanese common name *koji*. Kojic acid is a byproduct in the fermentation process of malting rice, for use in the manufacturing of sake, the Japanese rice wine. It is useful in patients who cannot tolerate hydroquinone, and it may be combined with a topical corticosteroid to reduce irritation. It can be found in many over-the-counter whitening products.

Other commonly used treatment modalities are highlighted in Table 17.3.

Table 17.4 summarizes the clinical trials that have been reported in literature on different topical treatment of PIH. It generally takes 1 to 6 months of topical treatments to see some improvement. All topicals may cause irritation or allergic contact dermatitis, so it is recommended to treat a test area for several days before applying to large areas. Hydroquinone has been the standard of treatment for years. However, a recent warning from FDA has put it under the spotlight. New data from laboratory research have shown some evidence of carcinogenicity in experimental animals, although such carcinogenicity has not been shown or established in humans. Leukoderma of the normal skin surrounding the treated areas and exogenous ochronosis after prolonged use may also occur. Because of this concern, the FDA is proposing that skin-bleaching products should be restricted to prescription use only, with users closely monitored under medical supervision.

Chemical peels and topicals work synergistically (Table 17.5). Chemical peels not only lighten skin, they can also allow better penetration of other topical agents. When using chemical peels to treat PIH, it is recommended to pretreat patients with tretinoin and hydroquinone.[17]

Q-switched ruby laser was not effective in treating PIH or melasma by itself.[19] Lee et al.[20] recommended a combination of Q-switched alexandrite laser and 15% to 25% trichloroactic acid (TCA) in treating melasma, PIH, or acquired bilateral nevus of Ota-like macules in Korean patients. In this study, all patients were

TABLE 17.4 ■ Topical Therapies of PIH

	Cause of PIH	Skin type	Dosage	Duration to see effect	Note
Single agent Tretinoin[4,13,15]	Acne, shaving, eczema, ingrown hair, folliculitis	Black	Once daily	4 weeks	Blinded, randomized
Tazarotene[10]	Acne	III to VI	0.1% cream daily	10 weeks	Blinded, randomized
Hydroquinone	Any type	II to VI	4%-8% cream daily	1-3 months	Watch for exogenous ochronosis
Azelaic acid	Any type	II to VI	Cream for dry skin, gel for oily skin	1-3 months	Irritation is the main side effect
Methimazole[13]	Acid burn	Iranian male	5% daily	6 weeks	One case report, nonmutagenic
Combination 4% HQ + 0.15% retinol[16]	Melasma and PIH	II to VI	Twice daily	12 weeks	Open label study
2% mequinol + 0.01% tretinoin (phase IV trial of Solagé) vs. 4% hydroquinone	PIH	African American	Daily to twice daily	12 weeks	Open-label, more effective than 4% cream of hydroquinone
Azelaic and glycolic acid[9]	Melasma (majority), PIH, idiopathic melanosis, drug-induced hyperpigmentation	III to V	Azelaic acid 20% cream and glycolic acid lotion versus hydroquinone 4%	24 weeks	Blinded, randomized, same efficacy, more burning with the acids

treated with the Q-switched alexandrite laser (755 nm) at fluences of 7.0 to 8.0 J/cm^2 with a pulse width of 100 ns using a 3-mm spot size. At the same session, the 15% to 25% TCA with or without Jessner's solution was used for chemical peeling. TCA was applied to the laser-untreated or -undertreated pigmentary sites, and Jessner's solution was applied to the whole face to blend treated and nontreated areas. All patients were instructed to avoid direct sunlight and to apply a sunscreen before any sun exposure. After a single treatment session, 63% of them considered the results as "clear, excellent, or good" in respect to the color and 54% of them assessed that the size of the lesion had cleared more than 50%. Major side effects included hyperpigmentation within the laser- or TCA-treated sites persisting longer than 3 months in three patients.

Interestingly, oral isotretinoin has been reported in one Asian patient to eliminate PIH because of acne. The patient had almost total disappearance of PIH after 60 mg of isotretinoin per day for 4 months.[21] Isotretinoin may or may not have any direct impact on melanogenesis, but it is such an effective treatment of acne that by preventing new lesions, it allows time for the old PIH lesions to disappear on their own.

DIRECTIONS FOR THE FUTURE AND CONCLUSIONS

We still do not have an ideal fast-acting, highly tolerated treatment of PIH. Promising basic research findings include an extract of *Lepidium apetalum* (ELA),[22] N-acetyl-4-cystaminylphenol (NCAP),[23] and gamma-tocopherol.[24]

L. apetalum (common name, peppergrass or pepperwort) is a wild annual or biannual flowering plant that is distributed in the Eurasia continent. ELA may be an effective inhibitor of hyperpigmentation caused by UV irradiation in animal studies, through a mechanism involving IL-6 (mediated downregulation of tyrosinase gene transcription rather than a direct inhibition of tyrosinase activity).[22]

NCAP is a new depigmenting agent that also acts through a different pathway than hydroquinone. It can decrease intracellular glutathione by stimulating pheomelanin rather than eumelanin. In a retrospective study of 12 patients with melasma using 4% NCAP, 66% showed marked improvement, and 8% showed complete loss of melasma lesions.[23] Changes of melanoderma were evident after 2 to 4 weeks of daily topical application of NCAP. It has not been studied in PIH.

TABLE 17.5 ■ Chemical Peels Used to Treat PIH

Peels	Skin type	Method	Frequency	Number of treatments needed	Notes
Spot peel[17]	Dark	TAC 25%, Jessner's solution, salicylic acid	Q month	Many	Spot application of skin-lightening agent
Salicylic acid[18]	Asian acne	30% SA in absolute ethanol	Bi-weekly 3 months	24	Not blinded or controlled, No other systemic or topical treatment used
Glycolic[8]	IV to VI	Glycolic peel with 68% maximum concentration	Q month	6	In addition to 2% hydroquinone/ 10% glycolic acid gel twice daily and 0.05% tretinoin cream at night.

A gamma-tocopherol (vitamin E) derivative was found to reduce UV-induced skin pigmentation in brownish guinea pigs if applied topically before and after UV exposure, through inhibition of tyrosinase activity and action of antioxidation.[24] Further clinical study is warranted to see if topical application of vitamin E derivatives may be efficacious in preventing photo-induced skin pigmentation in humans.

In summary, based on the current literature at the time of this writing, treatment of PIH requires tremendous trust and patience from both the patients and providers. Providers should have a large armamentarium of treatment options. Still, treatment of inflammation is the key.

REFERENCES

1. Nordlund JJ. Postinflammatory hyperpigmentation. *Dermatol Clin.* 1988;6:185-192.

2. Tomita Y, Maeda K, Tagami H. Melanocyte-stimulating properties of arachidonic acid metabolites: possible role in postinflammatory pigmentation. *Pigment Cell Res.* 1992;5:357-361.

3. Takiwaki H, Shirai S, Kohno H, Soh H, Arase S. The degrees of UVB-induced erythema and pigmentation correlate linearly and are reduced in a parallel manner by topical anti-inflammatory agents. *J Invest Dermatol.* 1994;103:642-646.

4. Bulengo-Ransby SM, Griffiths CE, Kimbrough-Green CK, et al. Topical tretinoin (retinoic acid) therapy for hyperpigmented lesions caused by inflammation of the skin in black patients. *N Engl J Med.* 1993;328:1438-1443.

5. Humphreys F, Spencer J, McLaren K, Tidman MJ. An histological and ultrastructural study of the 'dirty neck' appearance in atopic eczema. *Clin Exp Dermatol.* 1996;21:17-19.

6. Iwata M, Iwata S, Everett MA, Fuller BB. Hormonal stimulation of tyrosinase activity in human foreskin organ cultures. *In Vitro Cell Dev Biol.* 1990;26:554-560.

7. Orlow SJ, Chakraborty AK, Pawelek JM. Retinoic acid is a potent inhibitor of inducible pigmentation in murine and hamster melanoma cell lines. *J Invest Dermatol.* 1990;94:461-464.

8. Burns RL, Prevost-Blank PL, Lawry MA, Lawry TB, Faria DT, Fivenson DP. Glycolic acid peels for postinflammatory hyperpigmentation in black patients. A comparative study. *Dermatol Surg.* 1997;23:171-174.

9. Kakita LS, Lowe NJ. Azelaic acid and glycolic acid combination therapy for facial hyperpigmentation in darker-skinned patients: a clinical comparison with hydroquinone. *Clin Ther.* 1998;20:960-970.

10. Grimes P, Callender V. Tazarotene cream for postinflammatory hyperpigmentation and acne vulgaris in darker skin: a double-blind, randomized, vehicle-controlled study. *Cutis.* 2006;77: 45-50.

11. Chan HH, Alam M, Kono T, Dover JS. Clinical application of lasers in Asians. *Dermatol Surg.* 2002;28:556-563.

12. Chan H. The use of lasers and intense pulsed light sources for the treatment of acquired pigmentary lesions in Asians. *J Cosmet Laser Ther.* 2003;5:198-200.

13. Kasraee B, Handjani F, Parhizgar A, et al. Topical methimazole as a new treatment for postinflammatory hyperpigmentation: report of the first case. *Dermatology.* 2005;211:360-362.

14. Usuki A, Ohashi A, Sato H, Ochiai Y, Ichihashi M, Funasaka Y. The inhibitory effect of glycolic acid and lactic acid on melanin synthesis in melanoma cells. *Exp Dermatol.* 2003;12(Suppl 2):43-50.

15. Rafal ES, Griffiths CE, Ditre CM, et al. Topical tretinoin (retinoic acid) treatment for liver spots associated with photodamage. *N Engl J Med.* 1992;326:368-374.

16. Grimes PE. A microsponge formulation of hydroquinone 4% and retinol 0.15% in the treatment of melasma and postinflammatory hyperpigmentation. *Cutis.* 2004;74:362-368.

17. Roberts WE. Chemical peeling in ethnic/dark skin. *Dermatol Ther.* 2004;17:196-205.

18. Ahn HH, Kim IH. Whitening effect of salicylic acid peels in Asian patients. *Dermatol Surg.* 2006;32:372-375.

19. Taylor CR, Anderson RR. Ineffective treatment of refractory melasma and postinflammatory hyperpigmentation by Q-switched ruby laser. *J Dermatol Surg Oncol.* 1994;20:592-597.

20. Lee GY, Kim HJ, Whang KK. The effect of combination treatment of the recalcitrant pigmentary disorders with pigmented laser and chemical peeling. *Dermatol Surg.* 2002;28:1120-1123.

21. Winhoven SM, Ahmed I, Owen CM, Lear JT. Postinflammatory hyperpigmentation in an Asian patient: a dramatic response to oral isotretinoin (13-cis-retinoic acid). *Br J Dermatol.* 2005; 152:368-369.

22. Choi H, Ahn S, Lee BG, Chang I, Hwang JS. Inhibition of skin pigmentation by an extract of *Lepidium apetalum* and its possible implication in IL-6 mediated signaling. *Pigment Cell Res.* 2005;18:439-446.

23. Jimbow K. N-Acetyl-4-S-cysteaminylphenol as a new type of depigmenting agent for the melanoderma of patients with melasma. *Arch Dermatol.* 1991;127:1528-1534.

24. Kuwabara Y, Watanabe T, Yasuoka S, et al. Topical application of gamma tocopherol derivative prevents UV-Induced skin pigmentation. *Biol Pharm Bull.* 2006;29(6):1175-1179.

Greg J. Goodman, MD

INTRODUCTION, ETIOLOGY, AND DEFINITION

Postacne scarring remains a challenge of therapy, no matter what the ethnicity of the subject. The skin behaves as if it had a tremendous memory of the depth and severity of the existing scarring and the skin requires an inordinate amount of therapy to alter and improve its appearance.

◼ Methods of Assisting Postacne Scars

There are only a limited number of ways that the scarred skin may be helped. Broadly and simplistically, one can act on the scar by following methods:

Cutting it out

This includes all methods of excising scars. This is necessary in a number of instances either when the scar is dystrophic, has a white base, or is in the middle of a bearded area (Figure 18.1A, B, C, and D). This category also includes a variety of "punch" techniques such as punch elevation, punch excision, and punch grafting. These techniques at utility in treating punched out and ice pick scars (Figures 18.2A and B).

Filling it up

This includes autologous (autologous collagen, dermal, and fat grafting) and nonautologous temporary, semipermanent, and permanent augmentation techniques, and agents (Figure 18.3).

Altering its color

Sometimes a scar is purely visible because of its color and sometimes the color makes an atrophic or hypertrophic scar more

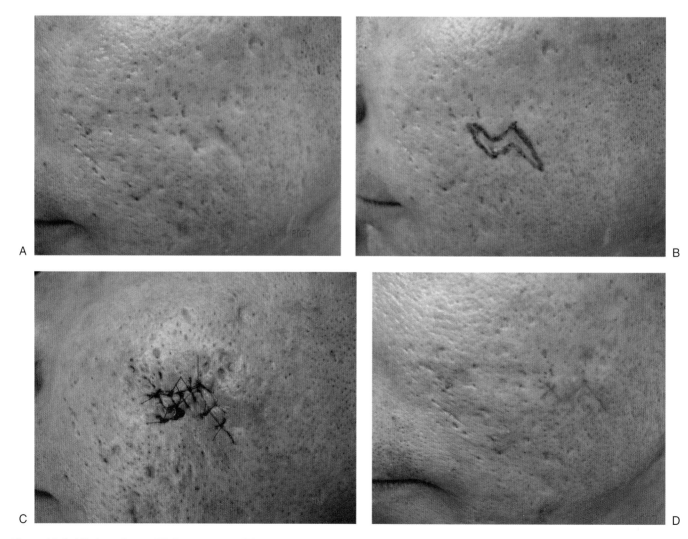

Figure 18.1 *W-shaped scar. (A) Pretreatment. (B) Outlined. (C) Immediately. (D) Three weeks postexcision*

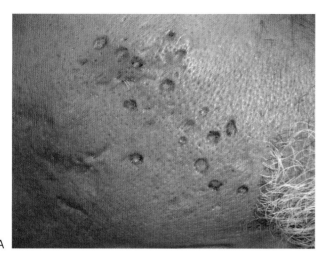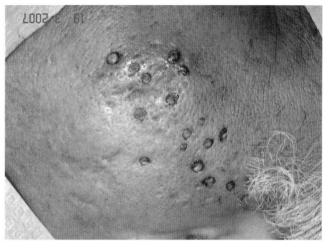

Figure 18.2 *Patient with type 4 skin immediately before (A) and immediately after (B) punch float technique*

visible. It depends on the color as to the technique utilized. For brown or hyperpigmented scars often this represents postinflammatory hyperpigmentation and is responsive to medical therapy with bleaching preparations and light chemical skin peeling (Figure 18.4). For erythematous scarring or marking home care, vascular laser and time may be all that is required (Figure 18.5). Hypopigmented marking is more difficult and may require pigment transfer techniques (Figures 18.6 and 18.7).

Inducing (or reducing) collagen (the most common methods utilized but usually AMONG the least efficient)

Inducing collagen formation is a common pathway used by all resurfacing techniques from the most minor home care through to superficial treatments such as microdermabrasion, light chemical skin peeling through to the deeper resurfacing techniques represented by medium and deep chemical peeling, dermabrasion, laser skin resurfacing, plasma skin resurfacing, and fractional resurfacing. It is with these techniques which are the least exact that patients of darker skin color may have variable outcomes (Figure 18.8).

All techniques relying on collagen remodeling have several things in common. The effect of therapy is often delayed for some months after the treatment, there is often a zenith and the drop away after any single therapy, the degree of collagen remodeling seems to be proportional to the severity of the injury, and there seem to be a reliance on multiple therapies or ongoing treatment to maximize the result.

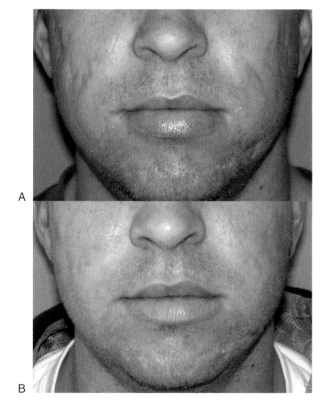

Figure 18.3 *Patient (A) before and (B) after subcision, fat transfer, and combined CO_2 and erbium laser resurfacing*

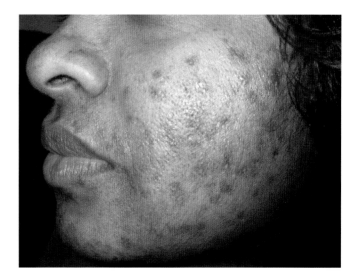

Figure 18.4 *Postinflammatory hyperpigmentation following acne misdiagnosed as postacne scarring*

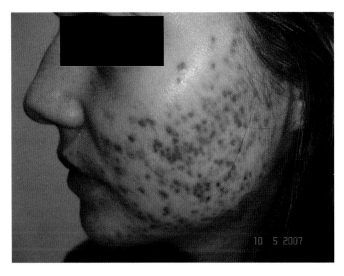

Figure 18.5 *Erythematous marking in a patient recovering from active acne*

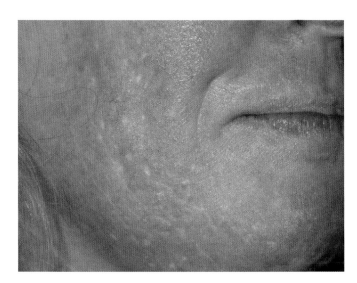

Figure 18.6 *Hypopigmented macular scarring*

Similar considerations, somewhat in reverse, seem to apply to hypertrophic scars with multiple and often periodically repeated therapies required to change the apparent "memory" of the excessive fibroblast produced dermal fibrosis.

Relaxing the region

This usually occurs on the forehead, chin, and lower jaw line and is because of excessive muscle activity on a scarred atrophic and compliant area of skin. By relaxing this skin puckering which is amplifying the scarring by the use of botulinum one may go a long way toward solving that problem albeit temporarily (Fig. 18.9A, B, C, and D).

■ Sun-Reactive Skin Types

Treatment of acne scarring in ethnic skin is a broad and deceptive topic. We are discussing ethnicity in a context of phototyping by sun burning reaction and immediate and delayed tanning responses to three minimal erythemal doses (MEDs) of skin as described by Thomas B. Fitzpatrick[1] (Table 18.1).

This scale described sun-reactive skin typing based on some inherent genetic traits and one's ability to withstand the ravages of short-term sun exposure. The ability to produce pigmentary change after procedural therapy for acne scarring differs; depending where one sits within the scale. Type 2 and type 3 skins may very well be

at risk of long-term hypopigmentation from ablative procedures whereas type 4 to 6 more likely to battle with hyperpigmentation. Scarring is said to be more common in darker skin patients but there are more reliable predictors for a person, the risk of scarring than skin coloring and as was written in 1993 "The myth that all black patients develop keloids or dyspigmentation after surgery should be dispelled."[2]

In this context, we are really discussing the skin types 4 to 6 (and maybe type 3), mainly those blessed with a deeper skin coloring which comes with a collection of benefits in regard to skin cancer and certain aging characteristics but with costs in terms of an increased rate of postinflammatory hyperpigmentation and possibly scarring when compared to those less replete with large melanosomes.

It is said that darker skin types differ from Caucasian skin not only in possessing increased epidermal melanin but also an increase in the stratum corneum cell layers, increased stratum corneum lipids, and increased recovery after tape stripping and numerous dermal fibroblasts.

Until comparatively recently many of the procedures for the treatment of acne scarring have been particularly difficult for patients with darker skin coloring. Technique-sensitive resurfacing (chemical peeling, dermabrasion, laser skin resurfacing, and plasma resurfacing) has been plagued by substantial morbidity and risk of adverse reactions.

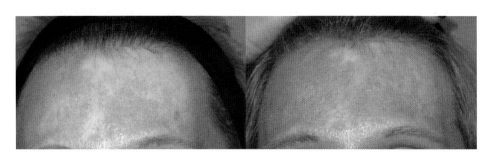

Figure 18.7 *Patient before and after autologous automated pigment cell transfer technique (ReCell ®)*

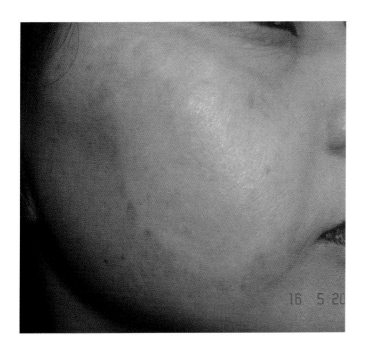

Figure 18.8 *Patient with long-term hypopigmentation following laser resurfacing*

More superficial wounding of the skin in darker individuals such as microdermabrasion, superficial skin peeling, and nonablative resurfacing seem to be comparatively safe. However, significantly deeper treatments such as medical skin rolling and fractional resurfacing also seem to offer a very good comparative safety.

LITERATURE REVIEW

Postacne scarring is a reasonably common disease and the treatment of this condition should start well before the scars are evident. One of the few epidemiological studies on the prevalence of postacne scarring suggests that the type and extent of scarring was in part correlated with the site of the acne, the previous acne severity, and its duration before adequate treatment. Facial scarring affected both sexes equally and occurred in 95% of cases. A time delay up to 3 years between acne onset and adequate treatment related to the ultimate degree of scarring.[3] As with many procedurally based topics in dermatology there are not many clinical trials either in acne scarring in general or in acne scarring in ethnic skin in particular.

There is a body of peer reviewed data written on acne scarring and a smaller amount more specifically looking at ethnic skin and

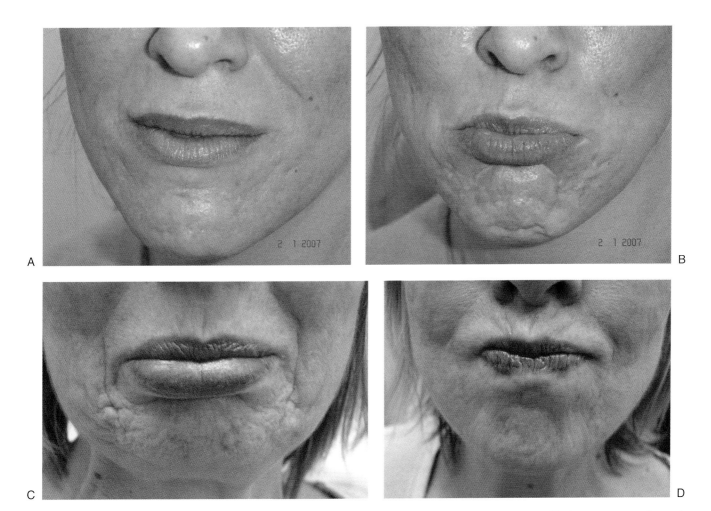

Figure 18.9 *(A) Patient at rest displaying chin scarring. (B) Same patient on animation displaying amplified appearance of scarring. (C) Another patient showing movement related dimpling and scarring. (D) Same patient attempting similar movements 2 weeks after botulinum toxin and hyaluronic acid injections*

TABLE 18.1 ■ **Reactivity of Human Skin to Solar Radiation Based on Skin Photo Types I-VI**

Skin Photo Type	Constitutive or Unexposed Skin Color Places (Buttock)	MED Range mJ/cm^2 of UVB	Reactivity or Sensitivity to UVR	Sunburn and Tanning History
I	Ivory white	15–30	Very sensitive or reactive ++++	Burns easily, strongly: never tans
II	White	25–40	Very sensitive or reactive +++/++++	Burns easily and tans minimally with difficulty
III	White	30–50	Quite reactive or sensitive +++	Burns moderately: tans moderately and uniformly
IV	Beige or lightly tanned	40–60	Moderately reactive ++	Burns minimally: tans easily and moderately
V	Moderate brown or tanned	60-90	Minimally sensitive +	Rarely burns: tans profusely (dark brown)
VI	Dark brown or black	90–150	Least sensitive − +	Never burns: tans profusely (deep brown or black)

its problems. The intersection between these two topics is less well covered, however, it probably is the quality rather than the quantity that is at issue.

Critical reviews and meta-analysis studies are generally lacking in the acne scarring literature.

No truly randomized prospective comparative studies (level A) exist. Studies tend to lack validity because of flawed design (no severity data, no emphasis on intention to treat, uncertainty reblinding observers or patients, and inadequate power).

Some articles are prospective, some retrospective but usually are descriptive case reports and case series,[4,5] descriptions of procedures without a formal study being conducted (level C evidence). Most studies on postacne scarring have been uncontrolled, unblinded, and not randomized even if prospective.

Some limited comparative studies have been described for lasers and acne scarring (level B).

• The difficulty in the evaluation of acne scarring is manifold.

There is no simple clinically reproducible method for evaluating the volume of deficiency or excess of a single acne scar or an acne scarred area.

Devices to measure specific lesion volume such as silicon profilemetry or 3D photography, confocal microscopy or cutaneous ultrasound are outside the abilities of usual practice. Some are unable to measure more than limited areas with some difficulty in reproducibility. Others are cumbersome, difficult to use, impractical, or too expensive.

Photography has often been poorly taken with respect to uniformity of the normal camera variables of using the same camera, same settings, same backdrop, same lighting, same patient angle distance, and magnification. Even if these parameters are followed, photography, which inherently is a two-dimensional tool, has trouble estimating the volume of scarring which is very much a three-dimensional issue. Turning the patient's profile ever so slightly will

completely alter the ability of the observer, no matter how blinded to determine improvement.

Often studies resort to analyze patients over time trying to estimate a percentage subjective or objective improvement. Often baseline photographs are compared subjectively or objectively or the patient asked just to estimate their percentage improvement. Often a relatively simple grading system is used such as 0% no improvement, 25% mild improvement, 50% moderate improvement, 75% excellent improvement, 100% complete eradication or similar scale. Yet, what this percentage improvement refers to is rather ill-defined (depth of scar, number of scars, change of scar type, and global cosmetic improvement). Patient satisfaction rating is another scale used and probably has been arguably as accurate and more important as any objective method utilized, yet this is open to many biases making it a less than desirable benchmark.

Long- term follow-up studies are required with many of the ablative technologies in regard to long-term efficacy and complications such as hypopigmentation but these studies are largely missing from the literature.

Adequate classifications exist for acne morphology and severity. Unfortunately, there remains no agreed classification on the morphology or severity of acne scarring.

Limited inroads have occurred over recent years on morphological description of acne scarring with various attempts at describing different scar types. However, the lack of consensus in morphological description remains a concern as it interferes with one's ability to compare articles discussing a patient's scar type and response to therapy.

Even less defined is any attempt in the literature to define the burden of disease of postacne scarring. There has been no agreed objective quantitative or qualitative scoring system of global severity to allow discussion and comparison of patients and their response to therapy (or that of a cohort) and for the purposes of further comparative studies.

Without adequate classification and measure of disease, it is hard to perceive how we may compare different patients, their response to treatments, and studies performed by different practitioners or investigating units.

Evidence for Ablative and Fractionated Resurfacing Technologies for the Treatment of Postacne Scarring in Darker Skin Patents

Laser skin resurfacing (Figures 18.3 and 18.10)

Despite the above comments, there has been an excellent systematic review of the treatment of postacne scarring by laser resurfacing.[6] In this analysis, the authors identified no controlled studies and only 16 case series, illustrating the effects of CO_2[7–19] or erbium:YAG lasers[20,21] or a combination of CO_2 and erbium lasers[22] for the treatment of postacne scarring patients. The authors could find no studies of reasonable quality. In terms of temporary morbidity, they did find that pigmentation as a side effect was common being evident, even transiently, in up to 44% of patients. The duration of pigmentary change was said to range between 1 and 6 months with CO_2 laser and 2 to 3 weeks with erbium laser. The length and erythema in the 14 studies averaged out for CO_2 laser at 6 to 16 weeks and for erbium laser 1 to 3 months. The mean improvement in scarring varied between 25% to 81% for the CO_2 laser and between 50% and 70% for the erbium:YAG laser. Measurements of improvement will usually be photographed with desparate attempts at blinding observers.

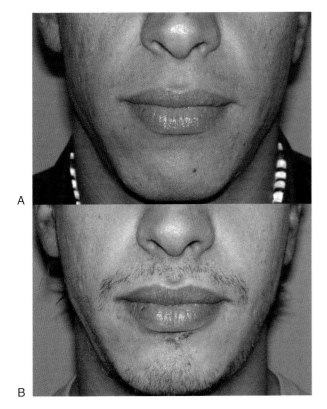

Figure 18.10 *Patient (A) before and (B) 3 weeks after CO_2 and erbium laser resurfacing showing typical delayed resurrection of pigmentation in a thin type 4 patient*

Two of these studies[13,18] and one subsequently[5] have discussed the use of ablative lasers in the skin of color.

In one of these studies[18], 36 patients skin of types 2 through 5 were resurfaced with CO_2 laser and followed for a period of 6 months. Although nine patients developed hyperpigmentation this had completely settled by the 3-month postoperative visit. Two patients developed focal erythema but no scarring developed. Although this was termed a prospective study, the improvement was graded by the patients at the 6-month follow-up visit.

Another study of 25 patients of Asian and Hispanic background included patients treated primarily for acne scarring.[13] Again, hyperpigmentation maximal at 6 weeks and present in some for 3 to 4 months appear to be the main postoperative concern. The authors stated that acne scar treatment with the lasers appeared less effective than that for rhytides and improvement appeared to average out at approximately 25%.

In a third small study[5] of 16 patients (13 of whom had acne scarring) of predominantly skin type 3 and 4, erythema was present in all the subjects but gradually faded over 6 months. Pigmentation was present at 3 months in 33%. At 6 months, one patient had residual pigmentation. Only one patient developed mild minimal hypopigmentation at 6 months, which cleared at 12 months. Another patient developed hypopigmentation at 12 months.

Dermabrasion

Although a number of authors have suggested that dermabrasion is less likely to cause pigmentary sequelae.[23,24] I could find no actual studies or case series to illustrate the effect of dermabrasion on skin of color neither prospective nor retrospective. Since it was suggested that the cold injury caused by the cryoanaesthesia was partly at issue in causing pigmentary abnormalities, a case series of sequential patients utilizing tumescent anaesthesia were presented in an attempt to limit this injury (Figure 18.11).[25] There were experimental reports of experienced physicians suggesting that morbidity associated with dermabrasion is predictable in all skin types.[26,27]

Chemical peeling

A number of case series have been presented on the use of medium and deep chemical peeling in the treatment of postacne scarring.[28,29] Again, this technique is followed by a portion of patients developing postinflammatory hyperpigmentation that seems to settle in most patients more than the first 3 months. One paper utilizing a modified phenol peel on 46 Asian patients[28] (11 of whom had acne scarring as their prime indication) suggested that this treatment was effective with seven of these patients improving by 51% or more. More than 74% of all patients developed postinflammatory hyperpigmentation. In 11% of patients postoperative erythema lasted longer than 3 months and there was also one case each of scar formation and long-term hypopigmentation.

Another paper utilizing a medium-strength trichloroacetic acid peel in 15 patients with dark skinned individuals with acne scarring showed improvement in all but one patient and moderate or marked improvement in nine of these patients.[29] Seventy-three percent suffered from transient hyperpigmentation. The authors concluded that this is a safe and effective modality in dark skin patents for the treatment of postacne scarring.

A variation of chemical peeling involving the use of 60% to 100% trichloroacetic acid[30,31] (termed the CROSS technique,

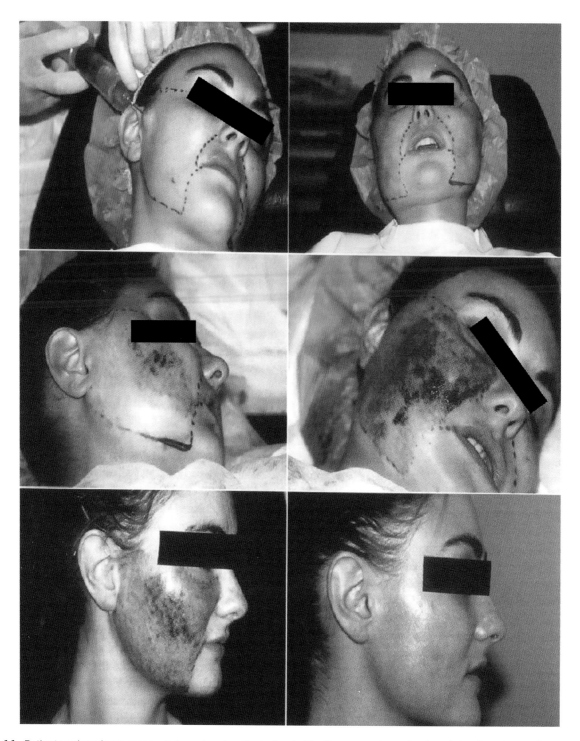

Figure 18.11 *Patient undergoing tumescent dermabrasion illustrating infiltration, procedure, day 1 and day 5 postoperative appearance*

Figure 18.12) has excited interest in the treatment of smaller "ice pick" and poral type scars which have always been difficult. Basically, this modality scars the inside of the cylindrical scar, making it cosmetically more appealing. A similar concept was discussed with the use of high-energy CO_2 laser.[32] A very well conducted study of 65 patients initially used to describe this technique[31] divided into two treatment arms of 65% and close to 100% trichloroacetic acid in dark skin individuals of Fitzpatrick skin type 4 to 6. The study showed no significant incidence of complications.

Plasma skin resurfacing

At the time of this writing, there has been no manuscript in the literature on this new method of resurfacing in regard to acne scarring or in regard to treatment of darker skin patents. This technology utilizes a plasma cloud of electrons originating from nitrogen atoms and radio frequency stimulation of these atoms and from personal experience of the author it appears to have utility in postacne scarring and may be expected to be reported in the literature in the near future. Again, anecdotally, it appears that postinflammatory hyperpigmentation in darker skin patents may again be a feature of this technology.

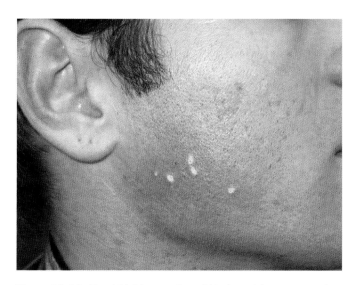

Figure 18.12 *Focal trichloroacetic acid to ice pick scars are close to 100% concentration*

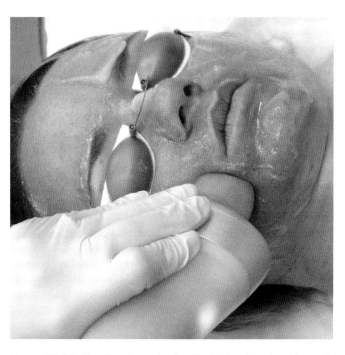

Figure 18.13 *Fractional resurfacing illustrating blue tracking optical guide*

Fractional resurfacing

A recently introduced laser technology employing the concept of "fractionated photothermolysis" produces small vertical zones of full thickness thermal damage by a midinfrared laser (Figures 18.13 and 18.14).[33] This is akin to sinking posts or drilling holes of thermal damage with areas surrounding these posts left free of damage. This is a method of ablative resurfacing without the patient having to experience a pronounced healing phase.

There have been a number of recent studies suggesting its efficacy in postacne scarring. One important recent study in Asian skin[34] showed that increased density of the small vertical zones of damage cause more swelling, redness, and hyperpigmentation as against higher fluences or energy of these zones. Patient satisfaction was seen to be higher when treated with higher fluences but not higher densities.

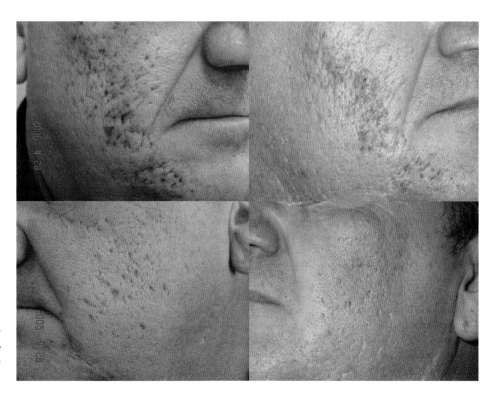

Figure 18.14 *Patient with Fitzpatrick skin type 4 showing improvement in severe ice pick and dystrophic scarring with fractional resurfacing*

An excellent prospective case series of 53 patients[35] with atrophic acne scarring using blinded observers showed 51% to 75% improvement and 90% of patients. Adverse events included no incidence of dyspigmentation or scarring. Importantly, clinical response rates were independent of age/gender photoskin type.

A number of smaller studies and case reports have also looked at acne scarring, hypopigmented, and postsurgical scarring[36–38] also suggesting satisfactory outcome although not concentrating on darker skin patients.

This technology may allow treatment for extra facial scarring which has not been accessible with other resurfacing technologies.

■ Evidence or Efficacy and Safety of Nonablative Technologies for Atrophic Acne Scarring

Manual skin needling or rolling

In a concept not dissimilar to fractionated resurfacing, manual needling or skin rolling may be used when expensive machinery is not available. In its simplest form one may employ a 30-gauge needle introduced into the skin to a controlled depth with the aid of a small artery forcep held at approximately 2 to 3-mm from the tip to stab the skin repeatedly, but this is only appropriate for small areas of scarring. For larger areas a tattoo gun without pigment may be used or a needle studded rolling pin[39] may be rolled over the face or extrafacially. The dermal trauma heals with collagen remodeling and this is responsible for any improvement in atrophic scarring (Figure 18.15). It can be readily added to other procedures such as dermal augmentation or fat transfer.

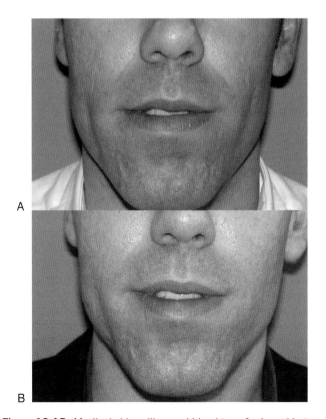

A

B

Figure 18.15 *Medical skin rolling and blood transfer in a skin type 3 patient (A) before and (B) 3 months after treatment*

Adequate studies into this technology are entirely lacking at this point in time.

Nonablative resurfacing

Nonablative lasers appear to have a role in the treatment of minor atrophic acne scarring. This topic seems to have been studied more methodically than the ablative lasers. Although still prospectively based case series dominate, there seems to be more thought put into the outcome measurements. Some true comparative studies between laser systems have been performed[40] and different conditions utilizing the same laser system also being compared.[41,42] The major lasers for this purpose have been the midinfrared lasers at wavelengths of 1320 nm, 1450 nm, and 1540 nm appropriately cooled to protect the epidermis while targeting dermal water.[40–45] These lasers used, conducted heat from the chromophore to produce a diffuse dermal injury heating to above 50°C inducing collagen remodeling. Repeated treatments are required and longevity of result is still largely unknown.

This technology seems safe when it has been studied in Asian skin[41,45] although postinflammatory hyperpigmentation can be seen if blistering occurs. There appears to have a reasonable level of patient satisfaction and perception of efficacy[42] but objectively and on histology there may be somewhat less efficacy.[41]

■ Evidence for Augmentation and Similar Procedures in Atrophic Postacne Scarring

Autologous blood transfer

Among autologous agents, blood transfer is a possible option for patients with milder atrophic acne scarring. It relies on stimulation of the implanted chromophore (autologous blood) by relatively low-level vascular laser or intense pulsed light (IPL). Blood is injected immediately after drawing by simple injection with a 1-mL syringe with attached 30-gauge needle high up in the dermis distending the scar giving a bleb with a bruised appearance. This bruise is then targeted as any blood vessel would be, but with approximately 50% to 75% of the usual fluence. A single case series suggested that treatment may be repeated at monthly intervals until adequate correction is attained.[46] It is most often performed in combination with other procedures such as fat transfer and subcision in the deeper scars (Figure 18.16).

Fat transfer

For grossly atrophic disease with destruction of the deeper tissues, fat remains the optimal replacement agent (Figures 18.3 and 18.16). Fat is an excellent deeper augmentation material. It is cheap, readily available, and will neither be rejected nor suffer allergic reactions. It is easy to work with and is without risk of communicable disease. The issue of permanence has gradually been resolved[47] and it is just as effective and safe in any ethnicity. However, despite some anecdotal reports of its efficacy,[48,49] at this time there are no adequate studies to illustrate its efficacy in postacne scarring.

Subcision

Subcision of scars appears to work by breaking up the attachments of atrophic acne scars, releasing the surface from the deeper structures. Successive treatments appear to produce further improvement.[50,51] The technique usually involves the insertion of a sharp

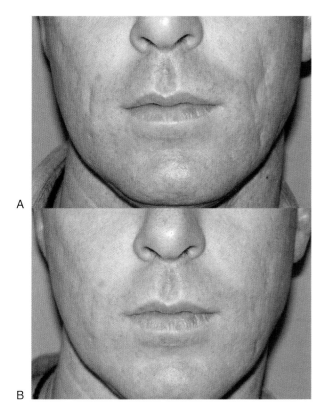

A

B

Figure 18.16 *Patient (A) before and (B) 3 weeks after combined treatment with blood transfer, fat transfer, and subcision*

hypodermic needle. The depth of the probe insertion depends on the type of scar being treated with intradermal insertion for small superficial scars while deeper dermal undermining is performed for more severely bound down scars. It has become a first-line

treatment for many isolated moderate bound down atrophic scars. This is despite a lack of controlled studies although, one interesting split face designed study utilizing subcision on one side alone, compared to a nonablative laser combined with subcision on the other side was used to show the relative efficacy of the combined side[52] suggesting a synergistic effect between these two modalities.

Dermal grafting

Dermal grafting may be used for recent deep focal or linear scars.[53–55] Despite some case series, there have been no controlled studies or comparative studies. This technique is somewhat limited by cyst formation and the requirement for a donor site to be prepared by either dermabrasion or laser skin resurfacing and the dermis harvested.

Punch techniques

Punch techniques such as punch excision,[56] grafting[57] and elevation, or float techniques[58] have been useful and probably remain the gold standard for punched out scars probably up to 3 to 4 mm in width (deep "box car" and larger "ice pick" scars). These techniques are all old ones and have not been studied with any scientific rigor (Figure 18.17).

Nonautologous tissue augmentation

For patients with few atrophic scars, there is now quite an array of injectable fillers including human collagen and hyaluronic acid among the short-term agents and many agents of a longer term nature with the reintroduction of silicon and variations of polyacrylamides for longer correction. However, there are no controlled trials in acne scarring, neither in the general population nor in darker skinned patients. A very elegant prospective double-blinded randomized placebo-controlled study of 145 evaluated patients treated with autologous cultured fibroblasts in a phase 3 clinical

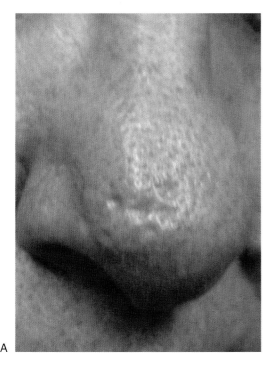

A

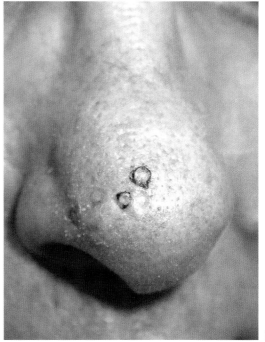

B

Figure 18.17 *Patient (A) before and (B) 1 week after punch float technique to the nose*

trial showed particularly good results in the 50 patients treated for acne scarring. The response rate at 6 months was 48.4% compared to 7.7% for placebo.[59] Unfortunately, it would appear that this product is no longer available.

■ Evidence for Cytotoxic and Vascular Laser Therapy in the Treatment of Hypertrophic Postacne Scarring

Cytotoxics

Traditionally, high-strength corticosteroids have been used for the intralesional drugs of choice in the treatment of hypertrophic and keloidal acne scars. However, there has been recent interest in the intralesional use of the cytotoxics fluorouracil[60–62] and bleomycin[63,64] and mitomycin[65,66] as treatments of hypertrophic and keloidal scars. Fluorouracil is usually utilized at a concentration of 50 mg/mL and has been mixed 80:20 with low-strength intralesional steroid (Figure 18.18). However, it may be used alone.[67] Usually, approximately 1 mL is utilized in each session and often 0.1 to 0.3 mL is all that is required for an individual scar. Recently, the molecular basis of the action of Fluorouracil (5-FU) has been elucidated.[68] 5-FU appears to be a potent inhibitor of TGF-beta/SMAD signaling, capable of blocking TGF-beta-induced, SMAD-driven up regulation of COL1A2 gene expression in a JNK-dependent manner.

Vascular lasers

In 1995, it was reported that Flashlamp-pumped pulsed dye tunable laser was useful in the treatment of keloid sternotomy scars with improvement in scar height, skin texture, erythema, and pruritus in the laser treated scars.[69] This initial work has been borne out by more recent studies.[70,71]

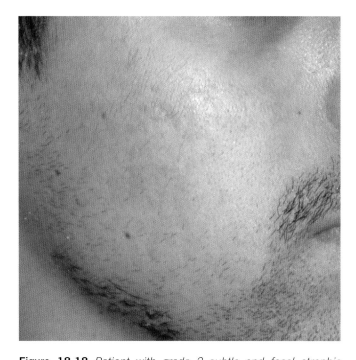

Figure 18.18 *Patient with grade 2 subtle and focal atrophic postacne scarring on the midright cheek*

CLINICAL EXAMINATION AND PATIENT HISTORY

Table 18.2 summarizes the important points that must be gleaned from the patient's history and examination before proceeding with the planning of the patient's therapy.

■ Preoperative Patient Education

The patient should be educated as to what type of scars they have and what types of treatment are available for that particular scar type. There will usually be a number of different possibilities that need to be explained to the patient along with their potential adverse effects and complications. The use of computer aids such as PowerPoint or similar presentations with embedded videos is an extremely useful educational tool for discussing different alternatives for treating their condition.

Printed information should also be supplied on any discussed techniques, including the possible risks of these procedures and a further appointment made to discuss any further queries. It should also be remembered that if the physician's and patient's first language is not the same, then reasonable efforts must be made by inclusion of family members or interpreters or printed information in the patient's language.

Often there will be a number of different techniques that will be combined to treat the particular condition at hand and the timing of these procedures need also to be spelt out to the patient.

Possible risks and likely benefits both need to be addressed for every procedure discussed.

In particular, acne scarring is not a condition that usually improves rapidly after therapy (aside from excision and augmentation procedures) and often is an incremental improvement over time with a number of procedures being required especially when alterations in collagen are being required.

The patient must be assessed from both the psychological and physical points of view and should be guided to accept a realistic outcome from the available treatments.

The patient needs to be assessed according to the types of scars as well as their severity and their extent.

■ Contraindications

The patient should be one who has an appropriate awareness of their disease severity and their likely outcome. A lack of such awareness would be considered a contraindication to ongoing therapy.

■ Particular Advice and Procedures for the Darker Skin Patient

The particular problems of darker skin patient undergoing treatment for postacne scarring really revolve about the probability of prolonged erythema, pigmentary change, and a higher risk of hypertrophic scarring. The patient needs to be made aware of this and to take these risks on board and to prepare themselves for a prolonged postoperative recovery. There are procedures which carry no further risk independent of photoreactive skin type such as dermal and subcutaneous, autologous and nonautologous fillers,

TABLE 18.2 ■ Patient History and Examination Details

Parameter	What Needs to Be Done
Activity of associated acne	Treat acne before beginning treatment for scarring
Patient Fitzpatrick skin type	In skin types 3 to 5, one should be concerned about postinflammatory hyperpigmentation. In skin type 6 (black skin) there is usually only a short-term issue with pigment which seems to be normalized faster than in the less pigmented olive skin types. Certain procedures with better safety margins in darker skin patients are usually chosen
Gender	Males do not wear make-up readily. Females do not have beard to hide demarcation lines
Age	Be concerned about treating the very young (maturity) and the very old (concomitant illness, motivation)
Psychological and physical health	Make sure it is appropriate to proceed with suggested course of action Ensure adequate understanding of the limitations of the procedure
Social constraints	Ensure adequate care is available in the postoperative period and the patient is able to report for follow-up appointments. Payment needs to be discussed especially if there is to be a long process involved or expensive equipment used
Burden of disease	The treatment required will vary according to how much disease load is present. Severe scarring may require a number of procedures and even hospitalization while with milder disease this is less likely. However, milder disease patterns by no means is assured to reach patient expectations and may still need multiple if less morbid procedures
Type of scarring	Certain types of scarring (e.g., ice pick, gross atrophy, erythematous macular marks to raise a few) may need their own specific treatments
Site of scarring	Certain sites of scarring (neck, chest, and back) carry more risk of issues such as pigmentation and hypertrophic scarring.

and subcision. There are also some procedures that carry minimally more risk such as light skin peels, microdermabrasion, skin rolling, and fractional resurfacing. However, the one that need special explanation are any of the technique-dependant resurfacing procedures such as dermabrasion, laser skin resurfacing, and medium and deep chemical peeling.

GENERAL TREATMENT APPROACH

When seeing a patient for the first time with postacne scarring, it is most useful to determine both the severity of their disease (see Table 18.3) and the type of scarring present (see Table 18.4A, B, C, and B).

A PROCEDURAL GUIDE FOR THE PERPLEXED

There is a continuing battle between the safety of the patient and efficacy of the procedure in many cases of postacne scarring. There are no methods of totally removing acne scarring, hence everything is a compromise. Hence, it behooves the physician to do a number of things when addressing the problem of postacne scarring (in conjunction with Table 18.2).

Manufacture for the patient a set of realistic expectations. It is vital that the patient realizes the impossibility of complete removal of the scars.

Listen to the patient. Try to understand the relative importance of a temporary but useful and may be very accurate result produced by such agents as a temporary filler as against procedures such as

TABLE 18.3 ■ Graded Severity or Burden of Disease of Postacne Scarring

Grade	Characteristics
1: Macular disease	Erythematous, hyper- or hypopigmented flat marks visible to patient or observer at any distance.
2: Mild disease	Mild atrophy or hypertrophy that may not be obvious at social distances of 50 cm or greater and may be covered adequately by make-up or the normal shadow of shaved beard hair in males or normal body hair if extrafacial
3: Moderate disease	Moderate atrophic or hypertrophic scarring that is obvious at social distances of 50 cm or greater and is not covered easily by make-up or the normal shadow of shaved beard hair in males or body hair if extrafacial, but is still able to be flattened by manual stretching of the skin (if atrophic)
4: Severe disease	Severe atrophic or hypertrophic scarring that is obvious at social distances greater than 50 cm and is not covered easily by make-up or the normal shadow of shaved beard hair in males or body hair, if extrafacial and is not able to be flattened by manual stretching of the skin

TABLE 18.4A ■ **Grade 1 Abnormally Colored, Macular Disease**

Definition	Examples of Scars	Treatment Plan
Erythematous, hyper- or hypopigmented flat marks visible to patient or observer at any distance.	Erythematous flat marks (Figure 18.5)	***Time and optimized home skin care (retinoids, topical anti-inflammatories), often supplemented by vascular lasers
	Hyperpigmented flat marks (postinflammatory marks) (Figure 18.4)	***Optimized home care (bleaching, sun protection, etc.) and light strength peels +/− microdermabrasion supplemented by **pigment lesion lasers or IPL, only if required
	Hypopigmented macular scars (Figures 18.6 and 18.7)	***Pigment transfer procedures (blister grafting, autologous cell transfer) maybe fractional resurfacing

**Acceptable treatment modalities in olive and dark skinned patients.
***Safe treatment modalities in olive and dark skinned patients.

TABLE 18.4B ■ **Grade 2 Mildly Abnormally Contoured Disease**

Definition	Examples of Scars	Treatment Plan
Mild atrophy or hypertrophy that may not be obvious at social distances of` 50 cm or greater and may be covered adequately by make-up or the normal shadow of shaved beard hair in males or normal body hair if extrafacia	Mild rolling atrophic scars (Figures 18.18 and 18.19)	If localized: ***Consider combination of blood transfer, skin needling or rolling or microdermabrasion, and/or superficial dermal fillers
		If generalized: ***Multiple treatments of nonablative lasers, fractional resurfacing often complimented by the localized treatment modalities either simultaneous or as follow-up treatments
	Small soft papular (Figure 18.20)	**Fine wire diathermy (FWD). May be fluorouracil injections if FWD unsuccessful

**Acceptable treatment modalities in olive and dark-skinned patients.
***Safe treatment modalities in olive and dark-skinned patients.

TABLE 18.4C ■ **Grade 3 Moderately Abnormally Contoured Disease**

Grade 3	Examples of Scars	Treatment Plan
Moderate atrophic or hypertrophic scarring that is obvious at social distances of 50 cm or greater and is not covered easily by make-up or the normal shadow of shaved beard hair in males or body hair if extrafacial, but is still able to be flattened by manual stretching of the skin (if atrophic)	More significant rolling, shallow "box car" (Figures 18.21 and 18.22)	If generalized: ***Medical skin rolling or fractionated resurfacing; **If unavailable consider ablative lasers or dermabrasion or *plasma skin resurfacing
		If localized: ***Dermal fillers or subcision
	Mild-to-moderate hypertrophic or papular scars (Figure 18.23)	***Intralesional corticosteroids and/or fluorouracil and/or vascular laser. Combine with silicon sheeting

*Relatively less safe treatment modalities.
**Acceptable treatment modalities in olive and dark-skinned patients.
***Safe treatment modalities in olive and dark-skinned patients.

TABLE 18.4D ▪ Grade 4 Severely Abnormally Contoured Disease

Definition	Examples of Scars	Treatment Plan
Severe atrophic or hypertrophic scarring that is obvious at social distances greater than 50 cm and is not covered easily by make-up or the normal shadow of shaved beard hair in males or body hair if extrafacial, and is not able to be flattened by manual stretching of the skin	Punched out atrophic (deep "box car"), "ice pick" (Figures 18.12, 18.14, and 18.17)	***If very numerous, deep, and small consider focal trichloroacetic acid (CROSS technique) maybe combined with fractional resurfacing ***If fewer and broader but still < 4 mm in diameter consider punch techniques (float, excision grafting), with or without subsequent fractional or **ablative resurfacing techniques
	Bridges and tunnels, dystrophic scars (Figure 18.1A, B, C,and D)	*Excision
	Marked atrophy (Figures 18.3, 18.24, and 18.25)	***Fat transfer, *stimulatory fillers such as PLA, hydroxyapatite, silicon (if fat not feasible), occasionally rhytidectomy, if acquired cutis laxa
	Significant hypertrophy or keloid (Figure 18.26)	***Intralesional corticosteroids steroids or fluorouracil and/or vascular laser

*Relatively less safe treatment modalities.
**Acceptable treatment modalities in olive and dark-skinned patients.
***Safe treatment modalities in olive and dark-skinned patients.

excision or punch techniques which may be less accurate but more permanent. Understand the limitations of the patient's budget, intellect, social circumstances, work requirements (including the ability to stay out of the sun during any required healing phase), and capacity for accepting complications if they were to occur. Even predictable morbidity can be difficult for a patient who is not anticipating this and often despite information both written and ver-

bal patients often underestimate the postoperative phase of even relatively mild procedures.

Educate the patient about the nature of acne scarring, the apparent "memory" that the skin as to the position, and severity of scarring and its seeming reluctance to alter with therapy. This is most apparent with techniques that rely upon "collagen remodeling." As a group, this includes almost all active skincare, space

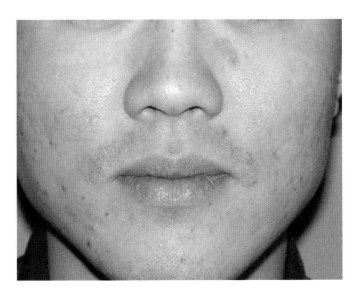

Figure 18.19 *Patient with rate to generalized mildly atrophic post acne scarring*

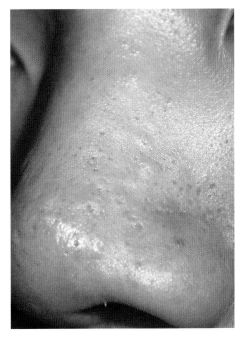

Figure 18.20 *Patient with mild papular nasal acne scars*

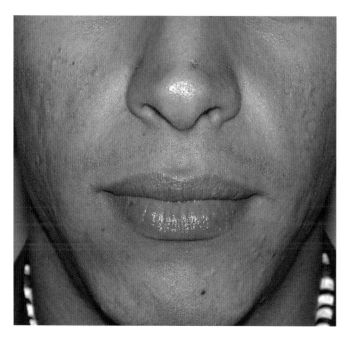

Figure 18.21 *Fitzpatrick skin type 4 patient with grade 3 moderate atrophic acne scarring*

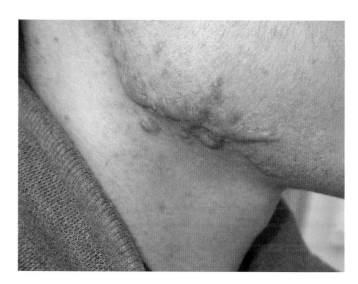

Figure 18.23 *Patient with grade 3 moderate to severe right jaw line hypertrophic scar*

surface treatments such as microdermabrasion and light skin peels as well as nonablative and ablative resurfacing techniques. Incomplete results and the requirement for multiple treatments and ongoing therapies categorize this group of techniques and processes.

Some patients will desire a single therapeutic intervention and often this is unachievable in a condition such as acne scarring. Instead, the patient should be educated to accept a number of therapeutic interventions to achieve optimal results. A carefully mapped out plan of action is required in most patients with an understanding that a "one size fits all" model is not satisfactory for most cases. This requirement increases with the complexity of the scar types and the disease burden of the patient.

Particularly relevant for this chapter, the most efficacious procedure may not be practical or may be too likely to produce unsatisfactory complications or excess morbidity. This may have to be passed over in favor of a less effective treatment if the patient skin type is inappropriate for a more aggressive one.

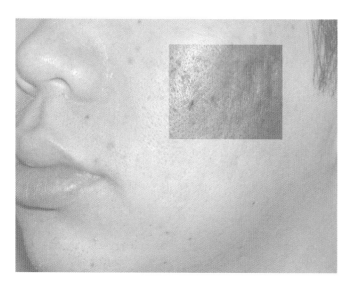

Figure 18.22 *Patient with focal (outlined) grade 3 moderate atrophic acne scarring*

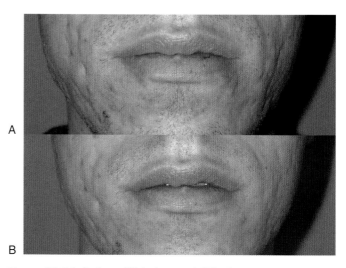

Figure 18.24 *Patient (A) before and (B) after two treatments of polylactic acid injections*

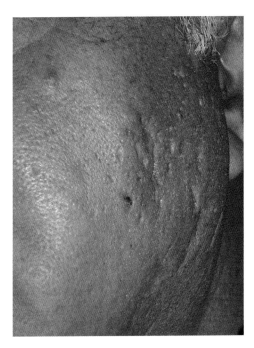

Figure 18.25 *Fitzpatrick skin type 5 patient with grade 4 punched out atrophic postacne scars*

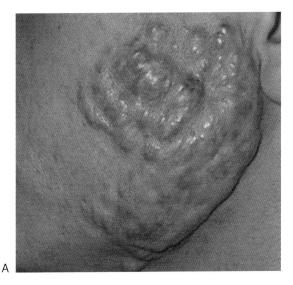

A

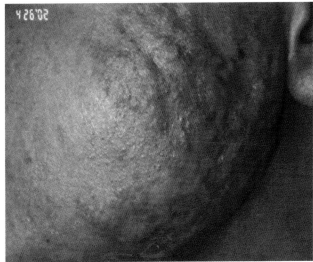

B

Figure 18.26 *Patient with very severe keloidal postacne scarring on the left jaw line (A) before (B) and after multiple fluorouracil treatments*

It is also important for the physician to realize his own or her own limitations. If the patient's condition requires expertise in an operation that is outside the physician's capability or requires equipment that the physician does not have, then referral should occur to a more appropriate clinic.

In Table 18.5A and B, look at the comparisons of different techniques according to practical parameters of cost, longevity, efficacy, and safety which the patient should appreciate before embarking on the journey of treatment.

▨ Tabulated Treatment Plans

The first rule, I feel, is to give patients hope that their condition can be improved, but not false hope that their scars can be completely abolished. Patients require a treatment plan together with an understanding of their condition will take time and patience and possibly multiple therapies to settle.

DIRECTIONS FOR THE FUTURE AND CONCLUSIONS

The treatment of acne scarring is evolving and doing so in a way that is comforting to both the patient and the practitioner. It is

TABLE 18.5A ▪ **Methods of Scar Improvement not Relying on Collagen Remodeling—Excisional and Filler Technologies**

Method of Scar Improvement	Temporary Dermal Augmentation	Fat Transfer	Semipermanent/ Permanent Filler	Excision of Scar Including Punch Techniques
Morbidity	+	+	+	+ +
Longevity result	+	+ + +	+ +/+ + +	+ + +
Relative cost	+ +	+ +	+ +/+ + +	+
Efficacy	+ + +	+ + +	+ + +	+ + +
General safety	+ + +	+ + +	+	+ +
Safety for darker skin	+ + +	+ + +	+	+ +

TABLE 18.5B ■ **Scar Revision Techniques Reliant on Resurfacing or Similar Technologies of Collagen Remodeling**

Method of Scar Improvement	Dermabrasion	Deep and Medium Chemical Peeling	Laser Skin Resurfacing	Fractionated Resurfacing
Morbidity	+++	+++	+++	+
Longevity result	+++	++/+++	++/+++	+++
Relative cost		++	++/+++	+++
Efficacy	++	++	++	+++
General safety	++	+/++	++	+++
Safety for darker skin	+	+	+	?+++

becoming safer for all ethnicities. As useful as they have been, ablative technologies are on the wane as a result of a relative intolerance to the twin evils of downtime and adverse events. For a short while, attempts to replace these technologies resulted in treatments best described as similar to the nursery story "the emperor has no clothes" with results that may have obeyed Hippocrates first rule but gave no meaningful improvement to the patient. The advent of first manual skin rolling, focal TCA peeling, and then fractional resurfacing have been major advances but one should not forget very useful techniques from the past such as punch techniques, excisional surgery, and subcision.

Pendulums swing and mildly ablative resurfacing is making a comeback in the form of plasma skin resurfacing and mid-range erbium laser resurfacing. These ablative technologies are trying to occupy the halfway house between downtime and complications on one hand and efficacy on the other. They offer more rapid healing and more limited morbidity and may have a place in the future.

Fractional resurfacing without doubt seems to be the most useful new technology and new fractional wavelengths will be added over the coming years. We will probably see a convergence between these technologies pushing the boundaries of patient tolerance and efficacy. It has also added an ability to treat unusual forms of scarring gleaned from the experience of treating postacne scarring (Figure 18.27).

Dermal augmentation and our understanding of what can be achieved with it is now increasing exponentially and one could envisage safer, longer term, and elegant materials to work with in the future for the correction of focal atrophic acne scarring disease.

The treatment of hyperplastic postacne scarring continues to be disappointing and we await an improved understanding of its pathogenesis. However, some improvements have been made in this treatment such as new cytotoxic therapies but we still have a long way to go.

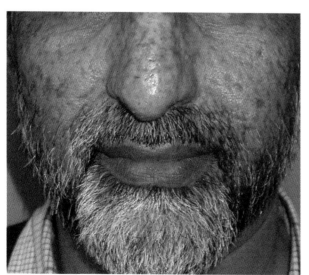
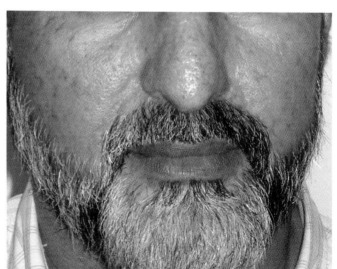

A B

Figure 18.27 *Patient with small pox scarring (A) before and (B) after laser skin resurfacing and multiple fractional resurfacings*

The future always looks brighter than the past and this is certainly true when one looks at this hitherto very difficult disease of postacne scarring and especially its treatment in skin of color.

REFERENCES

1. Fitzpatrick TB. The validity and practicality of sun-reactive skin types I through VI. *Arch Dermatol.* 1988;124:869-871.

2. Grimes PE, Hunt SG. Considerations for cosmetic surgery in the black population. *Clin Plast Surg.* 1993;20:27-34.

3. Layton AM, Henderson CA, Cunliffe WJ. A clinical evaluation of acne scarring and its incidence. *Clin Exp Dermatol.* 1994; 19:303-308.

4. Chua SH, Ang P, Khoo LS, Goh CL. Nonablative 1450-nm diode laser in the treatment of facial atrophic acne scars in type IV to V Asian skin: a prospective clinical study. *Dermatol Surg.* 2004;30:1287-1291.

5. Goh CL, Khoo L. Laser skin resurfacing treatment outcome of facial scars and wrinkles in Asians with skin type III/IV with the unipulse CO_2 laser system. *Singapore Med J.* 2002;43(1): 28-32.

6. Jordan R, Cummins C, Burls A. Laser resurfacing of the skin for the improvement of facial acne scarring: a systematic review of the evidence. *Br J Dermatol.* 2000;142:413-423.

7. Bernstein LJ, Kauvar AN, Grossman MC, Geronemus RG. The short- and long-term side effects of carbon dioxide laser resurfacing. *Dermatol Surg.* 1997;23:519-525.

8. Alster TS, West TB. Resurfacing of atrophic facial acne scars with a high-energy pulsed carbon dioxide laser. *Dermatol Surg.* 1996; 22:151-154.

9. Apfelberg DB. Ultrapulse carbon dioxide laser with CPG scanner for full-face resurfacing for rhytids, photoaging, and acne scars. *Plast Reconstr Surg.* 1997;99:1817-1825.

10. Apfelberg DB. A critical appraisal of high-energy pulsed carbon dioxide laser facial resurfacing for acne scars. *Ann Plast Surg.* 1997;38:95-100.

11. Apfelberg DB. The ultrapulse carbon dioxide laser with computer pattern generator automatic scanner for facial cosmetic surgery and resurfacing. *Ann Plast Surg.* 1996;36: 522-529.

12. Bernstein LJ, Kauvar AN, Grossman MC, Geronemus RG. Scar resurfacing with high-energy, short-pulsed and flash-scanning carbon dioxide lasers. *Dermatol Surg.* 1998;24:101.

13. Ho C, Nguyen Q, Lowe NJ, et al. Laser resurfacing in pigmented skin. *Dermatol Surg.* 1995;21:1035-1037.

14. Rubach BW, Schoenrock LD. Histological and clinical evaluation of facial resurfacing using a carbon dioxide laser with the computer pattern generator. *Arch Otolaryngol Head Neck Surg.* 1997;123:929-934.

15. Shim E, West TB, Velazquez E, et al. Short-pulse carbon dioxide laser resurfacing in the treatment of rhytides and scars: a clinical and histopathological study. *Dermatol Surg.* 1998;24: 113-117.

16. David LM, Sarne AJ, Unger WP. Rapid laser scanning for facial resurfacing. *Dermatol Surg.* 1995;21:1031-1033.

17. Garrett AB, Dufresne RGJ, Ratz JL, Berlin AJ. Carbon dioxide laser treatment of pitted acne scarring. *J Dermatol Surg Oncol.* 1990;16:737-740.

18. Ruiz-Esparza J, Barba GJ, Gomez de la Torre OL, et al. Ultrapulse laser skin resurfacing in Hispanic patients. A prospective study of 36 individuals. *Dermatol Surg.* 1998;24: 59-62.

19. Ting JC. Carbon dioxide laser treatment of facial scars. In: ISCLS Abstracts. American Society for Dermatologic Surgery. 1998, 118 (Abstr.).

20. Kye YC. Resurfacing of pitted facial scars with a pulsed Er:YAG laser. *Dermatol Surg.* 1997;23:880-883.

21. Drnovsek-Olup B, Vedlin B. Use of Er:YAG laser for benign skin disorders. *Lasers Surg Med.* 1997;21:13-19.

22. Weinstein C. Computerized scanning erbium:YAG laser for skin resurfacing. *Dermatol Surg.* 1998;24:83-89.

23. Jackson BA. Lasers in ethnic skin: a review. *J Am Acad Dermatol.* 2003;48(Suppl 6):S134-S138.

24. Harmon CB, Mandy SH. Dermabrasion. In: Nouri, K, Leal-Khouri, eds. *Techniques in Dermatologic Surgery.* New York, NY: Mosby; 2003.

25. Goodman GJ. Dermabrasion Using Tumescent Anaesthesia. *J. Dermatol Surg Oncol.* 1994;20:802-807.

26. Pierce HE. Cosmetic surgery of black skin. *Derm Clin.* 1988;6: 377-385.

27. Yarborough JM. Dermabrasive surgery: state of the art. *Clin Dematol.* 1987;4:75-80.

28. Park JH, Choi YD, Kim SW, Kim YC, Park SW. Effectiveness of modified phenol peel (exoderm) on facial wrinkles, acne scars, and other skin problems of Asian patients. *J Dermatol.* 2007;34:17-24.

29. Al-Waiz MM, Al-Sharqi AI. Medium-depth chemical peels in the treatment of acne scars in dark-skinned individuals. *Dermatol Surg.* 2002;28:383-387.

30. Yug A, Lane JE, Howard MS, Kent DE. Histologic study of depressed acne scars treated with serial high-concentration (95%) trichloroacetic acid. *Dermatol Surg.* 2006;32:985-990.

31. Lee JB, Chung WG, Kwahck H, Lee KH. Focal treatment of acne scars with trichloroacetic acid: chemical reconstruction of skin scars method. *Dermatol Surg.* 2002;28:1017-1021.

32. Koo SH, Yoon ES, Ahn DS, Park SH. Laser punch-out for acne scars. *Aesthetic Plast Surg.* 2001;25:46-51.

33. Manstein D, Herron GS, Sink RK, Tanner H, Anderson RR. Fractional photothermolysis: a new concept for cutaneous remodeling using microscopic patterns of thermal injury. *Lasers Surg Med.* 2004;34:426-438.

34. Kono T, Chan HH, Groff WF, et al. Prospective direct comparison study of fractional resurfacing using different fluences and densities for skin rejuvenation in Asians. *Lasers Surg Med.* 2007;39:311-314.

35. Alster TS, Tanzi EL, Lazarus M. The use of fractional laser photothermolysis for the treatment of atrophic scars. *Dermatol Surg.* 2007;33:295-299.

36. Hasegawa T, Matsukura T, Mizuno Y, Suga Y, Ogawa H, Ikeda S. Clinical trial of a laser device called fractional photo-thermolysis system for acne scars. *J Dermatol.* 2006;33:623-627.

37. Glaich AS, Rahman Z, Goldberg LH, Friedman PM. Fractional resurfacing for the treatment of hypopigmented scars: a pilot study. *Dermatol Surg.* 2007;33:289-294.

38. Behroozan DS, Goldberg LH, Dai T, Geronemus RG, Friedman PM. Fractional photothermolysis for the treatment of surgical scars: a case report. *J Cosmet Laser Ther.* 2006;8:35-38.

39. Fernandes D. Skin needling as an alternative to laser. Delivered paper IPRAS, San Francisco, CA, 1999.

40. Tanzi EL, Alster TS. Comparison of a 1450-nm diode laser and a 1320-nm Nd:YAG laser in the treatment of atrophic facial scars: a prospective clinical and histologic study. *Dermatol Surg.* 2004;30(2 Pt 1):152-157.

41. Chan HH, Lam LK, Wong DS, Kono T, Trendell-Smith N. Use of 1320-nm Nd:YAG laser for wrinkle reduction and the treatment of atrophic acne scarring in Asians. *Lasers Surg Med.* 2004;34:98-103.

42. Bhatia AC, Dover JS, Arndt KA, Stewart B, Alam M. Patient satisfaction and reported long-term therapeutic efficacy associated with 1320-nm Nd:YAG laser treatment of acne scarring and photoaging. *Dermatol Surg.* 2006;32:346-352.

43. Kim KH, Geronemus RG. Nonablative laser and light therapies for skin rejuvenation. *Arch Facial Plast Surg.* 2004;6:398-409.

44. Sadick NS, Schecter AK. A preliminary study of utilization of the 1320-nm Nd:YAG laser for the treatment of acne scarring. *Dermatol Surg.* 2004;30:995-1000.

45. Chua SH, Ang P, Khoo LS, Goh CL. Nonablative 1450-nm diode laser in the treatment of facial atrophic acne scars in type IV to V Asian skin: a prospective clinical study. *Dermatol Surg.* 2004;30:1287-1291.

46. Goodman GJ. Blood transfer: the use of autologous blood as a chromophore and tissue augmentation agent. *Dermatol Surg.* 2001;27:857-862.

47. Coleman SR. Long-term survival of fat transplants: controlled demonstrations. *Aesth Plast Surg.* 1995;19:421-425.

48. Goodman G. Post acne scarring: a review. *J Cosmet Laser Ther.* 2003;5:77-95.

49. Goodman GJ. Autologous fat transfer and dermal grafting for the correction of facial scars. In: Harahap M, ed. *Surgical Techniques for Cutaneous Scar Revision.* New York, NY: Marcel Dekker; 2000:311-349.

50. Orentreich DS. Subcutaneous incisionless (subcision) surgery for the correction of depressed scars and wrinkles. *Derm Surg.* 1995;21:543-549.

51. Branson DF. Dermal undermining (scarification) of active rhytids and scars: enhancing the results of CO_2 laser skin resurfacing. *Aesthetic Surg.* 1998;18:36-37.

52. Fulchiero GJ, Parham-Vetter PC, Obagi S. Subcision and 1320-nm Nd:YAG nonablative laser resurfacing for the treatment of acne scars: a simultaneous split-face single patient trial. *Dermatol Surg.* 2004;30:1356-1359.

53. Swinehart JM. Pocket grafting with dermal grafts: autologous collagen implants for permanent correction of cutaneous depressions. *Am J Cosmet Surg.* 1995;12(4):321-331.

54. Abergel RP, Schlaak CM, Garcia LD, et al. The laser dermal implant: a new technique for preparation and implantation of autologous dermal grafts for the correction of depressed scars, lip augmentation, and Nasolabial folds using silk touch laser technology. *Am J Cosmet Surg* 1996;13(1):15-18.

55. Goodman GJ. Laser assisted dermal grafting for the correction of cutaneous contour defects. *Derm Surg.* 1997;23(2):95-99.

56. Grevelink JM, White VR. Concurrent use of laser skin resurfacing and punch excision in the treatment of facial acne scarring. *Dermatol Surg.* 1998;24:527-530.

57. Johnson W. Treatment of pitted scars. Punch transplant technique. *J Dermatol Surg Oncol.* 1986;12:260.

58. Orentreich N, Durr NP. Rehabilitation of acne scarring. *Dermatol Clinics.* 1983;1:405-413.

59. Weiss RA, Weiss MA, Beasley KL, Munavalli G. Autologous cultured fibroblast injection for facial contour deformities: a Prospective, Placebo-controlled, Phase III Clinical Trial. *Derm Surg.* 2007;33:263-268.

60. Fitzpatrick RE. Treatment of inflamed hypertrophic scars using intralesional 5-FU. *Dermatol Surg.* 1999;25:224-232.

61. Lebwohl M. From the literature: intralesional 5-FU in the treatment of hypertrophic scars and keloids: cinical experience. *J Am Acad Dermatol.* 2000;42:677.

62. Uppal RS, Khan U, Kakar S, Talas G, Chapman P, McGrouther AD. The effects of a single dose of 5-fluorouracil on keloid scars: a clinical trial of timed wound irrigation after extralesional excision. *Plast Reconstr Surg.* 2001;108:1218-1224.

63. Bodokh I, Brun P. Treatment of keloid with intralesional bleomycin. *Ann Dermatol Venereol.* 1996;123(12):791-794.

64. Espana A, Solano T, Quintanilla E. Bleomycin in the treatment of keloids and hypertrophic scars by multiple needle punctures. *Dermatol Surg.* 2001;27:23-27.

65. Bailey JN, Waite AE, Clayton WJ, Rustin MH. Application of topical mitomycin C to the base of shave-removed keloid scars to prevent their recurrence. *Br J Dermatol.* 2007;156:682-686.

66. Stewart CE, Kim JY. Application of mitomycin-C for head and neck keloids. *Otolaryngol Head Neck Surg.* 2006;135:946-950.

67. Gupta S, Kalra A. Efficacy and safety of intralesional 5-fluorouracil in the treatment of keloids. *Dermatology.* 2002;204:130-132.

68. Wendling J, Marchand A, Mauviel A, Verrecchia F. 5-Fluorouracil blocks transforming growth factor-beta-induced alpha 2 type I

collagen gene (COL1A2) expression in human fibroblasts via c-Jun NH$_2$-terminal kinase/activator protein-1 activation. *Mol Pharmacol*. 2003;64:707-713.

69. Alster TS, Williams CM. Treatment of keloid sternotomy scars with 585-nm flashlamp-pumped pulsed-dye laser. *Lancet*. 1995;345(8959):1198-2000.

70. Manuskiatti W, Fitzpatrick RE. Treatment response of keloidal and hypertrophic sternotomy scars: comparison among intralesional corticosteroid, 5-fluorouracil, and 585-nm flashlamp-pumped pulsed-dye laser treatments. *Arch Dermatol*. 2002;138:1149-1155.

71. Manuskiatti W, Fitzpatrick RE, Goldman MP. Energy density and numbers of treatment affect response of keloidal and hypertrophic sternotomy scars to the 585-nm flashlamp-pumped pulsed-dye laser. *J Am Acad Dermatol*. 2001;45: 557-565.

CHAPTER 19

Treatment of Keloids and Hypertrophic Scars in Ethnic Skin

**Voraphol Vejjabhinanta, MD, Keyvan Nouri, MD, FAAD,
and Asha R. Patel, BS**

INTRODUCTION, ETIOLOGY, AND DEFINITIONS

The integument system, also known as the human skin, is a vast organ of protection. It is the barrier that provides bodily defense between the internal and external environment. The skin's chief functions are to prevent invasion of pathogenic organisms and to keep a harmonious balance between the inside and outside of the body. When the skin is injured, it can repair itself via the mechanism called wound healing.

The normal wound-healing process can be divided into three principal stages (1) the inflammatory phase, (2) the proliferative phase, and (3) the maturation (or remodeling) phase. The inflammatory phase starts immediately at the time of injury with activation of the clotting cascade and release of certain cytokines. The release of chemotactic factors such as platelet-derived growth factor (PDGF, the major factor released by platelets during thrombus formation), prostaglandins, complement factors, and interleukins (e.g., IL-1) stimulates the migration of inflammatory cells such as neutrophils and monocytes/macrophages. The recruitment and involvement of inflammatory cells help to remove debris including bacteria and release specific growth factors. Macrophages play a role in secreting many cytokines, particularly transforming growth factors (TGF-β) and IL-6.[1] These specific cytokines initiate the formation of granulation tissue, proliferation of keratinocytes, fibroblast production, and an increase in endothelial cells in the proliferative phage. This increase in cell production and migration begins approximately 4 days after initial tissue injury. Fibroblasts play a major role in the formation of provisional matrix that is composed of collagen I, collagen III, fibronectin, elastin, and proteoglycans. The keratinocytes start the epithelialization process with reconstruction of the disrupted basement membrane zone. During the maturation phase, the collagen network and proteoglycans are also remodeled. Both collagen types I and III increase during the beginning of the wound-healing process. However, when remodeling takes place, the proportion of collagen type III to collagen type I is decreased and collagen fibers are cross-linked and oriented in a more parallel arrangement, toward the direction of mechanical stress.[2]

Hypertrophic scars and keloids are believed to be an abnormal response during the aforementioned wound-healing process.[3] Hypertrophic scars and keloids can occur in all races, but they occur much more frequently in ethnic skin, ranging from 3 to 18 times higher incidence, compared with Caucasians.[4-6] The incidence has been reported to be between 4.5% and 16% in African Americans, the Chinese, and Hispanics. Patients in their second to third decade of life are more commonly affected with the same prevalence in both sexes.

There are many predisposing factors that influence the formation of hypertrophic scars and keloids, such as disruption in the integrity of the skin, location on the body, race, and genetic background.[7,8] Common causes include surgery, ear piercing, tattoos, infection, vaccination, burns, and inflammatory acne. Locations that are especially prone are the jaw line, upper chest, and upper back; some patients report spontaneous scars and keloids arising in these specific locations without any history of injury or trauma.[9]

The precise mechanism has not yet been established. It is thought that hypertrophic scars and keloids may be caused by a disturbance in the natural wound-healing process. It may result from abnormal cytokine release, epithelial disruption, excessive matrix deposition, reduction in matrix degradation, or abnormal remodeling of excessive matrix.

Abnormal cytokines have been reported in the formation of hypertrophic scars and keloids[10] including TGF-β[11,12] and IL-6.[13,14] In an in vitro study, fibroblasts from keloids showed an abnormal response to stimulation, producing high levels of collagen, specifically collagen type I. On the other hand, fibroblasts from hypertrophic scars exhibited a normal response to growth factor with only a moderate increase in collagen synthesis. The linkage between TGF-β and IL-6 shows an increase in collagen synthesis and fibronectin deposition within hypertrophic scars and keloids. In the normal wound-healing process, during the maturation phase, angiogenesis usually regresses over time but keloids exhibit persistent hyperemia because of a constant presence of new vessels in the area. Other factors implicated in the development of hypertrophic scars and keloids are increased hyaluronic acid production,[15,16] decreased apoptosis rate of fibroblasts,[17] and presence of mast cells,[18] among others.

The treatment of hypertrophic scars and keloids is a challenging topic in regard to ethnic skin given that there is a high rate of recurrence, as high as 50% after surgical excision[19] and a high risk of complications after treatment, especially pigmentary alterations. Understanding the nature of hypertrophic scars and keloids is very important to achieve a successful outcome and to improve the quality of these scars with minimal to no side effects/complications from treatment.

CLINICAL EXAMINATION AND PATIENT HISTORY

Hypertrophic scars and keloids may arise anywhere on the body; however, those areas under constant pressure, movement, and stretching are commonly affected. Areas known to be frequently affected include the ear lobes, jaw line, clavicular area, shoulders, chest, nape of the neck, and upper back. The palms and soles are uncommon areas to be affected, but there are case reports in the literature describing keloids in these rare areas.[20–23]

Hypertrophic scars and keloids begin with the same clinical manifestations by becoming red, raised, and firm with a smooth and shiny surface. Pruritus and hypersensitive sensations are symptoms that patients frequently report. At the initial stage, they are difficult to distinguish between the two. However, we can distinguish hypertrophic scars from keloids by some other clinical manifestations and by the typical growth pattern.

Hypertrophic scars (Figure 19.1) have well-defined borders within the original injury site and remain confined to the site of injury. They usually occur within the initial weeks of healing. They begin with a pink to erythematous papule or plaque and stabilize for some time. Some of them may show cosmetic improvement over a period of time and either turn hyper- or hypopigmentated.

Keloids (Figure 19.2) can present as a nodule, tumor, papule, or plaque and they usually hyperpigment to a black/red/purple color. In some lesions, we can see prominent vessels and a claw-like projection of growth at the peripheral borders. They are usually more exaggerated than hypertrophic scars, and always proliferate well beyond the boundaries of the original injury. They can occur during the initial weeks of healing or may even develop many months after the initial healing process. They still remain active in growth, whereas hypertrophic scars tend to regress and flatten over time.

Normally, diagnoses of both hypertrophic scars and keloids are a clinical diagnosis and often straightforward; usually, a biopsy is not necessary. However, histopathology may be required to differentiate these from other skin lesions which present as a papule, plaque, nodule, or tumor. The differential diagnoses include inflammatory disorders (i.e., lichen planus, sarcoidosis), dermal lesions (fibrous tumors, dermatofibroma, dermatofibrosarcoma protuberans, dermal nevus), adnexal tumors, endothelial tumors (i.e., Kaposi's sarcoma), recurrent tumors arising in a surgical scar, and cutaneous metastasis (carcinoma en cuirasse).[24]

Histopathologically, hypertrophic scars (Figure 19.3) and keloids (Figure 19.4) prolong formation of new collagen and have a delay in the remodeling process. Collagen fibers tend to be thick, hyalinized, and arranged in a whorl or nodular pattern.[25] Specifically in keloids

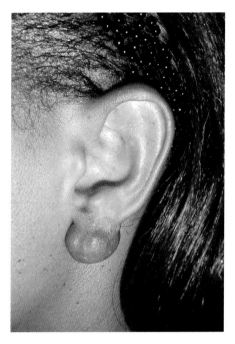

Figure 19.2 *A keloid at the left earlobe of an African American woman secondary to ear piercing (Image courtesy of Dr Heather Woolery-Lloyd, University of Miami)*

(Figure 19.4), the nodular pattern persists without relenting and they contain more thickened hypereosinophilic collagen bundles with some mast cells, more mucin, few elastic fibers, and adnexal structures. In hypertrophic scars (Figure 19.3), abnormal collagen fibers may become thinner and arrange into a parallel fashion near the surface of the skin.[26]

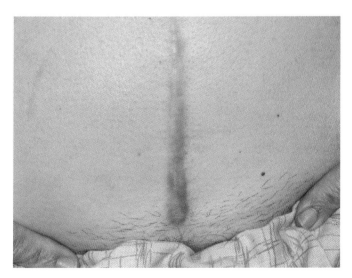

Figure 19.1 *A pink, smooth, shiny, and well-circumscribed linear hypertrophic scar at lower abdomen after transabdominal hysterectomy*

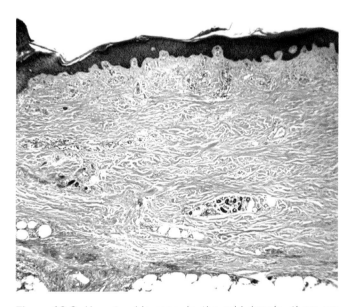

Figure 19.3 *Hypertrophic scar: in the mid-dermis, there are bands of sclerotic collagen bundles oriented parallel to the skin surface (Image courtesy of Dr George W. Elgart, University of Miami)*

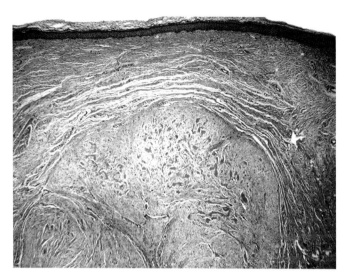

Figure 19.4 *Keloid: the reticular dermis is replaced by a whorl-like aggregate of thick, hyalinized, and eosinophilic collagen bundle (Image courtesy of Dr George W. Elgart, University of Miami)*

GENERAL TREATMENT APPROACH

Although hypertrophic scars tend to stabilize or regress spontaneously without treatment, we cannot predict how much they will regress or if they will recur. On the other hand, keloids show no tendency toward regression and tend to enlarge over time. Generally, it is very difficult to differentiate between the two at the beginning stages, and early treatment for both diseases results in a great outcome.

Overall, early treatment of these lesions is consistently much more successful than treating lesions at a later stage. Normally, in Caucasian skin, newly formed surgical scars that are erythematous may not need further treatment because of the probability of spontaneous resolution over time. However, in individuals with ethnic skin, who have a tendency to develop hypertrophic scars and keloids, early treatment of susceptible lesions is recommended and, if treated correctly, receive superior outcomes.

Patients usually seek treatment because of a cosmetically unfavorable result or associated symptoms such as pruritus, hypersensitive sensations, or impaired functions of the body, especially lesions that arise over joints or weight bearing areas like the back and plantar surfaces.

Although new hypertrophic scars respond well with early intervention, keloids by nature have a high recurrence rate even after treatment. Combining many treatment modalities should be entertained to get a better result. In regard to ethnic skin, many treatment options are not available in comparison to Caucasian skin because of a greater tendency of ethnic skin to develop side effects and complications from available interventions (i.e., pigmentary alterations or enlarging of the lesion).

To avoid unfavorable side effects and to achieve a suitable outcome, we recommend treating susceptible lesions as early as possible, especially in ethnic skin. The suggested methods should be less invasive, safe, and easy to perform and have minimal potential side effects.

In older lesions, albeit it is difficult to clear the entire lesion, treatments still are recommended to improve the quality of these lesions (i.e., reducing redness, volume of the scar, pliability, and relief of pain, itching, and hypersensitivity).

Our strategies to prevent the occurrence of such lesions and the treatment of existing lesions include the following (1) educate your patients with ethnic skin about what hypertrophic scars and keloids really are, (2) advise patients to avoid unnecessary invasive procedures (i.e., tattoos and piercings) on high-risk areas, especially in patients with family or personal history, (3) implement an early intervention plan to the site of injury (i.e., make the wound heal as fast as possible, close the wound by primary closure, use a graft and flap, and amend factors that can cause a delay in wound healing such as infection or poor nutrition), and (4) modulate wound healing by a recommended intervention (i.e., using a pulse dye laser for scar treatment or use of occlusive dressings).

For improvement of an existing lesion, there are many available modalities to treat these conditions such as surgical excision, laser ablation, nonablative lasers, radiation, compression, application of corticosteroids, injection of some chemotherapeutic agents (i.e., 5-fluorouracil, bleomycin, and mitomycin), interferon injection, and retinoic or imiquimod application.

Choosing a mode of treatment depends on your patient's needs and the nature of their lesions. Patient factors to consider include: (1) skin type (a higher Fitzpatrick skin type may develop more complications such as epidermal burns from laser/light treatments or pigmentary alterations posttreatment; a physician may choose a nonaggressive method or a low parameter on the laser setting in susceptible patients), (2) age and sex of the patient (there are a limitation of treatment modalities in children and in sexually active women who have tendency to get pregnant), (3) the patient's pain threshold, (4) economic status and financial restrictions (as these procedures may be viewed as strictly cosmetic and thus insurance will not provide coverage), (5) compliance of your patient as some treatments require multiple visits, and (6) patient education (as some lesions are best left untreated).

Choosing a modality of treatment also depends upon the actual lesion's factors some of which include: (1) age of the lesions (new vs. old), (2) color of the lesion (a very red and hypervascular lesion will lead to better results as the red color is a chromophore target for a vascular laser), (3) the nature of the lesion (stable versus active in growth), and (4) the location of the lesion (earlobe keloids respond well with surgical excision, whereas lesions at weight-bearing areas such the plantar surface or lesions at large joints need aggressive treatment to improve quality of life and function).

With overall assessment of patient factors, lesion factors, and physician discretion, the most appropriate method of treatment can be planned and executed. The following contains details on the practical interventions of keloids and hypertrophic scars in ethnic skin in order to receive a superior outcome with minimal complications.

■ Pulsed Dye Laser

Currently, the pulsed dye laser (PDL, 585 and 595 nm) is widely used and accepted as the laser of choice for improvement of the quality of hypertrophic scars and keloids.[27–29] The precise mechanism is not well known or discovered as of yet. Theories do exist; one being focused on microvascular destruction from selective absorption of hemoglobin in newly formed capillaries resulting in ischemia. This leads to deprivation of oxygenation and nutrition directly to the scar and consequently interferes in collagen production.

Other hypotheses include modulation of mast cells, reduction of expression of TGF-β1,[30] disulfide bond disruption from the super-heating process, and collagenolysis from collagenase stimulation via lactic acid production in the hypoxic tissue. This mainly causes collagen turnover and remodeling with the result creating a flatter scar and reduction of the red color. The ideal setting[31,32] is 585-nm PDL at 450 μs, using a spot size of 7 to 10 mm, with the fluence ranging from 3.5 to 7.5 J/cm^2. The interval for each treatment session is between 4 and 6 weeks. In ethnic skin, we prefer using a low fluence (3 to 3.5 J/cm^2 with a 10-mm spot size and 10% overlap) in order to reduce any complications from this procedure (Figure 19.5A and B). We suggest starting as early as possible because new lesions have numerous capillaries. This procedure can also improve surgical scar appearance, when performed on the suture removal day with 4-week intervals for at least three sessions, since the suture removal day.[33] However, old scars—greater than 1-year-old, do not show a good response to this treatment when compared with new scar treatments.

This laser procedure is performed in an outpatient clinic setting. It is usually well tolerated without requiring the use of any anesthesia. The patient may feel discomfort that is consistently compared to "a rubber band snapping" against their skin. Most patients report a low pain score of a 1 or 2 (of 10). After the procedure, patients may feel a burning or itching sensation in the treated area, which usually subsides within a couple of days. In high fluence settings, purpura is a commonly noted side effect, which usually appears immediately after the laser procedure and may persist for a long time in ethnic skin. To reduce complications of this treatment, we recommend using a low fluence setting, doing a "test spot," and judicious adequate cooling.

Corticosteroids

Corticosteroids, especially triamcinolone acetonide, are well known in the treatment of hypertrophic scars and keloids. Its actions inhibit migration of inflammatory cells, decreases cellular proliferation (fibroblasts) and collagen production, and cause significant decreases in the level of TGF-β1 and vasoconstriction. One can apply the medication to the lesions by topical form (clobetasol propionate 0.05% cream) with occlusion or intralesional injection (10 to 40 mg/mL). Although topical form is a very simple method and less invasive it is not recommended in ethnic skin as a result of high risk of side effects (steroid-induced acne, hypopigmentation, dermal atrophy of surrounding skin). Even though intralesional corticosteroid injections are more invasive, it is an effective technique and has a more predictable outcome than other methods available.

There are various concentrations of corticosteroids for the treatment of hypertrophic scars and keloids. A 40-mg/mL dosage is used for initial lesions which are large, hard, fibrotic, and active in growth. A 10 to 20-mg/mL dosage is for softer lesions and this dosage reduces the common side effects. This dosage is also used, when the physician wants to prevent recurrence of the lesion after

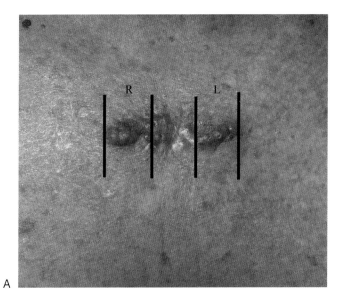

A

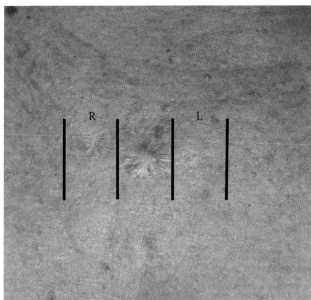

B

Figure 19.5 *(A) Female patient with a surgical linear scar on anterior mid-upper chest. The right section received 585-nm PDL with pulse duration of 450 μs, the middle remained as a control, and the left section received 585-nm PDL with pulse duration of 1.5 ms. (B) One month after the third PDL treatment. There was a significant clinical difference between the treated and the untreated sites*

surgery. However, this method can elicit a lot of pain. Topical anesthesia, cooling agents (ice packs, cool air), or a combination of the steroid with 1% lidocaine and epinephrine is recommended to reduce pain from this procedure. Using a 30-gauge needle on a 1-mL Luer-Loc syringe is the recommended vehicle for injection. Injections are repeated at intervals of 4 to 8 weeks with as many treatments as required. Over-treatment must be avoided to prevent permanent atrophy.

One must also be wary of superficial injections which can make the drug precipitate superficially on the lesions and consequently have white spots over the areas of treatment. Hypopigmentation and telangiectasia are common side effects for high concentrations of steroids or repetitive injections. Hypothalamic-pituitary axis suppression should be mentioned because prolonged use of high amounts of corticosteroid may cause this systemic complication. The use of corticosteroid can be used in conjunction with other available treatment modalities such as surgical excision, cryotherapy, or PDL.[34–36]

Surgical Excision/Combination with Other Modalities

In small and well-circumscribed lesions (keloids on earlobes), surgical excision of these lesions is suggested. However, a high rate of recurrence is documented when surgical excision is performed alone. Combination therapies with other modalities are highly recommended. Techniques for minimal recurrence are using low-trauma treatments and trying to close the defect with minimal skin tension. After removing the lesion, the skin that is covering the lesion may be excised and brought back to cover the wound as a skin graft. Other modalities which have been reported in the literature show a successful combination of surgical excision with intralesional steroid injections, postoperative radiation,[37–39] and application of imiquimod postoperatively.[40]

Silicone and Occlusion

These modalities are safe, painless, and easy to perform by patients. Improvements in a scar's appearance have been shown after application of a silicone sheet or silicone gel.[41–45] They are recommended for at least 12 hours a day for 2 to 4 months. Precise mechanisms are unknown, but it is believed that the occlusion effect increases hydration and static electricity during the use of the sheet and modulates abnormal matrix synthesis and the remodeling process. Even though these modalities are simple, skin irritation, allergies to these products, and their efficacy should remain concerns.

Pressure

Continuous scar pressure of at least 24 mm Hg can produce tissue ischemia which leads to an increase in lactic acid and results in increased levels of prostaglandin E_2 (PGE$_2$), collagenase (MMP-1), and gelatinase B (MMP-9) activity, which help remodel the scar. A pressure dressing is recommended for at least 18 hours a day for a minimum of 6 months.[46–49]

Chemotherapeutic Agents

Chemotherapeutic agents are currently being used for the treatment of hypertrophic scars and keloids. According to one theory of keloid formation, keloids develop from hyperproliferation of fibroblasts and capillaries. Therefore, any chemotherapeutic agent that can inhibit cell proliferation can decrease the growth of keloids. However, these substances understandably are associated with high risks and side effects which can lead to high morbidity and mortality. From the literature, the most common chemotherapeutic agents used for keloid treatment are 5-fluorouracil[50–52] and bleomycin.[53,54] They are always used in combination with corticosteroids (triamcinolone acetonide)

and the normal route of administration is via intralesional injection. The common side effects are pain, necrosis of lesions, and pigmentary alterations.

Other Modalities

There are other modalities which have been used for the improvement of the quality of hypertrophic scars and keloids; however, they are not as popular as the aforementioned treatments because of severe side effects in ethnic skin. Such side effects and treatments include dyspigmentation with cryotherapy,[55,56] dyspigmentation with interferon,[57,58] and low efficacy with topical retinoic acid application.[59,60]

DIRECTIONS FOR THE FUTURE AND CONCLUSIONS

The basic science regarding pathogenesis of hypertrophic scars and keloids are very essential to understand the necessary treatment for these lesions. Increasing our knowledge base about the wound-healing process can also apply to the treatment of hypertrophic scars and keloids.

Specific treatments that are tailored to a specific abnormality in the lesion can result in a favorable outcome. The parameter of the lasers, the type of lasers, the target of the lasers, and dosage of agents for treatment have to be precise and well studied in order to achieve the best outcome. Treatments that are to be used at home will be an important addition to therapeutic modalities in conjunction with treatments available in office.

The treatment of hypertrophic scars and keloids remain a challenging topic. Patients suffer greatly both in physical appearance and bodily function. Although there are many modalities for treatment, combination modalities are the most effective. When choosing any method, side effects and complications must be a top priority, especially in patients of ethnic skin.

REFERENCES

1. Ghazizadeh M. Essential role of IL-6 signaling pathway in keloid pathogenesis. *J Nippon Med Sch.* 2007;74(1):11-22.
2. Nouri K, Lanigan SW, Rivas MP. Laser treatment for scar. In: ed. Goldberg DJ, *Laser and Lights: Procedures in Cosmetic Dermatology,* series edited by Dover JS. Vol. 1. Elsevier Sauders, Phidelphia;2005:67-73.
3. Shaffer JJ. Keloidal scars: a review with a critical look at therapeutic options. *J Am Acad Dermatol.* 2002;46:S63-S97.
4. Alhady SM, Sivanantharajah K. Keloids in various races. A review of 175 cases. *Plast Reconstr Surg.* 1969;44(6):564-566.
5. Taylor SC. Epidemiology of skin diseases in people of color. *Cutis.* 2003;71(4):271-275.
6. Oluwasanmi JO. Keloids in the African. *Clin Plast Surg.* 1974;1(1):179-195.
7. Laurentaci G, Dioguardi D. HLA antigens in keloids and hypertrophic scars. *Arch Dermatol.* 1977;113(12):1726.

8. Chen D, Wang Q, Bao W, Xu S, Tang Y. Role of HLA-DR and CD1a molecules in pathogenesis of hypertrophic scarring and keloids. *Chin Med J (Engl)*. 2003;116(2):314-315.

9. Murray JC. Scars and keloids. *Dermatol Clin*. 1993;11(4):697-708.

10. McCauley RL, Chopra V, Li YY, Herndon DN, Robson MC. Altered cytokine production in black patients with keloids. *J Clin Immunol*. 1992;12(4):300-308.

11. Lee TY, Chin GS, Kim WJ, Chau D, Gittes GK, Longaker MT. Expression of transforming growth factor beta 1, 2, and 3 proteins in keloids. *Ann Plast Surg*. 1999;43(2):179-184.

12. Babu M, Diegelmann R, Oliver N. Keloid fibroblasts exhibit an altered response to TGF-beta. *J Invest Dermatol*. 1992;99(5):650-655.

13. Uitto J. IL-6 signaling pathway in keloids: a target for pharmacologic intervention. *J Invest Dermatol*. 2007;127(1):6-8.

14. Ghazizadeh M, Tosa M, Shimizu H, Hyakusoku H, Kawanami O. Functional implications of the IL-6 signaling pathway in keloid pathogenesis. *J Invest Dermatol*. 2007; 127(1):98-105.

15. Alaish SM, Yager DR, Diegelmann RF, Cohen IK. Hyaluronic acid metabolism in keloid fibroblasts. *J Pediatr Surg*. 1995; 30(7):949-952.

16. Alaish SM, Yager D, Diegelmann RF, Cohen IK. Biology of fetal wound healing: hyaluronate receptor expression in fetal fibroblasts. *J Pediatr Surg*. 1994; 29(8):1040-1043.

17. Ladin DA, Hou Z, Patel D, et al. p53 and apoptosis alterations in keloids and keloid fibroblasts. *Wound Repair Regen*. 1998;6(1):28-37.

18. Smith CJ, Smith JC, Finn MC. The possible role of mast cells (allergy) in the production of keloid and hypertrophic scarring. *J Burn Care Rehabil*. 1987;8(2):126-131.

19. Callender VD. Considerations for treating acne in ethnic skin. *Cutis*. 2005;76(Suppl 2):19-23.

20. Britto JA, Elliot D. Aggressive keloid scarring of the Caucasian wrist and palm. *Br J Plast Surg*. 2001;54(5):461-462.

21. Sandler B. Recurrent plantar keloid. *Cutis*. 1999;63(6):325-326.

22. Aslan G, Terzioglu A, CigSar B. A massive plantar keloid. *Ann Plast Surg*. 2001;47(5):581.

23. LeFlore I, Antoine GA. Keloid formation on palmar surface of hand. *J Natl Med Assoc*. 1991;83(5):463-464.

24. Mullinax K, Cohen JB. Carcinoma en cuirasse presenting as keloids of the chest. *Dermatol Surg*. 2004;30(2 Pt 1):226-228.

25. Linares HA, Larson DL. Early differential diagnosis between hypertrophic and nonhypertrophic healing. *J Invest Dermatol*. 1974;62(5):514-516.

26. Heenan PJ. Tumors of the fibrous tissue involveing the skin. In: Elder D, Lever WF, Elenitsas R, Johnson BL, Murphy GF, eds. *Liver's Histopathology of the Skin*. 8th ed. Philadelphia, PA: Lippincott-Raven;1997:881-882.

27. Alster TS, Tanzi EL. Hypertrophic scars and keloids: etiology and management. *Am J Clin Dermatol*. 2003;4(4):235-243.

28. Kono T, Erçöçen AR, Nakazawa H, Honda T, Hayashi N, Nozaki M. The flashlamp-pumped pulsed dye laser (585 nm) treatment of hypertrophic scars in Asians. *Ann Plast Surg*. 2003;51(4):366-371.

29. Nouri K, Vidulich K, Rivas MP. Lasers for scars: a review. *J Cosmet Dermatol*. 2006;5(1):14-22.

30. Kuo YR, Wu WS, Jeng SF, et al. Suppressed TGF-beta1 expression is correlated with up-regulation of matrix metalloproteinase-13 in keloid regression after flashlamp pulsed-dye laser treatment. *Lasers Surg Med*. 2005;36(1):38-42.

31. Manuskiatti W, Fitzpatrick RE, Goldman MP. Energy density and numbers of treatment affect response of keloidal and hypertrophic sternotomy scars to the 585-nm flashlamp-pumped pulsed-dye laser. *J Am Acad Dermatol*. 2001;45(4):557-565.

32. Alster TS. Laser treatment of hypertrophic scars, keloids, and striae. *Dermatol Clin*. 1997;15(3):419-429.

33. Nouri K, Jimenez GP, Harrison-Balestra C, Elgart GW. 585-nm pulsed dye laser in the treatment of surgical scars starting on the suture removal day. *Dermatol Surg*. 2003;29(1):65-73.

34. Mutalik S. Treatment of keloids and hypertrophic scars. *Indian J Dermatol Venereol Leprol*. 2005;71(1):3-8.

35. Boutli-Kasapidou F, Tsakiri A, Anagnostou E, Mourellou O. Hypertrophic and keloidal scars: an approach to polytherapy. *Int J Dermatol*. 2005;44(4): 324-327.

36. Patel IA, Hall PN. A technique to avoid atrophy in combined intralesional excision and steroid injection for keloids. *Br J Plast Surg*. 2000;53(2):174.

37. Sclafani AP, Gordon L, Chadha M, Romo T 3rd. Prevention of earlobe keloid recurrence with postoperative corticosteroid injections versus radiation therapy: a randomized, prospective study and review of the literature. *Dermatol Surg*. 1996;22(6):569-574.

38. Klumpar DI, Murray JC, Anscher M. Keloids treated with excision followed by radiation therapy. *J Am Acad Dermatol*. 1994;31(2 Pt 1):225-231.

39. Chaudhry MR, Akhtar S, Duvalsaint F, Garner L, Lucente FE. Ear lobe keloids, surgical excision followed by radiation therapy: a 10-year experience. *Ear Nose Throat J*. 1994;73(10):779-781.

40. Berman B, Kaufman J. Pilot study of the effect of postoperative imiquimod 5% cream on the recurrence rate of excised keloids. *J Am Acad Dermatol*. 2002;47(Suppl 4):S209-S211.

41. Li-Tsang CW, Lau JC, Choi J, Chan CC, Jianan L. A prospective randomized clinical trial to investigate the effect of silicone gel sheeting (Cica-Care) on post-traumatic hypertrophic scar among the Chinese population. *Burns*. 2006;32(6):678-683.

42. Chan KY, Lau CL, Adeeb SM, Somasundaram S, Nasir-Zahari M. A randomized, placebo-controlled, double-blind, prospective clinical trial of silicone gel in prevention of hypertrophic scar development in median sternotomy wound. *Plast Reconstr Surg*. 2005;116(4):1013-1020.

43. Majan JI. Evaluation of a self-adherent soft silicone dressing for the treatment of hypertrophic postoperative scars. *J Wound Care*. 2006;15(5):193-196.

44. Signorini M, Clementoni MT. Clinical evaluation of a new self-drying silicone gel in the treatment of scars: a preliminary report. *Aesthetic Plast Surg*. 2007;31(2):183-187.

45. Berman B, Flores F. Comparison of a silicone gel-filled cushion and silicon gel sheeting for the treatment of hypertrophic or keloid scars. *Dermatol Surg*. 1999;25(6):484-486.

46. Rockwell BW, Cohen IK, Ehrlich HP. Keloids and hypertrophic scars: a comprehensive review. *Scand J Plast Recon*. 1989;84:827-837.

47. Hassel JC, Roberg B, Kreuter A, Voigtländer V, Rammelsberg P, Hassel AJ. Treatment of ear keloids by compression, using a modified Oyster-Splint technique. *Dermatologic Surgery*. 2007;33 (2):208-212.

48. Reno F, Grazianetti P, Stella M, Magliacani G, Pezzuto C, Cannas M. Release and activation of matrix metalloproteinase-9 during in vitro mechanical compression in hypertrophic scars. *Arch Dermatol*. 2002;138(4):475-478.

49. Reno F, Grazianetti P, Cannas M. Effects of mechanical compression on hypertrophic scars: prostaglandin E2 release. *Burns*. 2001;27(3): 215-218.

50. Lebwohl M. From the literature: intralesional 5-FU in the treatment of hypertrophic scars and keloids: clinical experience. *J Am Acad Dermatol*. 2000;42(4):677.

51. Asilian A, Darougheh A, Shariati F. New combination of triamcinolone, 5-fluorouracil, and pulsed-dye laser for treatment of keloid and hypertrophic scars. *Dermatol Surg*. 2006;32(7): 907-915.

52. Gupta S, Kalra A. Efficacy and safety of intralesional 5-fluorouracil in the treatment of keloids. *Dermatology*. 2002;204(2): 130-132.

53. Naeini FF, Najafian J, Ahmadpour K. Bleomycin tattooing as a promising therapeutic modality in large keloids and hypertrophic scars. *Dermatol Surg*. 2006;32(8):1023-1029.

54. Saray Y, Gulec AT. Treatment of keloids and hypertrophic scars with dermojet injections of bleomycin: a preliminary study. *Int J Dermatol*. 2005;44(9):777-784.

55. Rusciani L, Paradisi A, Alfano C, Chiummariello S, Rusciani A. Cryotherapy in the treatment of keloids. *Drugs Dermatol*. 2006;5(7):591-595.

56. Fikrle T, Pizinger K. Cryosurgery in the treatment of earlobe keloids: report of seven cases. *Dermatol Surg*. 2005;31(12): 1728-1731.

57. Berman B, Duncan MR. Short-term keloid treatment in vivo with human interferon alfa-2b results in a selective and persistent normalization of keloidal fibroblast collagen, glycosaminoglycan, and collagenase production in vitro. *J Am Acad Dermatol*. 1989;21(4 Pt 1):694-702.

58. Hasegawa T, Nakao A, Sumiyoshi K, Tsuboi R, Ogawa H. IFN-gamma fails to antagonize fibrotic effect of TGF-beta on keloid-derived dermal fibroblasts. *J Dermatol Sci*. 2003;32(1): 19-24.

59. Janssen de Limpens AM. The local treatment of hypertrophic scars and keloids with topical retinoic acid. *Br J Dermatol* 1980;103(3):319-323.

60. Panabiere-Castaings MH. Retinoic acid in the treatment of keloids. *J Dermatol Surg Oncol*. 1988;14(11):1275-1276.

CHAPTER 20

Special Considerations in African American Skin

Cheryl M. Burgess, MD, FAAD

INTRODUCTION

People of color are increasingly seeking out products and procedures to fight the effects of aging, including surgical and nonsurgical cosmetic procedures. In fact, a survey by the American Society for Aesthetic Plastic Surgery (ASAPS) found that cosmetic procedures performed on racial and ethnic minorities represented 22% of the 11.5 million surgical and nonsurgical cosmetic procedures performed in the United States in 2006.[1] According to the survey, this market segment consisted of Hispanics (10%), African Americans (6%), Asians (5%), and other non-Caucasian individuals (1%). In addition, racial and ethnic minorities had a 2% increase in cosmetic procedures from 2005 and are among the fastest growing segment of the cosmetic procedures market. Consequently, a thorough understanding of the aging process in ethnic skin and nonsurgical treatment options for patients of color is required of dermatologists and cosmetic surgeons who will treat these patients.

Of the 11.5 million procedures in 2006, nonsurgical cosmetic procedures made up 83% of the total.[1] Not surprisingly, new products in this market continue to emerge at a brisk pace—all the more reason for clinicians to take a proactive approach to education and training. The following chapter provides an overview of differences between Caucasian skin and ethnic skin, focusing on structural and pathophysiologic differences, and corresponding treatment options for ethnic patients.

UNDERLYING MECHANISMS IN THE AGING FACE

In order to make the appropriate selection and application of cosmetic procedures, clinicians must acquire a thorough understanding of the underlying mechanisms in the aging face. As the face begins to age, fat atrophy and hypertrophy cause hills and valleys to develop, producing demarcations between the cosmetic units. Features become concave, characterized by loss of volume in the lips (mainly the upper lip), sunken temple and cheek, scalloped mandible, and increased shadowing among the resulting hills and valleys. With aging, the most significant change in appearance is the sagging of excess skin, which causes the conversion of primary arcs to straight lines. Reversing the effects of fat atrophy/hypertrophy cannot be adequately accomplished through conservative techniques. A comprehensive approach, that considers the entire face and all the underlying causes of aging is necessary. Volume must be restored in regions experiencing fat atrophy and excess fat, must be removed from regions where fat has accumulated. Correcting the distribution of volume throughout the face can help restore homogenous topography, eliminate demarcations between cosmetic units, and restore the primary arcs.[2]

STRUCTURAL AND FUNCTIONAL DIFFERENCES BETWEEN CAUCASIAN SKIN AND ETHNIC SKIN

The most evident difference between ethnic skin and Caucasian skin is epidermal melanin content. While no differences exist in the number of melanocytes, variations do exist in the number and size[3] and packaging and distribution[4] of melanosomes. Moreover, the epidermal melanin unit in skin of color contains more melanin overall and may undergo slower degradation.[3] These differences in melanin and melanosomes provide superior UV protection in ethnic skin. As a result, people of color suffer less photodamage than Caucasians.[4] In fact, one study of adults living in Tucson, Arizona, found that the epidermis of African American participants was largely spared the gross photodamage observed in Caucasian participants. Most of the Caucasian women of age 45 to 50 years, had wrinkles in the crow's feet and on the corners of the mouth, while none of the African American women of comparable age had obvious crow's feet wrinkles or perioral rhytids. The skin of African Americans also felt firmer, and the histology of the dermal elastic fibers in African American skin was similar to the appearance of these fibers in sun-protected Caucasian skin.[5] Although differences in the structure of ethnic skin can be beneficial, the photoprotection afforded by differences in melanosome and melanin characteristics also causes frequent hyperpigmentation in skin of color, and may be responsible for divergent responses observed in burn injuries.[6]

Individuals with darker skin experience frequent postinflammatory hyperpigmentation.[6] Indeed, one survey found that uneven skin tone was a chief complaint in more than one-third of black women, while another survey found that pigment disorders were the third most commonly treated dermatoses. In a survey of 100 women of color, complaints about dark spots reached 86%, while 49% of women complained of sensitive or very sensitive skin.[3] Causes of hyperpigmentation include melasma, postinflammatory hyperpigmentation, and dyschromia of photoaging.[7] Although, the underlying mechanisms of postinflammatory hyperpigmentation have not been well clarified, the intensity and duration of the disease is linked to darker skin hues and to dermatoses with disruption of the basal layer.[5]

Keloidal scarring is thought to occur 3 to 18 times more often in ethnic persons compared with Caucasian persons, because of differences in the composition of fibroblasts. Research suggests that fibroblasts are larger and binucleated or multinucleated in ethnic persons. Because keloid scarring can occur in ethnic patients as a result of invasive procedures such as full or partial facelifts, many patients and practitioners are uncertain of what to expect from non-invasive procedures, such as soft-tissue augmentation. In fact, patients with a history of hypertrophic scarring are likely to fear soft-tissue augmentation, because of a history of scarring and/or discoloration. Fortunately, techniques can alleviate the occurrence of hyperpigmentation in ethnic skin and lead to positive results for restoring a youthful facial appearance.[8] For example, pretreatment with hydroquinone can prevent this scarring in patients at risk for hyperpigmentation. Although I am very cautious with these patients in recommending any surgical procedures, patients with a more reactive collagen can benefit from the noninvasive cosmetic procedures such as fillers and skin-tightening procedures. Because these procedures stimulate collagen, most patients of color will experience a more enhanced response, requiring less treatment sessions than their Caucasian counterparts. One note of caution about managing the expectations of patients who are at elevated risk for postinflammatory hyperpigmentation: The marketing of cosmetic procedures may lead to overzealous expectations of patients being able to "immediately return to work" following the procedure. Contrary to the marketing claims, patients may require a short period of healing before they are comfortable with their appearance in public.

MOST COMMON NONINVASIVE COSMETIC PROCEDURES IN ETHNIC SKIN

In the past 10 years, the number of noninvasive cosmetic procedures has increased from 1.1 to 9.5 million. The increase has resulted as a benefit of improved efficacy and safety of procedures, combined with an ever-increasing baby-boomer market and emerging markets in ethnic populations. In 2006, the top five noninvasive cosmetic procedures were (1) botulinum toxin injection, (2) hyaluronic acid, (3) laser hair removal, (4) microdermabrasion, and (5) laser skin resurfacing. Among these procedures, soft-tissue augmentation has experienced the greatest growth, with an increase in procedures of more than 35% since 2004.[9] The leading soft-tissue fillers in 2006 were (1) hyaluronic acid, (2) collagen derived from human or bovine sources, (3) autologous fat, (4) calcium hydroxylapatite, and (5) poly-L-lactic acid (PLA). Trends in filler substances can shift quickly. For example, the soft-tissue filler experiencing the most dramatic growth from 2005 to 2006 was calcium hydroxylapatite—a 90% increase.[1] These statistics show a dramatic growth in demand that is subject to significant shifts in product trends. The combination of new products, growth in procedures, and increasing use of cosmetic procedures in ethnic markets points to exciting possibilities for dermatologists and plastic surgeons.

SOFT-TISSUE FILLERS

Soft-tissue fillers are commonly categorized by type of material or durability (Table 20.1). Any filler can be used alone or in combination for augmentation of all facial areas, except for the lips, which should only be injected with hyaluronic acid. Some newer hyaluronic acid fillers contain cross-linking with ester and ether linkages to stabilize the molecule for greater durability in dermal processes.[10] Some of the new filler materials have been injected into the lips with successful outcomes; however, dermatologists should avoid using these new fillers until more information is known about the activity of these substances in the mucosal areas.

PLA is distinct from other soft-tissue fillers, because of its mechanism of action, treatment plan, preparation of injection material, and injection technique.[11] The application of PLA in soft-tissue augmentation exploits a mechanism of action, not seen in any other soft-tissue filler. Although the injection of PLA causes an immediate effect by physically occupying space, this initial response is temporary and only lasts 1 week or less.[12] Once the carrier solution is absorbed, a delayed but progressive volumizing effect begins. The process of hydration, loss of cohesion and molecular weight, and solubilization and phagocytosis of PLA by the host's macrophages, slowly degrades PLA into lactic acid microspheres and eliminates CO_2 by way of respiratory excretion. Crystals are left behind to stimulate collagen and a granulomatous reaction. This inflammatory reaction elicits resorption and the formation of fibrous connective tissue about the foreign body, causing dermal fibroplasia that leads to the desired cosmetic effect.[13]

SOFT-TISSUE AUGMENTATION IN ETHNIC SKIN

In African Americans, differences in skin composition lead to less frequency of certain conditions experienced with white skin, such as perioral rhytids or wrinkling. However, African Americans experience a variety of other issues related to skin sagging and sinking. Based on the particular ethnic skin-type, some soft-tissue fillers will achieve better results than others will. For example, volumizers are generally more effective in ethnic skin, caused by the presence of sagging skin. Histologically, there is less thinning of collagen bundles and elastic tissue in this skin-type. As a result, fillers that stimulate collagen or elastin production or skin tightening are more effective in skin of color.

Soft-tissue fillers are excellent for minimizing cheek festooning, filling accentuated tear troughs, and for treating the prejowl sulcus and temples. Volumizing is accomplished in the infraorbital, upper cheek, and lateral cheek regions using either cross-linked or larger particle hyaluronic acid, calcium hydroxylapatite, or PLA. Longevity of the effect varies with the type of substance. Temporary or less-permanent fillers provide immediate or delayed effects that last 9 to 18 months. For example, PLA, which requires three sessions with 4 to 7 week periods between treatments, produces a soft-tissue augmentation that lasts between 18 months and 3 years.[10] Around the eyes, laxity of the upper/lower eyelid skin may develop; therefore, volume enhancement of the sub-brow region can be achieved by injecting a filler just below the eyebrow hair for an instant brow lift.

In the 1990s, the desire among Caucasian women for full, voluptuous lips began to stimulate the market for collagen injections used to enhance the appearance of lips. Most women have historically viewed full lips as an unattractive feature. However, over the years, the desire for full lips has gained widespread popularity and fueled the demand for lip augmentation. In African American women, changes in self-perception are motivating more of these women to emphasize the beauty of their lips. As a result, many African American women are now choosing procedures to rebuild an aging lip.[14]

Whereas the typical goal of lip augmentation in Caucasian women is to increase the lip size beyond the original volume, African American women generally seek augmentation to only restore the size of the lip to the original volume and appearance (Figure 20.1). Although the intrinsic aging process causes similar effects to the lips of African American and Caucasian patients,

TABLE 20.1 ▪ Soft-tissue Fillers

(A) Categorized by Material Type

Natural implants	Autologous materials
	Fat transfer
	Fat autograft muscle injection
	Cultured human fibroblasts
	Cadaver-derived materials
	Dermis and extracellular matrix
	Acellular allogeneic dermis
	Injectable microparticulate acellular allogeneic dermis
	Lyophilized human particulate fascia lata
	Collagen
	Bovine-derived collagen
	Human-derived collagen from tissue culture
	Hyaluronic acid
	Hyaluronic acid derived from rooster combs
	Nonanimal stabilized hyaluronic acid from bacterial fermentation
	Viscoelastic nonanimal hyaluronic acid derived from bacterial fermentation
Synthetic or pseudo-synthetic implants	Silicone oil
	Expanded polytetrafluoroethylene
	Dual-porosity expanded polytetrafluoroethylene
	Polymethylmethacrylate microspheres in denatured bovine collagen
	Poly-L-lactic acid
	Synthetic calcium hydroxylapatite microspheres suspended in aqueous polysaccharide gel
	Alkyl-imide gel polymer

(B) Categorized by Durability

Temporary fillers	Fat transfer
	Fat autograft muscle injection
	Dermis and extracellular matrix
	Acellular allogeneic dermis
	Injectable microparticulate acellular allogeneic dermis
	Lyophilized human particulate fascia lata
	Bovine dermal collagen
	Bovine collagen cross-linked with glutaraldehyde
	Human-based collagen isolated from human fibroblast tissue cultures
	Human-based collagen cross-linked with glutaraldehyde
	Nonanimal stabilized hyaluronic acid derived from bacterial biofermentation process
	Viscoelastic nonanimal hyaluronic acid gel
	Viscoelastic acid gel from rooster combs
	Poly-L-lactic acid
Semipermanent fillers	Synthetic calcium hydroxylapatite microspheres suspended in polysaccharide gel
	Expanded polytetrafluoroethylene
	Dual-porosity expanded polytetrafluoroethylene
	Alkyl-imide gel polymer
Permanent fillers	Silicone oil
	Polymethyl-methacrylate microspheres in denatured bovine collagen

some subtle differences are important to note. Whereas in Caucasian women, lip aging usually occurs relatively early in life, these effects typically occur later in African American women. In Caucasian women, rhytids develop above and below the vermilion borders, because of thinning of the dermis, volume loss, loss of vermillion border, and the overactivity of the perioral musculature.

The lips of Caucasian women appear thin, long, flat, and wrinkled, with down-turned corners of the mouth that appear sad or angry-looking. However, for African American women, rhytids occur predominantly below the vermilion border, in response to loss of volume of the upper lip. In addition, the lower lip usually maintains the same appearance; however, it sometimes becomes flat and more visible.

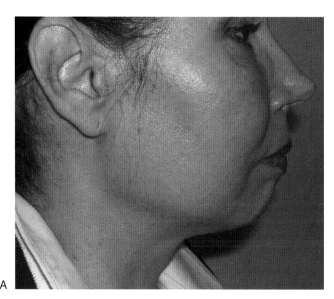
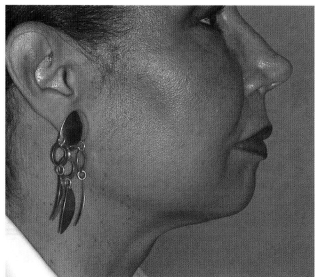

A   B

Figure 20.1 *(A) and (B) Lip enhancement using hyaluronic acid and radiofrequency procedure (Used with permission from Cheryl Burgess, MD.)*

Unlike Caucasian women, collagen enhancement of the vermilion border is rarely performed and therefore, the primary treatment consists of rolling the lip up using injections of hyaluronic acid. If there is overactivity of the peri-orbicularis oris musculature, botulinum toxin A is the preferred method to relax muscles perioral rhytids.[10]

BOTULINUM TOXIN

The formation of crease lines and rhytids is a natural component of the aging process that can lead to deep furrows and frown/scowl lines. Such furrows and frown/scowl lines are referred to as dynamic rhytids, because they arise when we laugh, frown, or smile. Dynamic rhytids are caused by the repeated forces generated by hyperkinetic muscles, including the frontalis (responsible for forehead furrows), corrugator supercilii (involved in frown/scowl lines), orbicularis oculi (crow's feet), and procerus and depressor supercilii (also involved in frown/scowl lines).[15] Although botulinum toxin has U.S. Food and Drug Administration (FDA) approval for treatment of the glabellar region of the face, it is often used off-label for relaxation of the upper and lower hyperkinetic facial and neck muscles. However, in ethnic skin, there is very little need to treat crow's feet, which rarely develops as seen in Caucasian patients.

The demand for botulinum toxin injections and other cosmetic procedures have continued to increase, fueled in part by growth in new sectors of the market. According to the ASAPS, the number of botulinum toxin injections increased 233% from 2000 to 2005. However, approximately 15% of these procedures were carried out in men in 2005, according to the American Academy of Cosmetic Surgery. In fact, some Internet sites have begun marketing these procedures directly to men. Large numbers of men are also seeking procedures for laser hair removal, microdermabrasion, hyaluronic acid, and laser skin resurfacing. It has been suggested that men typically follow the trends set by women.[9] The trend is also driven in part by the sheer number of men reaching the age at which they might want to appear younger. It is estimated that nearly 8000 people turned 60 years of age each day in 2006.[16]

RESTORING ELASTIN IN THE AGING FACE

Although several therapies have been developed to improve the loss of collagen that occurs in aging skin, until recently, no agent has been available to treat the loss of elastin function, which is a significant feature of chronologic aging and photoaging. Two recent studies have demonstrated favorable results by using a cream containing a zinc complex that penetrates the skin and stimulates elastin development through a myriad of molecular pathways. In both studies, the zinc complex cream was applied for 4 weeks. In the first study, improvement was evaluated by snap-test time, which determines the time needed for the skin to snap back to baseline after being pulled a specific distance. Response was also determined by measurement with a DermaLab[(r)] suction cup and blinded assessment by a dermatologist. After 4 weeks of treatment, there was a 40% improvement in snap time, significant improvement in vacuum as measured by the DermaLab suction cup, and improvement in skin roughness, fine and coarse lines, laxity, puffiness, dark circles, and crepey and sunken appearance. In the second study, there was a 29% decrease in the number and depth of fine lines and wrinkles around the eyes, following once-daily application for 4 weeks. Results of the study also found a 37% decrease in course wrinkles, 42% decrease in undereye laxity, 30% decrease and undereye puffiness, and a 21% decrease in undereye dark circles.[17] Restoration of elastin is likely to be especially effective in skin of color, because of the lower magnitude of elastin loss observed in the aging face of people of color.

SKIN TIGHTENING

Skin tightening can be accomplished through a number of heat-producing technologies, including radio frequency (RF), long wavelength laser, and broad-spectrum light sources (Figure 20.2). These technologies use heat-producing energy, which causes a cascade of molecular and mechanical effects that tighten skin without injury or removal of overlying epidermis.

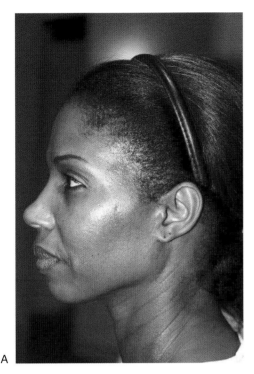
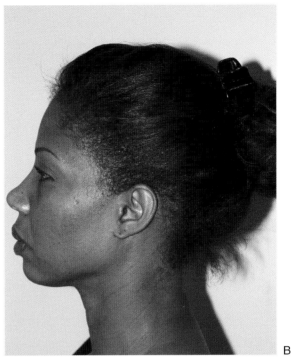

A   B

Figure 20.2 *(A) and (B) Treatment of skin tightening with RF (Used with permission from Cheryl Burgess, MD.)*

The result is direct and immediate contraction of collagen fibers, as well as a delayed wound-healing response.[18] While some FDA-approved devices use only one type of energy, other devices combine energy types; e.g., bipolar RF energy combined with diode laser energy or RF energy combined with both diode laser and intense pulse light energy.[19]

The various FDA-approved skin-tightening devices have demonstrated different results when used on different parts of the body, with reference to skin laxity, texture, firmness, and effects on volume reduction. For example, the multiple pass, low fluence treatment algorithm for lower face laxity has demonstrated favorable results with RF skin tightening.[20] In addition, the cost of procedure, associated adverse effects, and required treatment length and sessions are a consideration for both clinician and patient.[18–22]

Skin-tightening technology can be combined with other aesthetic modalities such as soft-tissue augmentation; the skin-tightening process can be applied either simultaneously or after receiving the other modality. The combination of modalities was recently tested in a study by England et al.[21] using an animal model. The study found that monopolar RF heating had no observed adverse effects on the filler collagen responses or persistence of the various filler substances, which included cross-linked human collagen (Cosmoplast™), hyaluronic acid (Restylane®), calcium hydroxylapatite (Radiesse™), polylactic acid (Sculptra™), and liquid injectable silicone (Silikon™). Further clinical studies are needed to study the effects on aesthetic outcome.

SUMMARY

People of color will soon comprise a majority of the international and domestic population. As the importance of ethnic markets continues to increase, dermatologists and cosmetic surgeons will require more expertise in the treatment of ethnic skin. People of color are increasingly seeking out products and procedures to reverse the effects of aging. Among nonsurgical cosmetic procedures, soft-tissue augmentation is experiencing the greatest market growth. Soft-tissue augmentation can be quite successful in patients with skin of color. However, when treating patients of color, important differences in the appearance of the aging face require different strategies and techniques. In addition, issues specific to ethnic skin such as skin sensitivity, hyperpigmentation, and keloid scarring require special consideration by clinicians. New agents and technologies for skin tightening and volumizing are producing excellent results in patients of color. As with patients of all skin colors, a comprehensive approach to assessment and treatment of the face is absolutely necessary. It is critical that clinicians receive specialized training for specific soft-tissue fillers before attempting to treat patients. With proper training and technique, clinicians can provide successful outcomes with little risk of adverse events to patients with pigmented skin.

REFERENCES

1. American Society for Aesthetic Plastic Surgery. Cosmetic surgery national data bank 2006 statistics. http://www.surgery.org/download/2006stats.pdf. Accessed June 15, 2007.

2. Donofrio LM. Fat distribution: a morphologic study of the aging face. *Dermatol Surg.* 2000;26(12):1107-1112.

3. Baumann L, Rodriguez D, Taylor SC, Wu J. Natural considerations for skin of color. *Cutis.* 2006;78(Suppl 6):2-19.

4. Kaidbey KH, Agin PP, Sayre RM, Kligman AM. Photoprotection by melanin—a comparison of black and Caucasian skin. *J Am Acad Dermatol.* 1979;1(3):249-260.

5. Stephens T. Ethnic sensitive skin: a review. *Cosmet Toiletries.* 1994;109:75-80.

6. Draelos Z. All skin is not the same. *Cosmet Dermatol.* 2006; 19:99-101.

7. Pigmentary Disorders Academy, by MedSense Ltd., on behalf of Galderma International. Pigment matters: Focus on pigmentary disorders. http://www.pigmentarydisordersacademy.org/pigmatters_summer.pdf. Accessed June 29, 2007.

8. Taylor SC. Skin of color: Biology, structure, function, and implications for dermatologic disease. *J Am Acad Dermatol.* Feb 2002;46(Suppl 2):S41-S62.

9. American Society for Aesthetic Plastic Surgery. Cosmetic surgery national data bank 2005 statistics. http://www.surgery.org/press/statistics-2005.php. Accessed June 15, 2007.

10. Burgess CM. *Cosmetic Dermatology.* Heidelberg, Germany: Springer; 2005.

11. Burgess CM, Lowe NJ. Newfill for skin augmentation: a new filler or failure? *Dermatol Surg.* 2006;32(12):1530-1532.

12. Mest D. Experience with injectable poly-L-lactic acid in clinical practice. *Cosmetic Dermatology.* 2005;18(2 S2):5-8.

13. Burgess CM, Quiroga RM. Assessment of the safety and efficacy of poly-L-lactic acid for the treatment of HIV-associated facial lipoatrophy. *J Am Acad Dermatol.* 2005;52(2): 233-239.

14. Ascend Media. Garries R. Restoring the fullness: lip rejuvenation in the African American female. http://www.plastic-surgeryproductsonline.com/article.php?s=PSP/2006/05&p=7. Accessed August 24, 2006.

15. Carruthers A, Kiene K, Carruthers J. Botulinum A exotoxin use in clinical dermatology. *J Am Acad Dermatol.* 1996;34(5 Pt 1): 788-797.

16. U.S. Census Bureau. Oldest baby boomers turn 60. http://www.census.gov/Press-Release/www/releases/archives/facts_for_features_special_editions/006105.html. Updated February 7, 2007. Accessed June 27, 2007.

17. Baumann L. Improving elasticity: the science of aging skin. *Cosmet Dermatol.* 2007;20(3):168-172.

18. American Society for Dermatologic Surgery. Technology Report: Tissue Tightening. Feb 2007. http://www.asds.net/Media/Position Statements/technology-tissuetightening.html. Accessed June 21, 2007.

19. Mayoral FA. Skin tightening with a combined unipolar and bipolar radiofrequency device. *J Drugs Dermatol.* 2007;6(2): 212-215.

20. Bogle MA, Ubelhoer N, Weiss RA, Mayoral F, Kaminer MS. Evaluation of the multiple pass, low-fluence algorithm for radiofrequency tightening of the lower face. *Lasers Surg Med.* 2007;39(3):210-217.

21. England L, Tan M, Shumaker P. Effects of monopolar radiofrequency treatment over soft tissue fillers in an animal model. *Lasers Surg Med.* 2005;37:356-365.

22. Sadick NS, Makino Y. Selective electro-thermolysis in aesthetic medicine: a review. *Lasers Surg Med.* 2004;34(2):91-97.

CHAPTER 21

Special Considerations in Asian/Far Eastern Skin

Henry Hin-Lee Chan, MD, FRCP,
and Stephanie G.Y. Ho, MBBS, MRCP

Skin of color is differentiated by the amount and epidermal distribution of melanin. Although there is no difference in melanocyte density among different racial groups, previous studies indicate that darker skin has larger melanocytes producing more melanin and melanosomes are distributed individually in keratinocytes.[1] This allows more effective absorption and deflection of ultraviolet light.

Because of the cultural and genetic differences, cosmetic dermatology in Asians differs from that in other racial groups of skin of color. In women from Far Eastern countries including Japan, Korea, China, and Singapore, light-colored complexion is widely considered to be beautiful. Asian females go to extreme measures of sun avoidance in order to have a lighter skin complexion. Such behavior is reflected by the nonmelanoma skin cancer prevalence among Japanese in Hawaii compared to Japanese in Japan, which differs by 45-fold. The use of sun protection, antioxidants, bleaching agents, and keratolytic preparations such as alpha-hydroxy acid forms an essential part of any skin care regimen.

The clinical presentation of photoaging differs between Asians and Caucasians in that pigmentary changes tend to occur with a greater incidence than skin wrinkling in Asians.[2,3] Chung et al.[4] more recently found both pigmentary changes and wrinkling to be major features of photoaging in Asians. However, moderate to severe wrinkling becomes apparent only at about 50 years, which is a decade or two later than in age-matched Caucasians.[5]

There are several acquired pigmentary conditions that are particularly common in Asians. Lentigines and seborrheic keratoses are frequent signs of photoaging among Asian. Melasma and Hori's macules are particularly common among Asian females. The use of appropriate laser or intense pulsed light (IPL) together with topical bleaching agents can significantly improve these conditions.

Laser or IPL sources for the treatment of these pigmentary conditions in Asians are not without risk given the fact that Asians have higher epidermal melanin content, which can lead to increased risk of postinflammatory hyperpigmentation (PIH). In addition, because epidermal melanin acts as a competing chromophobe, the light energy that reaches the targeted blood vessels or follicular melanocytes is reduced and higher fluences may be necessary to produce the desired effect. Besides sun avoidance and sun protection before and after laser/IPL treatment, topical bleaching agents are important as an adjunctive therapy. The appropriate use of laser/IPL parameters are also important including the use of skin cooling, longer laser pulse width to protect the epidermis, and longer laser/light source wavelength to reduce absorption by competing epidermal melanin.[6] All these measures can further enhance clinical outcomes as well as reduce the adverse effect of laser/IPL treatment.

Another important genetic variation is the incidence of melanoma among Asians is found to be significantly lower than Caucasians. Incidences of melanoma have been reported to be between 0.2 to 2.2 per 100 000 in Asians. From a Singapore study, the incidence of melanoma was reported to be 0.2 per 100 000 in the darker-skinned Indians and 0.5 per 100 000 in the fairer-skinned Chinese.[7] In Hong Kong, melanoma incidence was reported to be 1.1 per 100 000 women and 1.0 per 100 000 men.[8] The Japanese have roughly double the incidence of melanoma (2.2 per 100 000) compared to other Asian races.[9] Besides much lower incidences of melanoma, the distribution of melanoma also differs. In skin of color, the most common sites for the development of melanoma are nonsun exposed areas, such as palmar, plantar, subungual, and mucosal surfaces. In a study of 43 cases of melanoma in Chinese patients at the University of Hong Kong from 1964 to 1982, 56% of tumors arose from the foot, with 83% on the plantar surface.[10] A study from Japan also reported the foot as the most commonly affected area, with 50% being the acral lentiginous melanoma type. The implication is that the use of laser for the treatment of melanocytic lesions including melanocytic nevi can be considered as a safe procedure provided that the patient has no personal or family history of melanoma and the pigmented lesion is not located in the acral area[11] and that the patient has been evaluated by a dermatologist.

Besides pigment reduction, improvement of skin texture, pore size, and facial erythema are common requests among patients with moderate degrees of photoaging. The use of nonablative skin rejuvenation is particularly applicable to Asians given the lesser degree of wrinkling among this population (Figure 21.1).[6] Other advantages include lack of downtime and lower risk of adverse effects. A combination approach using multiple devices, with the intention to optimize the clinical outcome, has gained much popularity in recent years.[12] Such treatment includes the use of vascular lasers—infrared lasers and pigment lasers or IPL all in the same session. Vascular laser/IPL is used to reduce facial erythema, induce microvascular injury, and in doing so, promote new collagen formation. Infrared lasers heat up the dermis and promote collagen damage, therefore lead to new collagen formation.[13–15] To protect the epidermis, skin cooling is extremely important in Asians. Detailed treatment parameters are described in the chapter on dermal color improvement.

The delay in the onset of wrinkling in Asians also implies that more aggressive approaches for skin rejuvenation such as laser resurfacing, plasma skin rejuvenation (PSR) (Rhytec, Inc., Waltham, MA), or ablative fractional resurfacing are less applicable. However, these procedures can be useful in patients with acne scarring or in older age groups.[16] Treatment parameters for acne scarring in Asians depends on several factors. While a more aggressive approach can lead to a greater degree of improvement, the downtime and risk of PIH also increase. As a result, for patients who wish to have treatment and are not too concerned about the risk of PIH (e.g., young male with acne scar), we treat them with two passes of PSR (4 J/cm^2). In our experience, PSR leads to approximately 30% to 40% improvement (Figure 21.2).

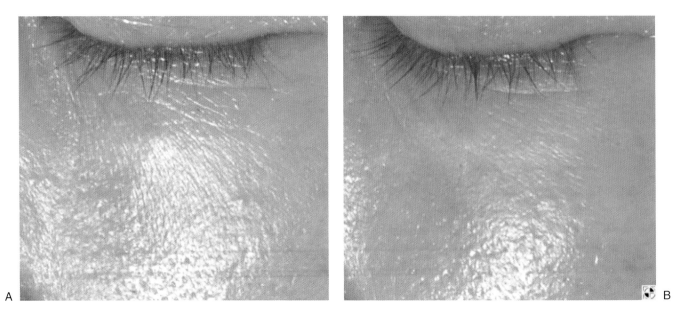

Figure 21.1 *Photorejuvenation using nonablative laser devices. (A) Pretreatment. (B) Posttreatment*

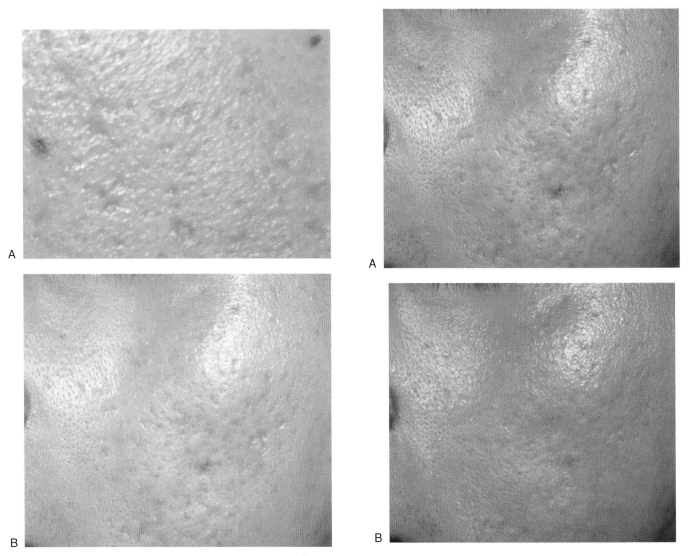

Figure 21.2 *Acne scar patient treated with PSR (4 J/cm². (A) Pretreatment. (B) Two months posttreatment*

Figure 21.3 *Acne scar patient treated with Fraxel II. (A) Pretreatment. (B) Posttreatment*

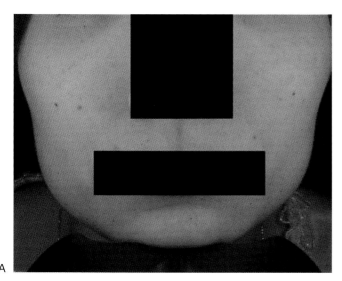 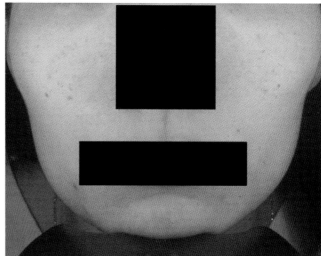

A B

Figure 21.4 *Square face. (A) Pretreatment. (B) After 60 units of Botox® per side*

Alternatively, high-energy fractional resurfacing (Fraxel Restore; Reliant Technologies, Mountain View, CA) can also be used (four monthly treatments, 70 mJ, treatment level 10 to 11, 8 passes), with approximately a 10% risk of PIH. Patients need more treatment sessions with swelling lasting approximately 2 to 3 days and redness lasting 7 days. The degree of improvement is better than PSR, at approximately 50% to 75%. For women who wish to avoid PIH, the treatment level is reduced to 5 with an energy of 50 mJ but more treatment sessions are required (6 to 10) (Figure 21.3).

Other aspects to consider in a cosmetic practice are the differences in physical features and cultural preferences. Narrow eyes, square face, and short, wide lower legs are considered undesirable. The use of botulinum toxin type A can significantly improve such features (Figure 21.4).[17,18]

Finally, besides cultural and genetic differences, geographical variation is another important factor to be considered. North Asian countries such as Korea, Northern China, and Japan have a much lower degree of UV exposure compared with Hong Kong, Singapore, or California. This can also have significant impact on treatment outcome. Cultural variation is another aspect that one has to bear in mind. Until recently, aesthetic procedures were generally less acceptable to Asians. Increase in media coverage on cosmetic surgery has changed this public view, at least in some Asian countries. Whether such trends continue remains to be seen.

REFERENCES

1. Szabo G. Pigment cell biology. In: Gordon M, ed. *Mitochondria and Other Cytoplasmic Inclusions*. New York, NY: Academic Press; 1959.

2. Griffiths CEM, Wang TS, Hamilton TA, Voorhees JJ, Ellis CN. A photonumeric scale for the assessment of cutaneous photodamage. *Arch Dermatol.* 1992;128:347-351.

3. Larnier C, Ortonne JP, Venot A, et al. Evaluation of cutaneous photodamage using a photographic scale. *Br J Dermatol.* 1994;130:167-173.

4. Chung JH. Photoaging in Asians. *Photodermatol Photoimmunol. Photomed.* 2003;19:109-121.

5. Chan HH, Jackson B. Laser treatment on ethnic skin. In: Lim HW, Honigsmann H, Hawk JLM, eds. *Photodermatology*. New York, NY: Informa Healthcare. 2007:417-432.

6. Chan HH. Effective and safe use of lasers, light sources, and radiofrequency devices in the clinical management of Asian patients with selected dermatoses. *Lasers Surg Med.* 2005; 37(3):179-185.

7. Koh D, Wang H, Lee J, Chia KS, Lee HP, Goh CL. Basal cell carcinoma, squamous cell carcinoma and melanoma of the skin: analysis of the Singapore Cancer Registry Data 1968-1997. *Br J Dermatol.* 2003;148:1161-1166.

8. Waterhouse J, Correa P, Muir C, Powel J, eds. *Cancer Incidence in Five Continents*. Vol 4. Lyon, France: International Agency for Research in Cancer; 1976.

9. Ishihara K, Saida T, Yamamoto A. Updated statistical data for malignant melanoma in Japan. *Int J Clin Oncol.* 2001;6: 109-116.

10. Collins RJ. Melanoma in the Chinese of Hong Kong: emphasis on volar and subungual sites. *Cancer.* 1984;54:1482-1488.

11. Chan HH. Laser treatment of nevomelanocytic nevi—can results from an Asian study be applicable to the white population? *Arch Dermatol.* 2002;138:535.

12. Lee MW. Combination visible and infrared lasers for skin rejuvenation. *Semin Cutan Med Surg.* 2002;21:288-300.

13. Chan HH, Lam LK, Wong DS, Kono T, Trend-Smith N. Use of 1320-nm Nd:YAG laser for wrinkle reduction and the treatment of atrophic acne scarring. *Lasers Surg Med.* 2004;34: 98-103.

14. Goh CL, Chua SH, Ang P, Khoo L. Efficacy of smoothbeam 1450-nm laser for treatment of acne scars in Asian skin. *Lasers Surg Med.* 2004;S16:76.

15. Fournier N, Dahan S, Barneon G, et al. Nonablative remodeling: a 14-month clinical ultrasound imaging and profilometric evaluation of a 1540-nm Er:Glass laser. *Dermatol Surg.* 2002; 28:926-931.

16. Chan HH, Manstein D, Yu CS, Shek S, Kono T, Wei WI. The prevalence and risk factors of postinflammatory hyperpigmentation after fractional resurfacing in Asians. *Lasers Surg Med.* 2007;39(5):381-385.

17. Kim NH, Chung JH, Park RH, Park JB. The use of botulinum toxin type A in aesthetic mandibular contouring. *Plast Reconstr Surg.* 2005;115(3):919-930.

18. Lee HJ, Lee DW, Park YH, Cha MK, Kim HS, Ha SJ. Botulinum toxin A for aesthetic contouring of enlarged medial gastrocnemius muscle. *Dermatol Surg.* 2004;30(6):867-871.

CHAPTER 22 Special Considerations in Indian/Near Eastern Skin

Joslyn N. Witherspoon, MD, MPH, Richard H. Huggins, MD, and Murad Alam, MD

INTRODUCTION

Treatment of cosmetic skin ailments in Indian and Near Eastern populations requires an understanding of the fragility of such skin, and its predisposition to hyperpigment and scar in response to aggressive procedures. Additionally, cultural and religious factors can modulate how Indian and Middle Eastern patients view their and others skin, and which diagnoses and treatments they consider most salient.

DISORDERS OF PIGMENTATION AND ALOPECIA

Skin diseases that alter skin complexion or color may be particularly worrisome for Indian and Middle Eastern patients.[1] For instance, melasma, vitiligo, and leprosy are associated with loss of self-esteem, social embarrassment, and depression.

Particularly in India, leprosy and vitiligo are stigmatizing conditions. Leprosy, in addition to the physical morbidity that results from the disease, is also considered a sign of moral fault in the afflicted. In some Indian religious texts, leprosy is said to result from a curse from God and serve as punishment for people who had committed a great offense in a past life. Social ostracism is further worsened by exaggerated concerns about how easily the disease can be spread. Individuals with vitiligo suffer much the same discrimination because the hypopigmented macules in vitiligo resemble those in leprosy. In ancient India, vitiligo was referred to as "Sweta Kushta," meaning white leprosy. Consequently, people suffering from vitiligo in India may have more psychosocial problems than sufferers in other countries.[1] These patients report depression and sleep disturbance at rates of 10% and 20%, respectively.[2] They are often considered unsuitable mates for marriage, and women who develop vitiligo after marriage have more marital problems and higher rates of divorce.[3] Women with vitiligo experience greater quality of life impairment than their male counterparts, according to a study by Borimnejad et al.[4] Though new treatment options for this disease continue to be developed, there is still no therapy that is effective in all patients. Surgical treatment is the recommended treatment for disease recalcitrant to medical therapy[5] and has been found to be effective in appropriately selected patients.[6]

Alopecia is another concern in Indian populations. Dalgard et al.[7] report that hair loss is a dominant complaint in men and women from the Indian subcontinent and Middle East/North Africa. Abundant hair is a marker of status for both men and women in many parts of the world, and reflects beauty and good health.

Other common cosmetic disorders in Indian populations include contact dermatitis, hyperpigmentation, hypopigmentation, contact urticaria, acneiform eruptions, hair breakage, and nail breakage.[8]

CULTURAL AND RELIGIOUS CONSIDERATIONS

Visible Scars

When treating patients with Indian skin in particular, it is important to be aware of cultural and religious differences. Indian women usually wear a saree, leaving the midriff uncovered and visible, so in cases such as liposuction of the abdomen, care should be taken to avoid visible scars in the central abdomen. Indian men often leave their chest open on ceremonial occasions such as during prayer, and care should be taken to avoid visible scars in this area as well.

Cosmetics

In India and other South Asian countries (Pakistan, Nepal, Tibet, Sri Lanka, Bangladesh), facial melanosis from cosmetics is well known. *Bindi* is a circular plastic disk applied to the forehead with adhesive containing substances such as t-butyl phenol and monomethylol phenol. Traditionally worn only by married Hindu women as a religious custom, the *bindi* spot is now regarded as a fashion accessory by unmarried women and even by non-Hindus. *Bindi* dermatitis has been shown to produce hypopigmentation or hyperpigmentation. *Sindoor* (vermilion) is a red powder sprinkled along the parting of the scalp hair to denote (female) marital status, and consists of lead oxide, *Kumkum* (alkalized turmeric powder), or commercial red dyes (Figure 22.1). *Surma* is a fine black powder containing 90% lead oxide which is usually applied to the eyelid margins, which are occasionally irritated and inflamed as a result.[9]

Keloids

The tendency for keloid formation is not as significant in Indian skin as in black skin, but a history of keloids should always be sought in Indian and Middle Eastern patients.[10] Keloids can often occur in areas of localized intentional trauma such as body piercings. In Near Eastern populations, numerous piercings are common and traditional adornments, especially among women, rather than signs of an alternative lifestyle. Ear piercings and nose piercings are among the most frequent, and piercings on the trunk are also seen.

Henna

Temporary natural henna painting for skin adornment and use of henna for hair dyeing is very common in several countries of the Indian subcontinent, Middle East, and North Africa (Figures 22.2 and 22.3). There have been reports of contact dermatitis to the paraphenylenediamine found in henna. Since henna-induced red-brown coloration fades over days to weeks, associated contact dermatitis is avoidable by refraining from future use of such dyes in susceptible patients.

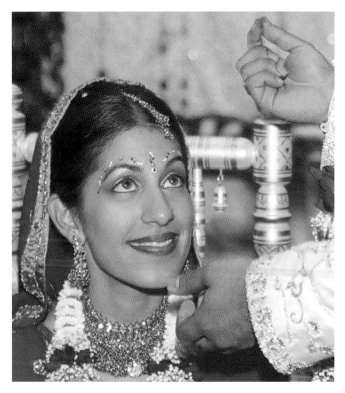

Figure 22.1 *Groom spreading kumkum powder along the parting of the bride's scalp hair to denote marital status (Used with permission from Sapna Patel, MD)*

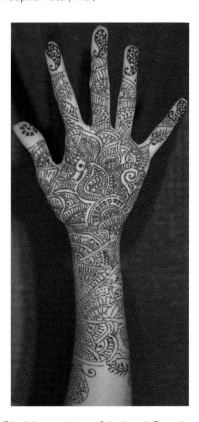

Figure 22.2 *Black henna tattoo of the hand. Paraphenylenediamine is a widely used dye that is added to the pastes in high concentrations to produce a darker shade. Some individuals may develop a contact dermatitis to the PPD (Used with permission from Sapna Patel, MD)*

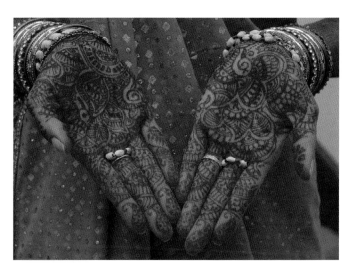

Figure 22.3 *Red-brown henna tattoo of the hands. (Used with permission from Sapna Patel, MD)*

▣ Nonstandard Therapy

Complementary, homeopathic, or traditional medicine also plays an important role in the Indian subcontinent and in the Middle East. Unusual dermatoses and pigmentation patterns may be cutaneous manifestations of nonstandard medical therapies. Obtaining a complete medication history, including herbal and homeopathic medications, may facilitate diagnosis and treatments of related skin conditions.

▣ Muslim Patients

For patients from predominantly Muslim areas of South Asia (Pakistan, Bangladesh, and parts of India), and from most of the Middle East, Islamic customs may impact the physician–patient relationship. Female patients may be reluctant to be examined by male physicians. If such examination is necessary, they may prefer to have a male relative present, and the examination may be limited to areas not usually covered by clothing. While Western physicians are taught that touching patients can relieve patient anxiety and build rapport, when examining female Muslim patients, unnecessary touching is best avoided. A request for a female physician should not be viewed as needlessly obstructive since this often emanates from a desire to be faithful to religious custom. It is not uncommon for adult women to present to the physician with their husband, and to allow the husband to convey their history and complaints; again, this is not necessarily a sign of oppression, but a traditional religious custom limiting female interactions with men who are not their relatives or their spouse. Of course, many Muslim women do not have any concerns about being examined, are able to speak for themselves, and do not wear restrictive, ritualistic clothing.

COSMETIC PROCEDURES IN SKIN OF COLOR

There are many topical agents and cosmetic procedures for treatment of pigmentation in Indian and Middle Eastern patients. These

TABLE 22.1 ▪ Key Cosmetic Dermatological Considerations in Indian/Near Eastern Skin

Increased social impact of disorders affecting pigmentation and hair.

Keloid formation and dyspigmentation secondary to therapeutic procedures and culture-specific cosmetics.

Contact dermatitis secondary to culture-specific cosmetics.

Cultural competency when interacting with female patients, particularly those of Islamic affiliation.

Unusual dermatoses secondary to alternative medical practices.

include topical bleaching agents, retinoids, chemical peels, microdermabrasion, botulinum toxin, and injectable fillers.[11] Topical hydroquinone remains the most common agent for treatment of postinflammatory hyperpigmentation (PIH) and melasma. Topical retinoids are indicated for the treatment of acne, textural changes, wrinkles, melasma, and PIH; these are generally better tolerated than in Caucasian patients. Indications for superficial glycolic or salicylic acid chemical peels in darker racial ethnic groups include melasma, PIH, acne, rough skin, enlarged pores and wrinkles. Microdermabrasion is also well-tolerated but should be used gently, without pinpoint bleeding, which can predispose to hyperpigmentation.[11] Botulinum toxin and injectable fillers are becoming more popular with Indian and Middle Eastern patients. While centrofacial atrophy and fine lines are less common among such patients than in Anglo-Saxon patients, dynamic forehead lines can be quite deep and noticeable. Fillers may be injected with linear threading technique instead of serial punctures so as to minimize the number of skin perforations and hence the risk of PIH.[11]

In a study conducted by Grover and Reddu,[12] 41 Indian patients with various skin conditions including acne, melasma, PIH, and superficial scarring, were treated with glycolic acid peels. It was shown that PIH occurred in two patients and suggested that glycolic acid induced hypopigmentation may have occurred in one patient in the melasma group.[12]

SUMMARY

In conclusion, patients from the Indian subcontinent and the Middle-East may be especially bothered by specific cosmetic concerns, including acquired pigmentation abnormalities and alopecia. Ailments like vitiligo or alopecia totalis may be stigmatized and lead to ostracism. Socially acceptable skin adornments including various dyes and adhesives, and also copious body piercings, may result in dermatitides or infections requiring treatment. For partially invasive procedures, such as excisional surgery, filler injections, or liposuction, minimizing the number and size of skin punctures will reduce the risk of postoperative hyperpigmentation and keloids. Treatment of hyperpigmentation is commonly with passive treatments, like topical hydroquinones, retinoids, and sun avoidance. Superficial chemical peels and microdermabrasion may be used gently and repeatedly for the same purpose (Table 22.1).

REFERENCES

1. Chaturvedi SK, Singh G, Gupta N. Stigma experience in skin disorders: an Indian perspective. *Dermatol Clin.* 2005;23: 635-642.

2. Sharma N, Koranne RV, Singh RK. A comparative study of psychiatric morbidity in dermatology patients. *Indian J Dermatol Venereol Leprol.* 2003;48:137-141.

3. Dogra S, Kanwar AJ. Skin diseases: psychological and social consequences. *Indian J Dermatol Venereol Leprol.* 2002; 47:197-201.

4. Borimnejad L, Parsa Yekta Z, Nikbakht-Nasrabadi A, Firooz A. Quality of life with vitiligo: comparison of male and female muslim patients in Iran. *Gend Med.* 2006;3:124-130.

5. Njoo MD, Westerhof W, Bos JD, Bossuyt PM. The development of guidelines for the treatment of vitiligo. Clinical Epidemiology Unit of the Istituto Dermopatico dell'Immacolata-Istituto di Recovero e Cura a Carattere Scientifico (IDI-IRCCS) and the Archives of Dermatology. *Arch Dermatol.* 1999;135:1514-1521.

6. Babu A, Thappa DM, Jaisankar TJ. Punch grafting versus suction blister epidermal grafting in the treatment of stable lip vitiligo. *Dermatol Surg.* 2008;34:166-178.

7. Dalgard F, Holm JO, Svensson A, Kumar B, Sundby J. Self reported skin morbidity and ethnicity: A population-based study in a Western community. *BMC Dermatol.* 2007;7:4.

8. Dogra A, Minocha YC, Kaur S. Adverse reactions to cosmetics. *Indian J Dermatol Venereol Leprol.* 2003;69:165-167.

9. Mehta SS, Reddy BS. Cosmetic dermatitis—current perspectives. *Int J Dermatol.* 2003;42:533-542.

10. Field LM. Cultural and ethnic differences in the acceptance or rejection of liposuction instrumentation entrance marks. *J Drugs Dermatol.* 2007;6(1):56-58.

11. Grimes P. *Cosmetic Approaches to Skin of Color.* New York, NY: Physicians Continuing Education Corp.; 2007.

12. Grover C, Reddu BS. The therapeutic value of glycolic acid peels in dermatology. *Indian J Dermatol Venereol Leprol.* 2003;69:148-150.

CHAPTER 23　Special Considerations in Latino Skin

Joseph F. Greco, MD, and Teresa Soriano, MD

The Latino population, comprising Hispanics and Latin Americans, is the fasting growing minority population in the United States. Latin Americans descend from the countries of the Western Hemisphere, south of the United States, that predominantly speak Spanish, Portuguese, or French while Hispanics are defined as persons of Spanish descent. Together, Latinos represent a beautiful and ethnically diverse population who are presenting in record numbers to dermatologists and plastic surgeons throughout the country for a variety of cosmetic procedures.

Over the past 10 years, the rate of cosmetic surgery procedures in ethnic patients has risen dramatically. Hispanic patients lead all ethnic groups in this trend and represent a sizable share of the market. In 2006, according to the American Society of Plastic Surgery, Hispanic patients had 932 410 cosmetic procedures performed, a marked increase from 552 638 procedures in 2004.[1] Hispanic patients accounted for 8.6% of total cosmetic procedures in 2006, an increase from 6.3% in 1999. The most commonly requested noninvasive cosmetic procedures among Hispanics were Botox®, injectable fillers, and chemical peels. With respect to invasive cosmetic procedures among Hispanics, breast augmentation, nose reshaping, and liposuction were the most frequently requested. The American Society for Aesthetic Plastic Surgery published similar statistics. In 2006, there were approximately 11.5 million surgical and nonsurgical cosmetic procedures performed in the United States, compared to 2.1 million in 1997.[2] Hispanics led all racial and ethnic minority groups undergoing 9.7% of the 11.5 million procedures, an increase from 6% in 1997.

Pigmentary disorders represent the predominant disturbances for which Latino patients seek cosmetic consultation.[3,4] Hyperpigmentation and facial melasma were among the top 10 most common skin diagnoses in a group of 2000 Latino patients treated in a hospital-based clinic.[4] The incidence of pregnancy-induced facial melasma among Mexican women has been reported to be as high as 50%.[4] Additionally, the mandibular type of melasma, associated with papillary dermal melanin accumulation, predominates in middle-aged females.[5]

Cosmetic consultation should be the prerequisite visit before any aesthetic procedure is considered. In addition to the standard medical and dermatologic history, a thorough understanding of the patients' concerns and expectations should be elicited. For example, pigmentary disorders particularly melasma and postinflammatory hyperpigmentation (PIH), cause significant psychosocial distress among Latinos, affecting their quality of life.[1,2] They often present at consultation hoping for immediate treatment and resolution. Additionally, Latino patients are presenting more frequently requesting the latest cosmetic treatments for photoaged skin including laser and light source therapies. The greatest risk posed to these patients would be a rush to treatment. Often times, the best and most cost-effective treatment options are time and

observation. Patient education on their skin type and perioperative care is important component of the cosmetic consultation. This typically includes a discussion on the increased risk of dyspigmentation with even the mildest irritation in darker skin types (Figure 23.1). In addition, counseling on proper sun avoidance and sun protection strategies is essential, as many ethnic-skinned patients falsely believe their skin is naturally protected from the dangers of ultraviolet radiation. Once patients thoroughly understand their skin behavior patterns and potential risks with treatment, they typically welcome a slower, directed, and safe treatment plan.

Topical bleaching agents are the mainstay of first-line therapy for the treatment of pigmentary disorders in ethnic skin and play a primary adjunctive role in the perioperative period of cosmetic procedures such as chemical peels, laser and light sources. For pigmentary disorders, including melasma, fixed combination products with a bleaching agent, retinoid, and topical steroid have been the most efficacious when used in conjunction with a sunscreen.[8] Hydroquinone and azelaic acid, alone or in combination are effective as well.[8] Pretreatment with 4% hydroquinone once to twice for at least 2 weeks prior to all chemical peels, laser, and light source therapies can suppress melanogenesis and minimize the potential risk for PIH (Figure 23.2).

In the past, laser and light source therapy were limited in the ethnic skin population because of a high likelihood of developing postinflammatory dyspigmentation and scarring. In general, the

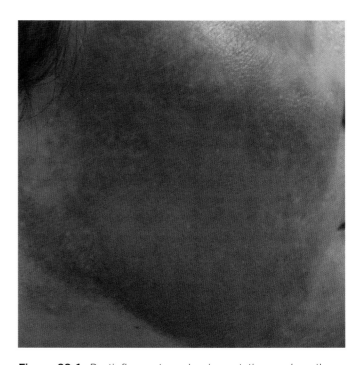

Figure 23.1 *Postinflammatory dyspigmentation and erythema after TCA 25% peel treatment of melasma in a Puerto Rican woman*

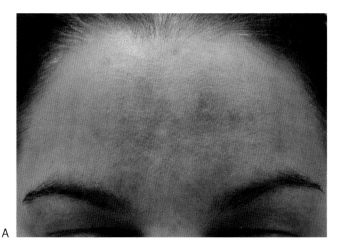

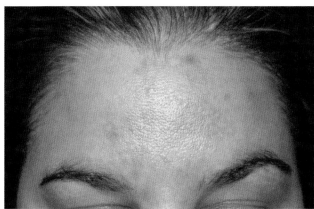

Figure 23.2 *Melasma and PIH on forehead of a Mexican woman. (A) Baseline and (B) after pretreatment with hydroquinone 4% cream and two Erbium Fraxel treatments*

treatments are followed when treating Latino patients compared to Caucasian patients. Performing test spots prior to performing laser procedures such as hair and tattoo removal and the treatment of pigmented lesions is recommended particularly in darker-skinned Latino patients.

Treatment approach with respect to botulinum toxin and injectable dermal fillers are identical in Latino patients as compared to non-Latino patients. However, it should be noted that each injection may induce a local inflammatory response capable of leaving residual PIH at the site of insult. Although this is rare, using the smallest caliber needle and the minimum number of injection sites needed to achieve the optimal cosmetic result is preferred in this situation.

Posttreatment considerations focus on minimizing the inflammatory response. Measures include the local application of ice packs immediately after treatment with dermal fillers and some lasers and the use of mild to moderately potent topical corticosteroids after chemical peels, lasers, and light sources twice daily for 3 to 5 days. In rare cases, a short course of prednisone may be warranted if a high degree of inflammation is suspected. However, the authors always caution against performing a procedure in ethnic skin patients when a significant inflammatory response is possible. Maintenance therapy with proper sun protection strategies is crucial to preventing PIH and the progression of pigmentary disorders. A broad-spectrum sunscreen covering UVA and UVB with an SPF of 30 or higher is recommended. Continuation of topical bleaching agents should be determined on an individual basis based on success of the current therapy and perceived benefits of future use.

With increasing popularity and access to minimally invasive aesthetic procedures, Latino patients continue to strengthen their position as the leading ethnic group presenting for cosmetic procedures. Consequently, understanding the potential variability in cutaneous reaction patterns of this population is paramount in providing cosmetic procedures for these patients.

development of lasers with longer wavelengths, longer pulse durations, and improved cooling mechanisms has allowed safe treatment of darker skin types for cosmetic concerns such as hair removal and photoaging. In addition, the advent of newer technologies, such as fractional photothermolysis, has permitted the safe and effective use of laser energy in the Latino population for treating melasma and acne scarring.[9–11] Through microscopic columns of thermal coagulation, dermal and epidermal pigment, sun damaged collagen, and scar tissue may be safely removed with relatively low energy settings.[10,11] By permitting only a fraction of the skin surface to be treated in a single session, islands of normal skin quickly repopulate and heal the thermally damaged tissue without eliciting a marked inflammatory response. More recently, combination laser and light source therapy has become popular with the idea that two distinct mechanisms of action will have an additive effect in treating photodamaged skin. The authors' experience in a few selected Latino patients thus far has been promising using a combination broadband light source followed immediately by an erbium:YAG microlaser peel for the treatment of dyschromia, redness, fine lines, and surface irregularities. In general, lower energy settings, longer pulsewidths, and longer intervals between

REFERENCES

1. American Society for Plastic Surgeons. 2006 Plastic surgery statistics. http://www.plasticsurgery.org/media/statistics/index.cfm. Accessed May 30, 2007.

2. American Society for Aesthetic Plastic Surgery. 2006 Cosmetic surgery statistics. http://www.surgery.org/press/statistics.php. Accessed May 30, 2007.

3. Taylor SC. Epidemiology of skin diseases in ethnic populations. *Dermatol Clin.* 2003;21:601-607.

4. Sanchez MR. Cutaneous diseases in Latinos. *Dermatol Clin.* 2003;21:689-697.

5. Mandry PR, Sanches JL. Mandibular melasma. *P R Health Sci J.* 2000;19:231-234.

6. Hexsel D., Arellano I, Rendon M. Ethnic considerations in the treatment of Latin-American patients with hyperpigmentation. *Br J Dermatol.* 2006;156(S1):7-12.

7. Downie JB. Esthetic Considerations for Ethnic Skin. *Semin Cutan Med Surg.* 2006;25(3):158-162.

8. Rendon M, Berneburg M, Arellano I, Picardo M. Treatment of melasma. *J Am Acad Dermatol.* 2006;54(S2):S272-S281.

9. Munavalli GS, Weiss RA, Halder RM. Photoaging and nonablative photorejuvination in ethnic skin. *Dermatol Surg.* 2005; 31:1250-1260.

10. Geronemus R. Fractional photothermolysis: current and future applications. *Lasers Surg Med.* 2006;38(3):169-176.

11. Rokhsar CK., Fitzpatrick RE. The treatment of melasma with fractional photothermolysis: a pilot study. *Dermatol Surg.* 2005;31(12):1645-1650.

12. Grimes PE. The safety and efficacy of salicylic acid chemical peels in darker racial-ethnic groups. *Dermatol Surg.* 1999; 25(1):18-22.

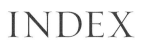

INDEX